Gendering Disability

Gendering Disability

EDITED BY
BONNIE G. SMITH
BETH HUTCHISON

Rutgers University Press
New Brunswick, New Jersey, and London

305.90816
G325g

Library of Congress Cataloging-in-Publication Data

Gendering disability / edited by Bonnie G. Smith and Beth Hutchison.
  p. cm.
"Based on scholarship presented at a three-day conference . . . organized by the Institute for Research on Women (IRW) at Rutgers University, March 1–3, 2001"—Ack.
Includes bibliographical references and index.
  ISBN 0–8135–3372–4 (alk. paper)—ISBN 0–8135–3373–2 (pbk. : alk. paper)
Women with disabilities—Congresses. 2. Sociology of disability—Congresses. I. Smith, Bonnie G., 140—II. Hutchison, Beth.
HV1569.3.W65G46 2004
305.9'0816—dc21
                                                                    2003007034

British Cataloging-in-Publication data record for this book is available from the British Library.

The publication program of Rutgers University Press is supported by the Board of Governors of Rutgers, The State University of New Jersey.

Manufactured in the United States of America

CONTENTS

v

ACKNOWLEDGMENTS

This collection is based on scholarship presented at a three-day conference, "Gender and Disability Studies," organized by the Institute for Research on Women (IRW) at Rutgers University, March 1–3, 2001. The impetus for the conference was a series of conversations with Rosemarie Garland-Thomson and Cathy Kudlick about the possibilities for an exchange among scholars whose work focuses on disability studies and women and gender. It is a pleasure to thank them for their provocative suggestions and enthusiasm.

Plans for the conference were further stimulated by conversations and work presented at the weekly graduate student-faculty seminar convened by the IRW and cosponsored by the Institute for Women's Leadership at Rutgers. Our deep appreciation to the Ford Foundation for a grant to the Institute for Women's Leadership in support of the seminar and to the Rockefeller Foundation, which enabled us to present the conference in conjunction with our grant for residential fellowships in the humanities, "Gender-Race-Ethnicity: Rearticulating the Local and the Global."

Marlene Importico, the IRW's irreplaceable office manager, managed logistical arrangements and supervised a staff of graduate student employees and volunteers led by Tara Wisniewski. Much of the success of the three-day conference was thanks to their tireless efforts.

Marlie Wasserman, the director of Rutgers University Press, was an early and consistent proponent of the book; her colleagues at the Press, particularly Nicole Lokach Manganaro and Michele Gisbert, have been insightful and patient collaborators. Many thanks to them, as well as to Kathleen Paparchontis, our indefatigable copyeditor and indexer.

We would especially like to thank all the conference presenters and participants for creating a unique environment of scholarly engagement in an atmosphere that acknowledged our differences while enabling productive exchanges that continue to inform our research and teaching. Those three days together remain an inspiring memory of what truly feminist work should be. We hope this collection will help to deepen and extend those conversations.

Gendering Disability

INTRODUCTION

BONNIE G. SMITH

The coming together of disability and gender studies provides exponential intellectual excitement, advancing the scholarly leadership that these two fields have displayed over the past decades. Beginning as separate enterprises that followed activist and scholarly paths, both gender and disability studies have reached a point where they look across boundaries for a better vision of a common landscape that can provide room for new growth. The sense that each discipline, in its uniqueness, has nonetheless much to offer the other is inescapable. Whether from a perspective in the humanities, social sciences, sciences, or arts, the shared subject matter—the body, inequity, identity, and sexuality—insistently calls for a deeper conversation. The chapters in this volume work to initiate forays across the borders of these contiguous fields.

Disability, a term that has heretofore been so clear-cut to the public, is becoming increasingly polymorphous in the light of a new politics and scholarship. It can suggest a set of practices, kinds of embodiment, interactions with the built environment, an almost limitless array of literary types, frames of mind, and forms of relationships. Gone are the days of a simple and dominant physiological or medical definition of disability. Instead, people have come to see an art of disability—poetry, music, song, literature—and a politics of disability that has accomplished path-breaking legislation and effected social change. In the university, disability has yielded disability studies, a field based on curricular offerings and research and scholarship into the many facets of disability including its history, economics, and theories. This multifaceted cultural and social phenomenon, operating from the statehouse, industry, the academy, and everyday life, has traced a new axis of attention, enriching thought and human action.

The chapters in this book bring gender into the orbit of disability studies. The complexity of disability is compounded when set in dialogue with issues of gender, which today is also seen as a complicated set of practices, ways of being, sexualities, politics, and artistic and social visions. No longer does the term *gender* refer to one's biological sex nor does it serve as a synonym for women or feminism. Instead, over the past three decades, the term *gender* has evolved to designate identities for men and women that come into being in relationship to one another. The social and cultural role of "men" can fluctuate according to norms for femininity; men can enact masculinity in a variety of ways. Cultural meanings help produce what it is to be a man or women—that is, cultural meanings produce gendered social actors.

Disability scholars such as Rosemarie Garland-Thomson have said that the fit between disability studies and gender studies is a good one. Issues of the body, social and cultural hierarchy, identity, discrimination and inequality, representation, and political activism have been central to both fields. The cultural meanings of disability, like the cultural meanings of gender, produce human actors, who act out all the rules and themes of disability and likewise the rules of gender. Simultaneously, the lived social environment of work, politics, and sociability may be hostile to the disabled as it may be to women. Moreover, both fields have an acute awareness of difference and have developed questions about difference in their scholarship. Over the past three decades, gender and women's studies, for instance, have stopped talking about "women" as if they constituted a unified category of social actors. Instead, the differences among women have become all-important to understanding society and the nature of political activism. Similarly, scholars in disability studies are now mining the social outcomes of differences among the disabled and investigating the cultural force and resonance of those differences. Moreover, difference is a relative term: thus, the concept of disability takes much of its meaning from the coordinate concept of able bodied, as femininity derives its meaning in relationship to masculinity. One can investigate a range of differences that come together along the axis of disability and gender, including those among disabled and able-bodied women. A desire for enhancing both fields through mutual dialogue thus unites the chapters in this book.

The chapters in this volume also address issues of advocacy that often infuse both disability and gender studies. These issues focus on questions of how researchers making strong advocacy claims can best accomplish their aims. How, it can be asked, does one present data in a way that would help advance the cause of those for whom one wanted to advocate. For instance, because both disability and gender studies are often devalued by many who see them as useless, minor, or partial, how do we validate the findings of these fields, especially when those findings have an aura of being less reliable and less important—like the disabled, like women. How do advocates, scholars have tried to determine, circumvent the lower prestige society assigns these two groups. Other advocacy concerns involve the neutrality of scholarship. The disabled and women are seen as highly political as teachers and scholars, while other researchers—those representing powerful groups such as able-bodied men—are seen as neutral and removed from an advocacy role. Among researchers and teachers of disability and gender studies, their subjects particularly need advocacy because of the generally lower economic and cultural standing of both women and the disabled.

The intellectual and institutional barriers seem high nonetheless, and even in the field of disability activism, one finds the presence of race, gender, and class discrimination. This coming together of types of discrimination, often called "intersectionality" by current theorists, is aptly demonstrated in the chapter by disabilities activist Corbett O'Toole.

For these reasons, disability and gender scholars take strong positions in this volume, particularly questioning their circumstances both as social actors and as individuals. The theorist Adrienne Asch chronicles a situation in which people cannot interact with the disabled as they would with humans in general, insisting instead in their interactions on discussing disabilities or on being allowed to give assistance. Rather than relating to others on the basis of her disability, Asch asks for a relationship based on the full range of her humanity—her love of music for instance is something that is written out of her persona. Instead, to most people, disability stands for her entire being and most important human trait. Disability, Asch maintains, is so looming that philosophers such as Peter Singer also disbelieve the humanity of the disabled and advocate that they be aborted instead of born. The "genocide" of the disabled comes into stark view in Asch's discussion.

Many in disability studies endorse the ability of this new field to explore the rich life of the disabled not only as an affirmation but also as part of a political process to stop both the killing of disabled fetuses and the mutilation through surgery of disabled adults and children. In this vein, they take an advocacy position congruent with that of the intersexed, who may or may not be considered disabled by society at large. Doctors, government officials, and service providers are among those who prefer gender identity to follow certain norms, thus leading them to determine that those with various biological sexual characteristics be "fixed"—that is, corrected through surgical or hormonal intervention to conform to a gender standard that follows textbook biology and social ideology. Disability studies takes a position against "normate" ideas of bodies and gender, encouraging us to think outside and in-between categories.

Championing in-betweeness can entail attention to various categories of the intermediate. An example in this volume involves investigating the position of interpreters for the deaf. Where do they position themselves in the social spectrum and the spectrum of power? Whose side are they on? Given that women throughout history have not only been translators and interpreters, the power involved in such an in-between positioning among the disabled raises insistent questions helpful to women's and gender studies. Positionality takes on new complexity when one imagines the lesser social power gender conveys and the greater social power able bodies hold.

Identity has lost its fixed, stable definition over the past decade of scholarship, leading to understandings of what used to be called human nature as a composite of characteristics such as gender and class or nationality and race. Under new theories of identity, one performs the rules of being a woman or the characteristics of being able bodied, and one may be acting more like a woman at one moment, more like a Kenyan or German at another, and more like a Muslim at still another. Like other identities, those of gender and disability are produced, displayed, and constructed by a host of forces including external ones such as cultural codes or internal ones such as desire. For instance, as one chapter shows, the identity of young men afflicted by a disease such as polio took shape in the 1950s around messages that one needed to fight the debility like a soldier or an athlete. However, as the body aged and as post-polio syndrome afflicted many, such cultural messages, especially those demanding the repression of emotions in the cause of physical prowess, no longer did their work, leading to crisis and the quest for a renewed identity. Simultaneously, disabled men, whether in the case of their own physical health or in their mental and sexual health, have proved able to devise new practices, including new sexualities.

In other instances, identity is acted out in relationships, seen at one point in this volume in the relationship between women amputees and male devotees. On one hand, these relationships may seem to vivify traditional gender roles, with the able-bodied male serving as a chivalrous knight to a fragile and feminine amputee. Disability facilitates in this case normative gender roles. Yet on the other hand, disabled women often appeal as powerful and independent, even providing strength for devotees who can be beaten down by society for their sexual preferences. Identity is less normatively gendered, less transparent to feminist and other theorists, than acted out on a case-by-case basis and in terms of a localized desire. Not only in the present but also in the past, disability has worked its way along the axis of gender with both of these precarious and transformative categories. In eighteenth-century France, even as the philosophes of the enlightenment were agitating for a reasoned attitude toward blindness and other disabilities, marriages of the disabled themselves, as the chapter on a blind merchant demonstrates, both sustained and undid gendered expectations. Partners in marriages, as in the devotee/amputee couple, could both enact and undo the ordinary terms of both gender and disability.

In cultural terms, plasticity of identity makes it so that the disabled often are seen as women are—to be either too embodied or too frail and wispy to be a real presence. Their status in the arts becomes problematic, especially given the cultural control exercised by able-bodied masters-of-the-universe type men. Neither the disabled and women, nor disabled women qualify for narrative plenitude of the type accorded able-bodied heroes. Instead, a character's disability and femininity serve to indicate a terrifying or defeated situation; such characters may also serve as a contrast to the richness, fascination, and strength of masculinity. Portraying themselves, however, the disabled can make important interventions in the discourse of the body, femininity, and normality, as the painting of Frida Kahlo demonstrates. Imaginings and artistic recreations, as in the fictionalized and humorous memoir of Helen Keller's teenage romance, depict transgressions and sly agency. These works bring the body and sexuality to the fore, uniting disability and gender as never before and demonstrating the rich harvest of aesthetic insights gained from juxtaposing perspectives from both fields.

The writing of Audre Lorde, conveying the intensity of women's sexual relationships, adds race to the equation. For in her sensual accounts of love between lesbians, disabled and passionate and black, Lorde raises the issue of what has been done to the bodies of women, of women of color, of lesbians, of the disabled, and she uses her account of the body's pleasures to heal the damage. The body—disabled, black, lesbian, female—is a recuperative one, as the powerful analysis of Lorde's work demonstrates.

Art may advocate through its aesthetic, but the social sciences often make a more direct approach in the presentation of evidence on the persistence of inequalities in the public sphere, the market, and the commercial world for the disabled. The disabled and women have particular concerns about the realization of their rights as citizens and consumers—roles that carry enormous weight in the contemporary world. When gender is taken into account, disability activism itself seems to participate in the discriminatory world in which race and masculinity are privileged. Of forty-two activists asked to participate in a disability oral history, the group was virtually all white and male. Responses to a detailed questionnaire bringing together disability, gender, employment, and political participation provide confirmation of the woman activist's own sense of the masculine and white hegemony within the disability movement. Although women with disabilities are poorer, less likely to be well employed, and less politically active than either men with disabilities or women without disabilities, employed women with disabilities and women with disabilities who belong to groups tend toward political activism. In addition to lobbying legislators and other public officials, they address discrimination in the workplace more often than do men with disabilities. Moreover, they are more likely to ask for help when needed to resolve workplace issues. If the public world seems less likely to earn the efforts of women with disabilities, the marketplace is similarly designed for those without disabilities. For instance, the color-coding associated with labels indicating dangerous products or sizes does not work for women lacking the ability to discriminate colors. The difference between caffeinated and decaffeinated eludes them, and there are many other ways in which they have difficulty providing for their families unless they rely on the help of others. Norms of marketing work to benefit people with certain kinds of visual capacities and to disadvantage others.

In the final analysis, the conversation among gender and disability scholars and activists provides fresh, sometimes shocking, findings not only about the discrimination practiced against both the disabled and women but also about a parallelism that can be put to productive use. These can range from a sudden understanding of the ways in which the built environment privileges the able bodied and the male to a comprehension of the cultural fusion of the disabled and female in representation and social policy. The conversation can also make for unease among those who might assume a total commonality of interest. Among these will be those who disagree with the disabled perspective that abortion is a genocide routinely practiced against them. Concomitantly, the conversation can provoke an awakening in those who have never seen the way the privileging of masculinity has worked to shape and intensify the special rights and privileges of the able bodied. Because of the cognitive importance of emotion and embodied voices, this collection tries to preserve the special qualities, including immediacy, of the authors' work. The anthology hopes to show that the activists' voice has as much to tell readers as the scholars' research does. Working the borders of contested terrain is never an easy task, but we believe that the chapters in this volume have successfully done so, showing the possibilities for crossdisciplinary hybridity and for intellectual and activist growth.

PART I

♪♪

Positions

Critical Race Theory, Feminism, and Disability

REFLECTIONS ON SOCIAL JUSTICE AND PERSONAL IDENTITY

⚜

ADRIENNE ASCH

Introduction

[I]ndividuals with disabilities are a discrete and insular minority who have been . . . subjected to a history of purposeful unequal treatment, and relegated to a position of political powerlessness in our society . . . resulting from . . . assumptions not truly indicative of the . . . ability of such individuals to participate in, and contribute to, society.[1]

These words form part of the findings and purposes section of the Americans with Disabilities Act (ADA), the 1990 law that is intended to protect people with disabilities from discrimination in, and promote their access to, employment, governmental services, and public accommodations. In the more than ten years since its passage, the law has been subject to analysis and critique from proponents and detractors[2] as well as significant challenge in the courts.[3]

The writings of many critical race theorists suggest that what disability scholars, activists, and legal advocates find so discouraging in court decisions, lackluster agency enforcement,[4] and public opposition is exactly the institutional response that should be expected. Central to critical race theory (CRT) is the view that racism is not aberrant but rather the natural order of American life. Describing the major points of the theory, Richard Delgado writes: "Because racism is an ingrained feature of our landscape, it looks ordinary and natural to persons in the culture. . . . [W]hite elites will tolerate or encourage racial advances for blacks only when they also promote white self-interest."[5]

There are many valuable messages to be gained from post-civil-rights-era CRT and feminist writing, and thus this chapter can examine only a few topics with resonance for disability. To summarize my principal contentions, let me suggest the following: Much of the message of CRT is skeptical about achieving the kind of social transformation that would enable historically excluded groups to achieve and maintain a valued place in American life. The early civil rights strategy of fighting for school integration, neighborhood integration, and affirmative action in employment was a strategy that, at best, could help only some people of color to improve their lives. Even for those who could gain material improvements, the dream of integration and a society without racial consciousness itself contained views that endangered the self-esteem and social cohesion of people of color. To the extent that this same message applies to the fight for social change for people with disabilities, I share some of the skepticism about whether the goals are attainable. However, I am not ready to abandon the quest for a society in which human beings are appreciated for abilities and talents; assisted based upon their needs; and where differences in skin color, gender, sexual orientation, and health status are not occasions for exclusionary or pejorative treatment. Like the integrated society discussed by Alan Freeman and the thought experiment of philosopher Richard Wasserstrom, but rejected by critical race theorists such as Gary Peller,[6] I am interested in achieving a society where eyesight is no more consequential for life chances than is eye color. The ideals I espouse here do not commit me to claiming that nonsocial consequences of being sighted or blind are identical to whether one has blue or brown eyes; however, they do commit me to putting forth an argument about disability and about social justice that appreciates similarities and differences among people with impairments and between people with impairments and people of other discriminated-against groups.[7]

Perspectives and Stories as Data

Critical race theory and feminism contend that the perspectives of the discriminated-against, oppressed individual or group must be better understood by the larger society and that the law should look not to wrongs of perpetrators but to helping those who have been victims of discrimination. In different words, Alan Freeman, Mari Matsuda, and Patricia Williams all contend that the public and the courts, as the representatives of society, must understand the experiences and responses of people who are regularly mistreated because of their "race."[8] Reading of Patricia Williams being denied the opportunity to shop at a department store, or of how her friend, also African-American, was ignored and then nearly arrested when she asked to have spoiled milk taken off her restaurant bill,[9] and of how their perspectives were discounted by others, I recoil with horror. I also recognize a painful similarity of small and large insults and of having those insults routinely discounted and reinterpreted by others so that I am wrong, I am too sensitive, or I am unfair to others "who are only trying to help." Much of the daily discrimination people with disabilities face is not the overt hostility of being shot at or lynched, although the institutionalization, involuntary sterilization, and school exclusion documented in *University of Alabama at Birmingham Board of Trustees v. Garrett* are blatant enough; rather, it is the experience of being denied the opportunity to play the social roles expected of one's nondisabled age-peers. Many commentators note that people with disabilities are expected to play no adult social role whatsoever;[10] to be perceived as always, in every social interaction, a recipient of help and never a provider of assistance;[11] and to be more disliked by nondisabled others if they are clearly competent than if they are perceived as incompetent at a task.[12]

Much personal narrative and social science writing about the experience of having a disability includes stories of indignities at the hands of strangers, neighbors, coworkers, friends, and family[13]—and then having to be told that your interpretation is always wrong.[14] The ADA may prevent a local health club or public pool from turning me away if I go to exercise or swim, but it will do nothing to help me persuade a group of new friends that I could join them for a carefree afternoon at a lake. To accomplish that, I must be prepared to provide my athletic credentials and convince them that they are not "responsible" for my safety. These indignities may be analogous to the unconscious racism captured poignantly in the writing of Charles R. Lawrence III, describing what it was like to be a five-year-old Black child amidst a White teacher and White classmates all enjoying the story of Little Black Sambo and then to have your daughter's four-year-old friend tell you, thirty years later, that the same story is his favorite.[15]

Like the academic feminists and CRT authors I cite, a growing number of professionals with disabilities, including myself, can point to professional recognition and the joys of doing work we love as well as its relative financial security and social status. Yet like these others, we have all-too-frequent reminders that we are unanticipated participants in workshops or conferences or unexpected guests at social gatherings. Sitting beside a stranger waiting for a lecture to begin at an academic conference, the stranger whispers loudly not "Hello, my name is Carol," but "Let me know how I can help you." What help do I need while waiting for the speaker to begin? Why not introduce herself rather than assume that the only sociability I could possibly want is her help? When I respond by saying that she can let me know if I can help her, she does not get the point, and I am all too well aware that the point is subtle; instead, she needs to be thanked for her offer and reassured that I will accept it—and then many pleasantries later perhaps we can discuss why we are at the lecture and whether we like it and what workshop we will attend that afternoon. When I complain of countless such incidents to most of my nondisabled friends and colleagues, I am told that I must understand how unusual it is to see a person with a disability in such a setting, that people are awkward, anxious, afraid of doing the wrong thing, only trying to be nice. My friends are right, and I will not get to know new people unless I tolerate these encounters and find ways to smile and be gracious and put people at ease.

But what of the people who have known me for years, who have considered themselves close friends but do not feel comfortable accepting my offers to pick up food as part of a dinner we plan to have; or find themselves reluctant to have me join them when they are meeting new people because they see me as a social liability; or who would prefer that a high-school-age stranger take care of their six-year-old son for an evening than have me do it, even though I have known their son and their home ever since his birth? Making new acquaintances is difficult enough, but recognizing the limits that others' perceptions of blindness place upon important and long-standing friendships is far more painful and discouraging.

The law can do nothing about the sorts of informal interactions described above that make up so much of the lives of people with disabilities lucky enough to have the education, jobs, and financial resources to be attending workshops and conferences or taking vacations where they meet new people. In order for the ADA and other anti-discrimination laws to help people with disabilities truly enter the mainstream, judges and juries will need to learn far more than they typically know about how people with disabilities manage their lives. Anita Silvers is right when she asserts that the burden of proof is high for anyone with a disability who claims that it is not a tragedy to live with an impairment.[16] However, it is more than that—the burden of proof is high to show that one can live competently at all.

Rights Theory and Models of Disability

Despite the skepticism of much of CRT about the philosophy of liberal civil rights, and despite the conviction that racial minorities would gain only what dominant society would grant,[17] CRT departs from many friends in the movement of critical legal studies (CLS) in asserting the importance of rights language and rights laws. Mari Matsuda captures the CRT message well when she says:

> How could anyone believe both of the following statements? (1) I have a right to participate equally in society with any other person; (2) Rights are whatever people in power say they are. One of the primary lessons CLS can learn from the experience of the bottom is that one can believe in both of those statements simultaneously, and that it may well be necessary to do so. . . .
>
> It is important to understand how claims to equality, procedural fairness, and political participation prove so compelling that human beings are willing to die for them.[18]

The organizations and individuals considered part of the disability rights movement clearly endorse the importance of rights rhetoric and rights laws as essential to their struggle for equality and social participation. Denied access to vote, education, employment, housing, transportation, marriage and parenthood, many people with motor, sensory, cognitive, and emotional impairments—along with an impressive group of legal advocates—have spent decades fighting for legal safeguards to citizenship and social life.[19] Using the rhetoric of other disenfranchised groups, disability activists and scholars began to describe their perspective as a minority group model of disability, as contrasted with the previously dominant medical views of having an impairment. According to the minority group view, the physical, cognitive, sensory, and emotional make-up of the individual was not the problem but was a problem only because social institutions and human-made environments were created without taking into account the characteristics of all people.[20] Without this bedrock conviction of the importance of legal rights as essential for any meaningful change in the position of people with disabilities, there would be not even the imperfect protections afforded by the patchwork of federal laws, including the beleaguered and imperfect Americans with Disabilities Act. No matter how court decisions chip away at its reach and no matter how poorly federal agencies enforce its provisions, the law provides a tangible assertion that the federal government believes in the moral equality and worth of people with disabilities and believes that people can benefit from, and contribute to, the common life of the society.

Recent scholarship argues that the minority group model is inadequate to the task of affording people with disabilities the conditions to turn legal rights into realities.[21] There are several reasons for replacing the minority group model with language that speaks of disability as a form of human variation and that calls for a universal design[22] and universalizing of disability. First, impairments are multiple and various; the same impairment may affect several individuals differently, depending upon other factors in their environments and in their own lives. The same impairment may affect the same individual differently at different times in life. Second, making notions of impairment equivalent to forms of human variation would reduce the need to decide who is "in" and who is "out" of the group of people counted as people with disabilities, which has become one of the major methods of denying people protection under the employment provisions of the Americans with Disabilities Act. Third, people with various conditions have a range of needs that influence their ability to take advantage of legal entitlements to education, employment, or public services. Without income to meet certain impairment-related expenses such as medications, transportation, personal assistance services, particular diet supplements, or items of clothing, for example, individuals may not flourish. Without the assistance of job coaches or other support staff, persons with emotional or cognitive impairments may not receive the individual assistance that permits them to manage the demands of typical schools or jobs. Without equipment or work schedules adjusted for rest or medical appointments, people with limited energy or with chronic pain may be unable to perform work for which they are otherwise well suited.

Scotch and Schriner argue:

[T]he minority group model cannot serve as the sole underpinning for disability policy. . . . [T]he commonly held notion of discrimination must be so stretched to include the various barriers faced by people with disabilities that the concept loses some of its precision and thus its utility as a guide to policy. It may be more useful . . . to look beyond discrimination to characterize the nature and consequences of a constructed environment that ignores the presence of people with disabilities. . . . [D]isability thus may be seen as an extension of the natural physical, social, and cultural variability of the human species. Disability could be defined as an extension of the variability in physical and mental attributes beyond the present—but not the potential—ability of social institutions to routinely respond. . . .

In this . . . human variation model of disability, the problems faced by people with disability might be seen as the consequence of the failure of social institutions (and their physical and cultural manifestations) that can be attributed to the institutions' having been constructed to deal with a narrower range of variation than is in fact present in any given population.[23]

Perhaps they are right in arguing that the concept of discrimination is "stretched" when it must incorporate concepts of "reasonable accommodation" in employment, or when such barriers as narrow doors have barred access to a service, lack of telephone relay systems, or needlessly inflexible work schedules are enforced. However, I want to argue that absent the pernicious belief that people with disabilities do not contribute to social or economic life and actually drain social resources, there would have been far more willingness prior to legislation to modify the social and built environment to include all the citizenry. I think that a "human variation" model has many advantages for people with a range of impairments, as I will discuss below, because it removes some of the pejorative specialness and exceptionality—some of the "us and them" quality—from disability and reminds everyone that human beings come in a variety of physical, mental, and emotional make-ups that change over time and may fit well into some sizes of clothing and some environments but not others unless we make more metaphorical and literal clothing sizes, styles of furniture, and methods of providing information to accommodate the range of physical, perceptual, and cognitive equipment that human beings possess.

What Matsuda, Bell, and other CRT writers contend, which I must concede, is that society will balk at making modifications that include everyone unless dominant members of that society can be perceived to benefit as a byproduct of these changes. How often, for example, are the proliferation of curb cuts, ramped entrances, and widened doorways hailed as a benefit for people who push shopping carts or for parents wheeling baby strollers! I applaud the fact that nondisabled persons may discover the convenience of these architectural changes, but they should not be justified as worthwhile because nondisabled people can enjoy them. They are worthwhile even if no substantial benefit accrues to the shopper or the parent and child using the stroller—which is, after all, an assistive device for young children to be mobile in the world—simply because they do benefit a portion of the population otherwise disenfranchised from our streets and public facilities.

In a small, but chilling example of societal resistance to complying with the legal requirements of providing access to mass transit to people with reading disabilities, the manufacturer of new technology told the following story to a convention of 2,500 members of the National Federation of the Blind: a device has been developed that, when installed on city buses, will verbally announce each stop, a great boon to anyone whose vision prevents the reading of street signs.[24] According to the regulations developed to implement existing law, bus drivers are expected to announce the stops, even without the device, but the device was developed because of well-known reluctance to do so and noncompliance with the law. However, the manufacturer of this technology revealed to the assembled convention-goers from every state in the nation that not even the installation of this technology was solving the problem of assuring that blind passengers could know where they were; bus drivers were turning off the device because they did not like having it as a routine part of their day.[25]

Exactly what prevents the drivers from calling out the stops themselves or from using the device developed and bought to get around their reluctance? Is it that they actually resent having nonreading passengers on the bus? Is it that the sound is more intrusive and monotonous than the same street signs? Is it that the environmental accommodation, the street sign usable by the visual reader, is considered ordinary, but the means that benefits the smaller number of passengers with visual, perceptual, or cognitive impairments is considered extraordinary, "special," foolish, or wasteful? Should such people not ride the public bus and use even more expensive segregated transit, or remain under constant supervision at even more expense, or simply not be abroad in the land? Will recalcitrant bus drivers call out the stops or at least tolerate the computerized announcements only when they are threatened with job loss or when "ordinary," nondisabled passengers tell them that they find the announcements convenient so that they need not continually look up from their newspapers or so they can be roused from dozing during a long ride?

Hearing this story, some people had the eerie feeling that perhaps Peter Singer, the bioethicist who believes that parents should be able to end the lives of "severely" impaired newborns if they do not want to raise them, might be right.[26] Perhaps the world really just does not want people with disabilities to be around after all. Until it is legitimate, respectable, and acceptable to be a person with a disability in the world, until the nondisabled majority recognizes how ubiquitous impairment is and how likely it is that everyone will experience it themselves or in someone they love, and until the nondisabled majority perceives that the millions of people with impairments are fully human and can contribute in meaningful ways to the economy and the family, that world will fight against every legal or moral claim made upon it to change institutions, cultural practices, and institutional and physical structures to become readily inclusive. Disability policy and politics must speak to the economic and emotional needs of the nondisabled majority to convince them that the accommodations made for people with disabilities in many ways can benefit them, if not directly, then indirectly. They must be persuaded that they, too, are accommodated in all manner of ways by social and architectural structures. As Susan Daniels, former Social Security Commissioner for Disability, is fond of pointing out, only those conferees using wheelchairs "bring their own chairs"; lights, microphones, and loudspeakers are environmental accommodations for those who obtain sensory input by sight or hearing.[27] Only when something like the Scotch and Schriner model of disability as human variation becomes widespread will it be possible for the majority to recognize that what they expect and demand as ordinary parts of institutional and physical life is no more required or reasonable than the changes that might make it possible for people with impairments to participate in routine activities.

Are All Impairments Created Equal?
Implications of the Variety of Impairments

Unfortunately, the very attempt to define a class of people called "disabled" under the Americans with Disabilities Act, and to indicate which members of the population could claim its protections, runs counter to the laudable goals of including people who have been disenfranchised by societal practices. Remember that the statutory definition of which persons can claim coverage under the Act as persons with disabilities defines a qualified individual in three ways: "(a) a physical or mental impairment that substantially limits one or more of the major life activities of such individual; (b) a record of such an impairment; or (c) being regarded as having such an impairment."[28] It thus differentiates between those who have "objective" departures from species-typicality, or what some people might consider "the truly disabled," and those who are inaccurately perceived as impaired by virtue of a record or of a misclassification.

For purposes of medical care and certain rehabilitative services, it is important to understand the nature of the departure from species-typicality to provide the correct medication or rehabilitation; for example, people with mobility impairments do not need Braille, and people who are blind do not need wheelchairs. For purposes of combating discrimination and unequal treatment that is the purpose of the Americans with Disabilities Act, there is no need to differentiate between the truly disabled and those merely "regarded as" disabled to determine whether there has been unlawful treatment by an employer, a restaurant, or a government agency.

Let me put forward the following, possibly radical, proposal: Instead of discussing which kinds of people have impairments or disabilities and which people do not, instead of saying that some members of society are disabled and others are not, we should consider which people cannot perform which activities in given environments and question how to modify the environments so that they are not disabling. Arguably, any person now living could, without any change in his or her physical, cognitive, sensory, and emotional make-up, be considered impaired by some employer, government service provider, place of public accommodation, or educational institution if the individual failed to meet particular standards for acceptance into a program or activity that the organization had established. Instead of discussing impaired individuals, attention should go to determining which environments—which social, physical, bureaucratic, and communication structures—could incorporate the widest array of individuals in all their diversity of capacities and then determine which environments were impairing and how they could be modified. When individuals complained that they were barred from an activity, program, or job because they were deemed outside the range of people the organization could accommodate, society could then decide on a case-by-case basis whether it wished the environment to change or wished to permit the exclusion of individuals because the environment found their characteristics unacceptable. Arguably, the most important prong of any definition of disability is that of being "regarded as" being impaired. Until society moves to evaluating the inclusiveness of environments, and as long as it insists upon evaluating which members of the population can fit into the existing ones, it would be better to recognize that all claimants under the ADA should be evaluated as having been "regarded as" impaired by the employer or other institution against which they are filing a complaint.

Readers may ask whether, on a "human variation" approach to disability, anyone might, at some point in life, believe that she or he should be able to use the Americans with Disabilities Act to claim a benefit, service, or job that they believed had been unfairly denied to them. Was the Americans with Disabilities Act intended for a particular "group" of people, or should it have been? Both disability rights advocates and ADA detractors have noted that many of the employment discrimination cases filed since the enactment of the ADA have not been brought by people commonly thought of as having disabilities, typically persons with visible impairments. In his preface to a group of articles devoted to the Americans with Disabilities Act, economist William Johnson writes:

> The ADA was clearly intended to provide entitlements to the persons represented by the advocacy groups, and little attention was given to the large number of persons who are identified as part of the disabled community by national surveys. . . .
>
> Information presented . . . demonstrates that the suits filed under the provisions of the ADA are more likely to come from the larger population than from the target group envisioned by the ADA's supporters. The larger group consists of persons, typically middle-aged or older, with nonvisible impairments, such as arthritis, cardiovascular conditions or chronic back pain that first occurred during adulthood.[29]

People familiar with cases filed under state and federal disability discrimination laws that existed prior to the enactment of the ADA should not have been surprised, since large numbers of state and federal cases of disability discrimination in employment had been brought by just such members of the population of those with disabilities.[30] I do not believe that this finding should trouble either disability rights advocates or give ADA detractors cause to contend that the law is being misused or being invoked to solve trivial problems. My nonlawyerly conviction accords with my understanding of ADA expert Chai Feldblum's discussion of the problems of definition in which the courts are now embroiled.[31] Instead of concluding that a person who uses eyeglasses or blood pressure medication is not a person with a disability for purposes of the Americans with Disabilities Act, it would be much more in keeping with the human variation approach to disability discussed above, and with the philosophy of nondiscrimination embodied in *Griggs v. Duke Power Co.*,[32] to permit such people to file complaints of employment discrimination as people who are "regarded as" having an impairment. The employer would then bear the burden of proving that the employee cannot, in fact, perform the essential functions of the job and that the employer's medical standards are job related. Permitting more people to claim protection from discrimination does not imply that their claims are correct, or that they can perform the essential functions of a particular job; nor does it suggest that employers are wrong in arguing that "reasonable accommodations" that might be needed by some people with certain conditions would impose an "undue hardship."[33] Such an approach simply calls for employers to ascertain which purported job requirements are truly necessary and which are the results of custom or convenience.

Along with other contemporary theorists of disability and of race, I conclude that what constitutes an impairment or disability, as what constitutes a racial category, is socially constructed.[34] Such a statement is not news; but law, society, and philosophy of race, sex, or disability are still working out the implications of the idea that formerly given categories are socially constructed. Saying that disability is socially constructed does not imply that the characteristics are not real or do not have describable effects on physiological or cognitive functions that persist in many environments. Just as the medical responses to different conditions are not identical, the social construction approach to disability does not imply that the social/psychological/nonmedical consequences of arthritis, muscular dystrophy, Down syndrome, hypertension, attention deficit disorder, or back pain are identical or that the accommodations, services, and responses to each condition need be identical.

Such factors as how observable an impairment is; what physical, sensory, or cognitive/emotional functions are affected; whether it is static or progressive; whether it is predictable or unpredictable in its manifestations; and whether it affects longevity all may influence the experience of disability for the person who has the condition, as well as for those around such an individual.[35] In different circumstances, the visibility of a characteristic—be it femaleness, weight, hair color, skin color, or navigating in a wheelchair—may influence someone's experiences. Persons with characteristics such as diabetes or asthma that may not be readily observable may sometimes find that their impairments affect a given set of activities and life decisions, whereas at other times they find life flowing smoothly with no thought to their medical label. Although appearing nondisabled when one first meets people professionally or socially may permit the person with diabetes or asthma to avoid the often adverse reactions of others to observable orthopedic, visual, or speech impairments, these so-called hidden disabilities may influence social life such as the food one eats, the places one visits, the activities one pursues for recreation, and so forth. Fearing the adverse reactions of others to the disclosure of a characteristic like diabetes, asthma, treated cancer in remission, a heart condition, or a history of mental illness produces its own psychological consequences; the stress of hiding may turn out to be as problematic as the feared responses from disclosure. A mother or father might be deeply shaken by learning that a child with cystic fibrosis could die in their thirties but might react with much less concern upon discovering that a child could expect an average lifespan but would have cerebral palsy. A different set of parents, on the other hand, might find the relative invisibility of a child's cystic fibrosis easier to incorporate into their lives than the more easily perceived, and thus possibly more stigmatized, condition of cerebral palsy.

My point here is that impairments impinge upon people differently from one another depending upon a host of psychological and social factors that all are external to the biomedical condition. Disability theorist Harlan Hahn characterizes disability as eliciting "existential and aesthetic anxiety" in others.[36] Notable in the history of governmental discrimination and segregation documented in the Garrett case is that people with only certain conditions received some of the most isolating and demeaning treatment.[37] The medical model of disability would explain this fact by contending that people with substantial departures from a notion of "species-typical" cognitive, orthopedic, hearing, and visual norms may be the only ones with genuine impairments. But from a social constructionist view, it is only that their characteristics were considered more difficult to incorporate into more environments. People who had such characteristics as ulcers, high blood pressure, or bad backs were more easily incorporated. As environments routinely incorporate members of society with historically stigmatized labels, the characteristics themselves could become as unremarkable as brown eyes or long hair. There is one such striking example on Martha's Vineyard in Massachusetts in the nineteenth century, as documented by Nora Groce in her book, *Everyone Here Spoke Sign Language*, in which she explained how common hereditary deafness ceased to be a disability because all island residents routinely used both sign language and speech for communication.[38]

Are there some environments that we do not wish to modify to admit a broader range of persons than now function within them? Should the rules of golf be modified to permit Casey Martin to use a cart to travel around the course,[39] or do we wish to maintain that playing golf requires a particular complement of physical capacities? We can choose. Can air carriers continue to have vision standards for pilots that preclude the wearing of glasses as the method of seeing the instruments? Reasonable people and experts on piloting and air safety may disagree among themselves about which physical, sensory, and cognitive abilities are crucial for successful control and navigation of an aircraft, but the debate about *Sutton v. United Air Lines, Inc.*[40] should have been on the grounds of business necessity, on essential functions of a demanding job, and not on the level of a particular person's impairment in some objective sense, abstracted from the circumstance in which capacity was at issue. Similarly, the Department of Transportation medical standard for truck drivers should be at issue in *Murphy v. U.P.S.*,[41] and not whether the individual had an impairment that prevented him from engaging in a substantial life activity. He was outside the environment that had been established for the job he sought; the relevance of the standard to the job, not his blood pressure in an abstract sense, should have been evaluated.

In these recent employment decisions, I decry the philosophy behind courts declaring that people are not sufficiently impaired to claim the statute's protection. Employers may successfully persuade courts to conclude that environments should not be more flexible with regard to a particular individual's characteristics. However, in the instance where an individual is denied a position because of measured blood pressure, for example, the employer should be asked to show why blood pressure of a certain reading disqualifies someone from performing the essential functions of a job and should not be able to argue that someone with blood pressure of a measured reading is not a person with an impairment under the meaning of the statute. Since the individual is alleging that employment was denied based on the blood pressure, the employer should be required to indicate either that the allegation is false or that it is true and that there is a legitimate, nondiscriminatory reason based on the requirements of the job.[42]

Are environments infinitely flexible? Each time environmental arrangements are challenged, society, as represented by courts and legislatures, must decide how flexible and inclusive it will be. To those unacquainted with how people with such characteristics as quadriplegia, autism, or limited ability to use or understand verbal language would study, work, or care for children, it may seem impossible; but people with such characteristics are now succeeding in these activities because they have found or constructed arrangements in which they can contribute based on their capacities and receive assistance with facets of life that are difficult. Arguably, that is what everyone does in life. Most lawyers do not repair their automobiles, but society does not degrade them for being dependent upon mechanics. There is no reason to devalue, patronize, or question the legitimacy of someone who obtains spoken information via an interpreter or real-time captioner, or who gets ready for work with the assistance of another human being who prepares meals or puts on clothes. Similarly, the man with limited verbal language who works with support staff to run errands and who invites others to his home for holidays, conducts customary adult activities of work, being a member of a household, and maintaining a social life. In these environments, he is not a person with a disability. If few environments will accommodate his mix of talents and needs, the problem may be the lack of imagination or the lack of will on the part of others.

If people labeled as mentally ill are filing complaints of discrimination in employment, it may derive from the existential anxiety occasioned by contact with someone whose behavior may be feared unpredictable, out of their or our control, or whose modes of social interaction startle those with the power to make employment decisions. Perhaps the difficulty they experience in finding employment should be attributed to managerial resistance to incorporating a person with particular characteristics into a fixed environment. People now thought unemployable in one setting may be employable in another setting that adapts to a greater level of human variation. If the social norm becomes one of trying to achieve an adaptive environment that can easily respond to a broad range of talents and needs, then we may be able to accept the occasional institution or setting with fixed standards of performance. Acting on Broadway may legitimately require more experience, skill, and versatility on the part of those who audition than acting in the community theater. Banks, restaurants, and the Internet should be open to all, accessible to and usable by virtually anyone. Most educational and employment situations should fall somewhere between the bank and the Broadway audition, and denials of employment should be based on an individualized assessment of why a particular applicant or employee was unsuitable for a particular job. Fluency with verbal and written language, for example, might be a skill basic to many positions in the contemporary economy. Anyone, who for any reason could not understand or express herself in words in any way would have limited work options; but employers who turned away people who could not communicate fluently should be able to demonstrate why this skill was required for the particular position and not resort to the statement that "all employees must be able to read and write and communicate at a sixth grade level."

I started the section by asking whether all impairments were equal and then proposed that instead of speaking of impairments at all, we should be speaking of environments. In noting that only some people who departed from the physical, sensory, cognitive, and emotional norms historically were subject to the most virulent forms of segregation, isolation, and neglect, I am acknowledging that historically and in contemporary society, the different forms of human variation called disabilities draw different responses. Children and youth with cystic fibrosis or diabetes, for example, are not typically isolated from others in their same grade in rooms for the disabled, but children with other characteristics deemed more challenging for the typical environment are still often educated in separate spaces. When they complete their education, those with cystic fibrosis or diabetes are likely to have an easier time finding work than someone with manual, but not linguistic or mathematical, skill. People who do not stand out by appearance or speech occasion no aesthetic anxiety in restaurants and movie theaters, and if they hide the fact of their epilepsy or back pain from others, they may go through much of their life without triggering the existential anxiety

Hahn describes as an explanation for the discriminatory treatment that the ADA is designed to combat. Within the large group of people who may not fit into existing environments and social arrangements, some have been and may continue to be considered more challenging to existing arrangements than others. But if we take the human variation model seriously, we should be questioning the arrangements for failing to include, rather than assuming that the arrangements are fine as they are and concluding that it is the personal deficiency that prevents certain people from participating.

Integration As a Goal?

In discussing the justifications for ending de jure and de facto segregation based on race, commentators from within critical race theory point out that implicit in the championing of "integration" was the idea that Black-White contact was good for Blacks because White-controlled institutions were self-evidently superior to those in the Black community.[43] Quoting Malcolm X, Peller points out that segregation and separation are not identical and that self-chosen separation sometimes can be necessary and valuable.

A segregated school system isn't necessarily the same situation that exists in an all-white neighborhood. A school system in an all-white neighborhood is not a segregated school system. The only time it's segregated is when it is in a community other than white, but at the same time is controlled by whites. So my understanding of a segregated school system—or a segregated community, or a segregated school—is a school that's controlled by people other than those who go there.[44]

Going on, Peller contrasts his own view with his description of the convictions of integrationists, who say that "race makes no real difference between people, except as unfortunate historical vestiges of irrational discrimination."[45] Peller makes a powerful argument for the value of community-controlled, strong institutions within the particular community. He argues that the goal of integration can never be truly achieved or that if it could, it would not be desirable for it would be a "total absorption and disappearance of the race—a sort of painless genocide."[46] Peller contrasts his own view with his understanding of a reigning 1960s liberal ideology "that race could be understood as just another example of the range of arbitrary social characteristics—like gender, physical handicap, or sexual preference—that right-thinking people should learn to ignore."[47]

He concludes his challenge to integrationist ideology:

[T]he construction of race reform as overcoming bias at the level of consciousness, overcoming discrimination at the practice level, and achieving integration at the institutional level has meant that tremendous social resources and personal energy have been expended on integrating formerly white schools, workplaces, neighborhoods, and attitudes. This program, . . . has had some success in improving the lives of specific people and in transforming the climate of overt racial domination. . . . Yet it has been pursued to the exclusion of a commitment to the vitality of the black community as a whole and to the economic and cultural health of black neighborhoods, schools, economic enterprises, and individuals.[48]

How does this apply to the situation of people with disabilities or to what is described as "the disability rights movement or the disabled community?" Most people who have disabilities acquire them in midlife and struggle to incorporate their changed bodies and minds into preexisting work and family arrangements. Even for those who acquire their conditions at birth or in childhood and young adulthood, most characteristics are not genetically transmitted, and thus, only a small fraction of the millions of people with disabilities grow up in a natural community of others with their same characteristic.

Lack of natural community, the variability among impairments, and the domination of medical services and philanthropic disability service organizations by nondisabled professionals have all mitigated against developing a strong, coherent, politically powerful community of people with disabilities. Nonetheless, these same people were kept out of schools and classes, workplaces, and sometimes neighborhoods and social life with nondisabled people of their age, sex, or ethnicity. If community formed at all among those with disabilities, it generally occurred along single-impairment lines, through residential schools for people who were deaf or blind, in institutions for people with intellectual or psychiatric diagnoses, or in the wards of rehabilitation centers.[49]

Here, many allies among the ranks of disability scholars may not share some of my views, perhaps because I formed my views of disability politics out of the very White integrationist views of the sixties.[50] Like others, I wholeheartedly endorse the integrationist, inclusionist philosophy behind the Individuals with Disabilities in Education Act (IDEA),[51] the *Olmsted v. L. C.* decision,[52] and the fight to keep people who need personal assistance services in their own families and neighborhoods and out of institutions or nursing homes. Voluntary associations for political or social purposes, controlled by people with disabilities, play crucial roles for many people and have championed the federal and state legislation that symbolizes acceptance into the nation's social and economic life. Deaf culturists, some members of the National Federation of the Blind, and some disability scholars, fed up with the social isolation and inadequate academic preparation of disabled students educated in the public schools since the passage of P.L. 94–142 in 1975, echo the views of Gary Peller and Malcolm X and call for a re-creation of separate schools that would give disabled youth strong academic skills, a life with potential friends, and a chance to develop ties to others with disabilities. Rather than support even a disability-controlled, disability-affirmative school, I urge our leaders and scholars to put our energies into promoting high expectations for the academic and social development of disabled youth in neighborhood schools. Genuine inclusion in schools along with nondisabled age-peers cannot come without environmental changes. Teachers must not refuse to give the schedule to a band member in a form she can read and thus reject her from the band because she can play the flute but cannot read the printed schedule.[53] As a first grade student, Amy Rowley was denied interpreter services in her classroom of hearing, non-signing students and teachers because she was reported to be passing from grade to grade despite her inability to obtain the same information as her classmates. She is now in her twenties, but the Supreme Court decision denying her the interpreter service has never been revisited.[54]

No wonder that Deaf community members would prefer to see today's deaf students be taught by people who could use American Sign Language and have classmates with whom they could communicate. Similarly, there is reason to fear that a classroom aide who functions as sole teacher and social contact, leaving the student isolated from the designated teacher and the other students, is segregating students with a range of disabilities within the public school and classroom.[55]

The same need to form political action groups or support groups that has fueled organizations like the National Federation of the Blind, Little People of America, People First, Disabled in Action, the Disability Rights Education and Defense Fund, and more may continue for many years and probably should include increased attention to disabled youth, much as churches and synagogues organize youth groups for their members. Until a teenager with cerebral palsy receives the message from his teachers, peers, and family that he should set his future goals based on interests and talents, and not ask himself "What can a boy with cerebral palsy do?" he is likely to need contact with older people with similarly atypical motor or speaking skills to assure him that there is a future. But these contacts, built around life with disability, should not be offered as his principal source of companionship, with the implication that he cannot expect equal-status friendship from among nondisabled members of his own school or class.

Race-Consciousness, Disability-Consciousness, and Identity Politics

While my dedication to the goal of social integration is tempered by my conviction that oppressed people, including those with impairments, will need to combat their situation by maintaining groups for social support and political action, the same dedication to the goal of integration leads me to hold each of the following views described respectively by Randall Kennedy, a professor who is African-American, and Duncan Kennedy, a professor who is a White critical race theorist. Randall Kennedy has stated: "I simply do not want race-conscious decision-making to be naturalized into our general pattern of academic evaluation. I do not want race-conscious decision-making to lose its status as a deviant mode of judging people or the work they produce. I do not want race-conscious decision-making to be assimilated into our conception of meritocracy."[56]

Taking issue with the world as ready for the meritocracy without reference to race that Randall Kennedy advocates, Duncan Kennedy responds:

> One index of a community's cultural subordination is its dependence on others to produce knowledge in areas where it would seem, at least superficially, that community interests will be affected by what that knowledge is. . . . Along with more scholarship on minority issues, there should be more scholarship on the implications for minorities of any issue currently under debate. In other words, Hispanic scholars working on the purest of corporate law questions within the most unquestionably Anglo scholarly paradigm are still, I think, more likely than white scholars to devote, over the long run, some time to thinking about the implications of law in their chosen technical area for the Hispanic communities.[57]

The two statements appear incompatible, yet I endorse both. In a society that still makes race, or sex, or sexual preference, or health status a basis for differential treatment in matters of life where the factor is irrelevant to the activity, members of "out" groups continue to share experiences Iris Young describes as five "faces" of oppression: exploitation, marginalization, powerlessness, cultural imperialism, and violence.[58] Absent family lineage or geographic concentration in neighborhoods outside of schools or treatment centers, disabled people with experiences of oppression have formed social and political organizations based on their shared experience—largely of being patronized, dismissed, misunderstood, in short, mistreated.

Do people with disabilities share positive experiences or see themselves as members of a cultural community with traditions to pass on and wisdom to teach? Many people in the Deaf community point to theater and poetry performed through ASL as examples of the richness of their cultural life.[59] Some longtime movement activists are bound together not only by their friendships and histories of political victories and defeats, but by the time spent in making disability politics the emotional centerpiece of their lives, much as any members of political movement groups or other causes might describe their passionate commitment as at the center of their lives and their psychological orienting point in the world.[60] How much is disability part of identity for members of the movement or for people who are not part of it? Whenever people with disabilities are surveyed by the Louis Harris organization, as they have been frequently since 1986, it turns out that pluralities, sometimes majorities, of respondents perceive disability status as akin to minority status and feel some commonality with people who have the same or different impairments.[61] Carol Gill, disability scholar and researcher on disability and identity, argues that in order for people with disabilities to function well in this oppressive society, disability should be a "positive and central" part of their identity.[62] Philosophers Anthony Appiah and Anna Stubblefield each have written valuable articles considering what it would mean to say that "race" or "sex" were a central component of identity. Appiah, for example, says that he could still be himself, recognizable to himself, were he to somehow wake up the next day not as a person of color. He suspects that:

> "Racial" ethical identities are . . . apparently less conceptually central to who one is than gender ethical identities. . . .
>
> Nevertheless, even for those for whom being African-American is an important aspect of their ethical identity, what matters to them is almost always not the unqualified fact of that descent, but rather something that they suppose to go with it: the experience of a life as a member of a group of people who experience themselves as—and are held by others to be—a community in virtue of their mutual recognition—and their recognition by others—as people of a common descent.[63]

Appiah, Anna Stubblefield, and Richard Wasserstrom are all philosophers who reject what Stubblefield calls "essentialism" about race.[64] Identity, essentialism, and community take on a particular significance when we remember the disability, unlike race or sex, is not usually shared by the members of one's biological or social family, notwithstanding genetic and chromosomal causes of some conditions. Most people with Down syndrome, cystic fibrosis, sickle cell anemia, spina bifida, diabetes, deafness, or blindness—even if manifest in early childhood—do not grow up with parents and siblings who share this characteristic. It is, in fact, the apprehensions about what raising a child with these conditions, and the belief that life for the child and the family will be more negative than positive, that fuel the increasing use of prenatal testing in today's developed nations. Unlike the African-American parent expecting to share bonds with their children that will provide love and community to be some refuge against racism in the outside world, the typical nondisabled prospective parents have no experience with or knowledge of life that includes disability, and they are generally counseled that raising a child with a disability will be an unhappy experience, likened by some to the "burden" of an unwanted child.[65] No pamphlets exist in inner-city clinics about the "dangers" of bearing and raising children, despite the fact that children raised in these circumstances are more likely than other children to experience poverty, exposure to drugs, arrest, or incarceration, poor schooling, and unemployment. Such pamphlets do not exist, and should not, because professionals recognize that society, and not biology, accounts for the problems and at least theoretically supports social changes to eradicate those problems. Professionals also are responding to the fact that inner-city prospective parents may fear these problems for their future children but may also imagine that love, family, and community make child-rearing worthwhile. Thus, the parents imagine a shared common identity and community with any future child, a marked contrast with the typical nondisabled prospective parent who fears that a future child's impairment will thwart parental hopes for a fulfilling family life.[66]

Contrast the views of disability as burdensome and disappointing to families expressed by many philosophers and physicians with the findings of recent research showing that most families who raise children with disabilities fare as well as others in overall life satisfaction and enjoyment of their children.[67] The words of a mother of a young child with a disability eloquently capture what many parents feel after having this experience, one that they may have previously feared or known nothing about:

> [P]arents of children with disabilities have often learned to see what is positive within their experience of parenting a disabled child. I would never trade my disabled son's infectious laugh, huge smiles, and enormous hugs for his sister's giftedness. This morning, my husband and I spent three hours at Children's Hospital watching him take aptitude tests and such. We have never taken so much pride in our children as when we watched him try his hardest and come up with answers that made sense in his very special world—which we had the fortunate opportunity to glimpse through his answers. . . . I don't know any parent of a disabled child who would trade that child in for a "better model" even if we were disappointed at some point to learn about our child's disabilities.[68]

To the extent that an increasing number of families successfully incorporate a child's, parent's, or spouse's impairment into their lives and relationships, they provide the evidence that community can be created by perceiving commonalties as well as differences, by recognizing that commonalties can transcend differences of health and disability status. Regrettably, the history of professional advice about how disabled children would harm families, as well as separate schooling and institutionalization of some members of the disabled population, means that many of today's people with disabilities do not perceive their families as allies or as including them in the family's community. If the social changes envisioned by the Americans with Disabilities Act transform schools and better include people with disabilities in the workforce and the world, perhaps people with disabilities will find more natural community in their family, religious, ethnic, or racial groups, those that traditionally nurture and sustain people facing the larger world. My reflections on disability-as-identity that follow are clearly affected by having been incorporated into family, school, and other meaningful groups throughout my life. As I ponder the Randall Kennedy and Duncan Kennedy assertions about race and affirmative action, along with these philosophical writings on race and sex as central components of identity, trying to draw analogies to my own experience of being a White, Jewish woman with a disability, I find that nothing I read quite captures my own understanding or my own desire for what I want identity to be.

Yes, I suspect that because characteristics like ethnicity, race, sex, and disability are all interwoven in my, or anyone's, experience, I can agree with all those writers who remind us that each characteristic is influenced by the others that make up our lives. Many sensitive people can and do teach and write eloquently about the experience of disability, although they do not themselves live as persons with disabilities or as family members of disabled persons. Although these same people teach excellent disability studies courses and have made significant contributions to the field of disability studies, they may not as easily or routinely infuse insights about disability into their thinking and writing in other topics. My own courses on motherhood, for example, include discussions of women with disabilities as mothers—something I have seen in none of the large numbers of recent books on the experiences of motherhood.[69] Thus, I suspect that perhaps Duncan Kennedy is right to believe that minority scholars will, whatever their topic, be alert to the implications of their work for minority communities. Bringing such insights into any curriculum constitutes an excellent intellectual argument for affirmative action in academia and elsewhere.

Christopher Nolan, author of a memoir about being an Irish boy with cerebral palsy growing up in the last quarter of the twentieth century, asked by interviewers how he would feel if he could one day get out of his wheelchair, replies that he would get right back in.[70] Like Nolan, I have had my disability of blindness from birth; I would not, however, give his answer. The possibility of sight is one I neither crave nor fear. Although it might be interesting, pleasurable, and convenient, I do not think it would markedly change my commitments, interests, passions, or how I think about the world, human relationships, work, or play. It makes great sense to work with other people who are blind or who have disabilities to combat oppression or to change society. It makes sense to check out reactions to perplexing instances of strained interactions around disability with others who have disabilities, as well as with others who do not. But save for getting advice about one or another piece of adaptive computing technology, I do not find blindness a source of discussion unless I am trying to deal with its misperception in the larger social world. My identity is defined by what I read, not by my means of reading it; Braille is a useful tool, but a taken-for-granted one, as print is to those who use it. The world can make disability central in certain contexts, if I have a day or week of especially assaultive or infantalizing encounters, but working for social change and inclusion necessitates being involved with all sorts of people who care about the intellectual and personal interests that define me—many of which concern topics other than disability.

My dream is much closer to Wasserstrom's dream of a society that makes no life option decisions based on race, sex, or disability status and thus leaves people freer than they are now to find how much of their lives are affected by any one of their many ascribed characteristics. Iris Marion Young, while not essentializing group identity, rejects this individualistic approach to identity-formation, saying:

> A person's group identities may be for the most part only a background or horizon to his or her life, becoming salient only in specific interactive contexts.

> Assuming an aggregate model of groups, some people think that so-
> cial groups are invidious fictions, essentializing arbitrary attributes.
> From this point of view problems of prejudice, stereotyping, discrimi-
> nation, and exclusion exist because some people mistakenly believe that
> group identification makes a difference to the capacities, temperament,
> or virtues of group members. This individualist conception of persons
> and their relation to one another tends to identify oppression with group
> identification. Oppression . . . is something that happens to people when
> they are classified in groups. Because others identify them as a group,
> they are excluded and despised. Eliminating oppression thus requires
> eliminating groups. . . .
>   This book takes issue with that position. . . . [I]t is foolish to deny
> the reality of groups. . . . [G]roup differentiation remains endemic. . . .
> Even when they belong to oppressed groups, people's group identifica-
> tions are often important to them, and they often feel a special affinity
> for others in their group. . . .
>   Though some groups have come to be formed out of oppression, . . .
> group differentiation is not in itself oppressive.[71]

Perhaps, despite embracing of disability activism and disability scholarship as a means of social change, I remain involved out of a sense of deep obli-
gation and not excitement. Perhaps the disability affiliation is for me only one
of friendships formed in the struggle for change, and although the friendships
as well as the work are positive and rewarding, I still do not find this facet of
my life and identity inherently interesting.

Paul Kenneth Longmore is eloquent in stating the positive learning and
values that, for him, can be attributed to living as a person with a disability when
he speaks of values that would change society for everyone if broadly adopted:
"not self-sufficiency but self-determination, not independence but interdepen-
dence, not functional separateness but personal connection, not physical autonomy but human community."[72] Many feminist theorists and critical race
authors could sign on to that list of values, coming, as they do, from learning to
survive and flourish as persons with little power who must work to glean connections, warmth, and intimacy from a world generally wary of acceptance and
welcome to those it sees as "different."

Survival and thriving will indeed be easier if we can move more and more
people to appreciate such values, but it will also be easier and more rewarding
if people discover and emphasize similarities and commonalities rather than announce their differences as armor to pierce or masks to remove. I draw much
solace in the generous writing of Martha Minow, who speaks my language as
she struggles with the dilemmas of overemphasizing or ignoring difference and
the pitfalls as well as values of identity politics.

> Identity politics tends to locate the problem in the identity group rather
> than the social relations that produce identity groupings. . . .

Judith Butler put the limitations of identity politics bluntly: "You can articulate your identity all you want; you need the damn resources in order to respond to the concrete problems of bodies in pain." To get the resources, you need to work with others; to care about other bodies in pain, you need to move beyond your own circumstances. . . . The potentially multiple, fluid qualities of any person's identity seem to evaporate in the assertion of a single trait.[73]

The human variation approach to disability and impairment could, if adopted, mute the notion of groups of people with disabilities as contrasted to people without them. If environments become more accepting of more members in the population, perhaps there will be less reason for excluded persons to form groups based on oppression because they will be increasingly welcomed into family, neighborhood, work, and interest groups. If people continue to find an impairment status worthy of embracing as a part of community membership, it could be out of whatever commonalities beyond oppression they find in that status.

Is there something about impaired capacities—less-than-typical hearing, motor coordination, strength, sight, or skill in understanding and communicating through language—that is unimaginably "neutral" or positive, no matter what the society? Philosophers and bioethicists with interests in disability rights are grappling with this question and as yet, I know of no emerging consensus on what remains of disability as a problematic status apart from an unwelcoming society. We are so far from achieving a welcoming society that it is about as fanciful as the thought experiments of racial identity and meaning discussed by Appiah, Stubblefield, and Wasserstrom above.[74]

For now, I cannot settle on an answer. I think about Gregory Williams's contribution to this symposium, a portion of which concerns his own musings on similarities and differences between race and disability:

I was challenged by a young man confined [sic] to a wheelchair as to whether his life had been harder than mine. I quickly agreed that, given the choice, I would have much preferred receiving the racial epithets hurled at me, the racial violence directed against me, and the doors closed to me because of my racial heritage than to live his life confined to a wheelchair.[75]

I think back to the first time, almost forty years ago, that I read an article questioning whether it was better to be a White, upper-class man who was blind, or to be any man who was Black in the North or South in the pre–Civil Rights Act 1960s. Comparing virulent racism to the limitations he found as a person who was blind, before the movement for Black civil rights had achieved its gains of the 1960s and before most people with disabilities were aware of any efforts to end their second-class status, Peter Putnam wrote:

Blindness is a confining handicap [sic], but it would not confine the boy to the life in the Negro ghettos that are the shame of our cities, North and South. If he had a Seeing Eye dog, he would be excluded for his dog, not for his skin. In blindness, he would know moments of humiliating helplessness [sic], but not so bitter as the practice of Jim Crow, the loss of civil rights, or the experience of police brutality Baldwin describes, not in the South, but in New York City.

Yet blindness is a genuine handicap. Blackness is not. The blind man has lost an important sense. The Negro has all his faculties. The handicap of blindness is intrinsic. The handicap of blackness comes from the outside, imposed by force or the threat of force. The handicap of the American Negro has been the American white.[76]

Putnam concludes his ruminations by saying that we should create a society in which it is "no longer a handicap to be black."[77]

When I first read those words as a high school student getting involved in the civil rights movement, it seemed to me that it was far easier to be a White, middle-class blind person than to be anyone who was Black. At that time, I had not yet encountered years of employment discrimination and social dismissal that would be part of my adult life. Putnam and myself, as people who are blind, and Gregory Williams, as a person who has self-identified as Black,[78] all were more comfortable with what we knew, with the problems we knew how to fight and survive, than with ones we could only imagine.

Perhaps social constructionists of disability will conclude with Putnam that even in a transformed society where racism, sexism, and disability discrimination are negligible portions of individual and social life, some aspects of life will nonetheless be more difficult or impossible if disabled, and that the human variations of race are easier to accommodate than the variations of differing health or ability. I believe it possible that disability is not entirely reducible to social construction, and that some forms of aesthetic experiences and some sorts of physical activities may be precluded by physiology alone. People who are deaf will not hear music, but they can have the aesthetic experiences of enjoying painting, and those who are blind will not see sunsets, but they can hear birdsongs and ocean waves; people who use wheelchairs will not run marathons even if they do race in them and cross the finish line before the runners. For now, as we struggle to retain the gains we thought we had won when the ADA became law, as we examine racism and sexism in a post–civil rights world where people of color still earn less than similarly educated Whites and where women in two-career families still perform more domestic work and childcare than their male partners, we can say that there is much work to do on all fronts. To quote Gregory Williams again on the race/disability comparison:

> However the more I thought about it, the more I realized that the issue was not who had the tougher life. . . . The issue was whether either one of our lives had been affected by external factors that should have had

absolutely no impact on our ability to live our lives to the fullest extent possible.[79]

Like feminists and CRT writers, I am not interested in changing my race, sex, or health/ability status; we all need to work with others to gain greater equality, more inclusivity, and greater appreciation of the complexity of humanity in all its variability. The goal is to create a society where it is irrelevant to be blind or Black.

Notes

Editor's Note: Professor Asch's paper was first presented at "Facing the Challenges of the ADA: The First Ten Years and Beyond," a symposium sponsored by the Center for Law, Policy and Social Science and Moritz Law School at The Ohio State University on April 7, 2000, in Columbus, Ohio, and published in *Ohio State Law Journal* 62, 2.

I wish to thank Ruth Colker for inviting me to examine the lessons of critical race theory and feminism for disability theory and policy. The invitation, and our several conversations as I grappled with these questions, have proved very provocative and stimulating for me, and I can only hope that this chapter captures some of what I have learned from our work together.

Many thanks go to Taran Jefferies, who not only provided superb logistical and research assistance and became a pro at Bluebook citation form but also provided intellectual stimulation through our discussion of these ideas and moral support that prevented me from deciding the task was too great to accomplish.

1. Americans with Disabilities Act, 42 U.S.C. § 12111(a)(7) (1994).
2. See generally *Berkeley Journal of Employment and Labor Law*, 22 (2000); *Annals of the American Academy of Political and Social Sciences*, 549 (1997); Leslie Pickering Francis and Anita Silvers, eds., *Americans with Disabilities: Exploring Implications of the Law for Individuals and Institutions* (New York: Routledge, 2000) (each containing articles analyzing and critiquing the ADA).
3. On February 21, 2001, as this chapter was being completed, the United States Supreme Court handed down its opinion in a case testing the extent of Congress's power to impose obligations upon the states. As reported in the *New York Times*,

> The Supreme Court today carved out a new area of immunity for the states from the reach of federal civil rights law, ruling that state employees cannot sue for damages for violations of the Americans With Disabilities Act.
>
> The 5-to-4 vote was the same by which the court, in a series of decisions over the past six years, has constricted the power of Congress and correspondingly expanded the sphere of state immunity to a degree unmatched in the modern era. . . .
>
> In overturning the appeals court's ruling today, Chief Justice William H. Rehnquist's majority opinion concluded that the effort to open the states to lawsuits exceeded Congress's authority.

Linda Greenhouse, "Justices Give the States Immunity from Suits by Disabled Workers," *New York Times*, February 22, 2001, A1.

At least as disturbing as the ruling is the majority's claim that, "[e]ven if it were to be determined that the half a dozen relevant examples from the record showed unconstitutional action on the part of States, these incidents taken together fall far short of even suggesting the pattern of unconstitutional discrimination on which § 5 legislation must be based." *Univ. of Ala. at Birmingham Bd. of Trs. v. Garrett*, No. 99–1240, 2001 U.S. LEXIS 1700, at *5 (February 21, 2001). This claim is vigorously disputed in Justice Breyer's dissenting opinion. *Garrett*, 2001 U.S. LEXIS 1700, at *38–42. Losing this case, as the amici curiae discuss, erodes the protection of people with disabilities from conduct by state governments that historically have been arguably as segregationist and discriminatory as Jim Crow laws were for African Americans in the pre–civil rights South. See Brief of Amici Curiae in Support of Respondents, *Univ. of Ala. at Birmingham Bd. of Trs. v. Garrett*, 193 F.3d 1214 (11th Cir.) (No. 99–1240).

It is also worth noting the majority's attitude toward people with disabilities as captured by the following remarks: "Thus, the Fourteenth Amendment does not require States to make special accommodations for the disabled, so long as their actions toward such individuals are rational. They could quite hardheadedly—and perhaps hardheartedly—hold to job-qualification requirements which do not make allowance for the disabled." *Garrett*, 2001 U.S. LEXIS 1700, at *4.

Fortunately, as Ruth Colker points out in this personal communication of October 11, 2000, it does not entirely preclude people with disabilities from winning suits against state governments:

> The correct technical explanation is that *Garrett* is about whether Congress has the authority to provide a private right of action for damages in actions brought by individuals against the state. Even if the plaintiff loses in Garrett, the federal government can still enforce ADA Title II. In addition, a private individual can still sue for injunctive relief. Finally, it is also the case that section 504 will still be fully available.

Letter from Professor Ruth Colker, Grace Fern Heck Faust Chair in Constitutional Law, The Ohio State University College of Law, to Adrienne Asch, Henry R. Luce Professor of Biology, Ethics and the Politics of Human Reproduction, Wellesley College (October 11, 2000; on file with author).

4. "Enforcement efforts seem more focused on 'micro,' individual cases. This means lost opportunities, because findings at the individual level often do not lead to an examination of larger systemic issues. Overall, the federal enforcement effort has been uneven, lacking in robustness, and suffering from low visibility in many areas." National Council on Disability, *Promises to Keep: A Decade of Federal Enforcement of the Americans with Disabilities Act* (Washington, DC: US GPO, 2000), 4–5.

5. Richard Delgado, ed., *Critical Race Theory: The Cutting Edge* (Philadelphia: Temple University Press, 1995), xiv. (hereinafter CRT: The Cutting Edge). The pervasiveness of disparate, unequal, and pejorative treatment of people with disabilities in the United States is documented not only in Congress's findings and purposes section of the Americans with Disabilities Act, but as applied to the actions of state governments particularly, in several amici curiae briefs submitted in the *Garrett* case. I will not try to further document the persistence of discrimination based on disability but will confine my discussion to the lessons to be learned from the legal scholarship of feminists and critical race theorists as they apply to disability.

6. Alan D. Freeman, "Legitimizing Racial Discrimination through Antidiscrimination

Law: A Critical Review of Supreme Court Doctrine," in *Critical Race Theory: The Key Writings that Formed the Movement*, edited by Kimberlé Crenshaw et al. (New York: New Press, 1995), 29, 35 (hereinafter *CRT: The Key Writings*):

"A second and slightly less extreme version of the utopia posits a society in which racial identification is still possible but no longer relevant to anyone's thinking or generalizations about anyone else. . . . Race would have become functionally equivalent to eye color in contemporary society. In yet a third version of the integrated society, racial identification persists as a cultural unifying force for each group, equivalent to an idealized model of religious tolerance. Each group respects the diverse character of every other group, and there are no patterns of domination or oppression between different groups"; Richard A. Wasserstrom, "Racism and Sexism," in *Philosophy and Social Issues* 11 (1980), cited in Anna Stubblefield, "Racial Identity and Non-Essentialism about Race," *Social Theory & Practice* 21 (1995): 341, 368 n.7; Gary Peller, "Race-Consciousness," in Crenshaw et al., *CRT: The Key Writings*, 127.

7. My discussion reflects only my own views on these very controversial topics. I represent no organization of people with disabilities in this chapter, nor do I claim that all of my views are likely to be shared by the majority of theorists of disability who might evaluate similarities and contrasts with critical race theory or contemporary feminism. Throughout this discussion, I attempt to indicate where I believe many other disability studies/disability rights theorists share my views and where I suspect that I am in a minority.

8. Freeman, "Legitimizing Racial Discrimination through Antidiscrimination Law"; Mari Matsuda, "Looking to the Bottom: Critical Legal Studies and Reparations," in Crenshaw et al., *CRT: The Key Writings*, 63; Patricia J. Williams, *The Alchemy of Race and Rights* (Cambridge, Mass.: Harvard University Press, 1991); I put the term "race" in quotation marks because the concept of race is itself a disputed one in critical race theory, as the concepts of "impairment," "disability," and "normality" are disputed among disability scholars as will be discussed later in this chapter.

9. Williams, *Alchemy of Race and Rights*, 44; Idem., 56–57.

10. See John Gliedman and William Roth, *The Unexpected Minority: Handicapped Children in America* (New York: Harcourt Brace Jovanovich, 1980), 261–263.

11. Michelle Fine and Adrienne Asch, "Disability beyond Stigma: Social Interaction, Discrimination, and Activism," *Journal of Social Issues* 44 (1988): 1, 3, 12.

12. Irwin Katz, R. G. Hass, and J. Bailey, "Attitudinal Ambivalence and Behavior toward People with Disabilities," in *Attitudes Toward Persons with Disabilities*, edited by Harold E. Yuker (New York: Springer, 1988), 47, 53.

13. Illustrative are the accounts of social interactions reported in the classic works: Erving Goffman, *Stigma: Notes on the Management of Spoiled Identity* (Englewood Cliffs, N.J.: Prentice-Hall, 1963); Alan J. Brightman, ed., *Ordinary Moments: The Disabled Experience* (Rockville, Md.: Aspen Publishers, Inc., 1984); Marilyn J. Phillips, "Damaged Goods: Oral Narratives of the Experience of Disability in American Culture," *Social Science and Medicine* 30 (1990): 849; John Hockenberry, *Moving Violations: War Zones, Wheelchairs, and Declarations of Independence* (New York: Hyperion, 1995).

14. Some examples of events that occurred during a two-week period while this chapter was my main intellectual focus and, therefore, causing me to be especially aware of the impact of routine events: I was asked by an examining physician whether, because I was blind, I needed her assistant to "come in and help you get dressed"; I was told by a bus driver and several passengers that I must sit down, even though

several other bus passengers were already standing on the crowded bus; I was pushed to the front of a line of customers at a bank, although blindness does not have any relationship to the ability to stand and wait one's turn in a bank line; I was spoken about rather than spoken to—"put her here" was said to a friend of mine as we walked into a crowded room to join a meeting; a friend was described by others not as my friend but as my "assistant" and my "guide"; a friend of more than twenty years explained to me that my distress, irritation, and frustration were unreasonable responses to people who were "trying to do the right thing."

15. Charles R. Lawrence, III, "The Id, the Ego, and Equal Protection: Reckoning with Unconscious Racism," in Crenshaw et al., *CRT: The Key Writings*, 235–236.

16. Anita Silvers, "Formal Justice," in *Disability, Difference, Discrimination: Perspectives on Justice in Bioethics and Public Policy*, edited by Anita Silvers, David Wasserman, and Mary B. Mahowald (Lanham, Md.: Rowman and Littlefield Publishers, 1998), 88.

17. See the following reprinted essays by Derrick A. Bell, Jr.: *"Brown v. Board of Education* and the Interest Convergence Dilemma," in Crenshaw et al., *CRT: The Key Writings*, 20; "Racial Realism," in Crenshaw et al., *CRT: The Key Writings*, 302; and especially, "The Civil Rights Chronicles: The Chronicle of the DeVine Gift," in Delgado, *CRT: The Cutting Edge*, 390; as well as the introductory essays in each book discussing Bell's insights and the review of Bell's book by Alan D. Freeman, "Derrick Bell—Race and Class: The Dilemma of Liberal Reform," in Delgado, *CRT: The Cutting Edge*, 458.

18. Matsuda, "Looking to the Bottom," 66.

19. Typically, people speak of the disability rights movement as developing out of the civil rights movement and the women's movement, in the late 1960s and early 1970s, with the creation of the Center for Independent Living in Berkeley, California, and the formation of Disabled in Action in New York City. See Joseph P. Shapiro, *No Pity: People with Disabilities Forging a New Civil Rights Movement* (New York: Times Books, 1994), 53–58. However, some segments of the population of people with disabilities began asserting their claims to protection from discrimination decades before. See Floyd W. Matson, *Walking Alone and Marching Together: A History of the Organized Blind Movement in the United States, 1940–1990* (Baltimore, Md.: National Federation of the Blind, 1990) (documenting the first fifty years of the National Federation of the Blind, as only one example of a single-disability group focused on acquiring rights to housing, travel, and employment); see also Jacobus tenBroek, "The Right to Live in the World: The Disabled in the Law of Torts," *California Law Review* 54 (1966): 841.

20. For some of the earliest such writings, see Frank Bowe, *Handicapping America: Barriers to Disabled People* (New York: Harper & Row, 1978); Frank Bowe, *Rehabilitating America: Toward Independence for Disabled and Elderly People* (New York: Harper & Row, 1980); Gliedman and Roth, *The Unexpected Minority*; Duane F. Stroman, *The Awakening Minorities: The Physically Handicapped* (Lanham, Md.: University Press of America, 1982); Harlan Hahn, "Paternalism and Public Policy," *Society* 20 (March–April 1983). 36. For a more recent scholarly discussion that usefully compares and contrasts the strengths and limits of medical, economic, and minority group models of disability, see Jerome E. Bickenbach, *Physical Disability and Social Policy* (Buffalo, N.Y.: University of Toronto Press, 1993).

21. Examples of calls for changing the conceptual framework include: Irving Kenneth

Zola, "Toward the Necessary Universalizing of a Disability Policy," *Milbank Quarterly* 67 (1989): 401; Jerome E. Bickenbach et al., "Models of Disablement, Universalism and the International Classification of Impairments, Disabilities and Handicaps," *Society for Science and Medicine* 48 (1999): 1173; Richard K. Scotch and Kay Schriner, "Disability as Human Variation: Implications for Policy," *Annals of the American Academy of Political and Social Sciences* 549 (1997): 148; and Chai R. Feldblum, "Definition of Disability Under Federal Anti-Discrimination Law: What Happened? Why? And What Can We Do About It?" *Berkeley Journal of Employment and Labor Law* 22 (2000): 91. Although these writers stress different reasons, I need not differentiate their reasons.

22. Adaptive Environments Ctr., Inc., Universal Design, available at *http://www.adaptenv.org/universal/default.asp*; retrieved February 27, 2001:

"Universal design is a worldwide movement based on the concept that all products, environments, and communications should be designed to consider the needs of the widest possible array of users. It is also known around the world as design for all, inclusive design, lifespan design. Universal design is a way of thinking about design that is based on the following premises:

- Varying ability is not a special condition of the few but a common characteristic of being human and we change physically and intellectually throughout our lives
- If a design works well for people with disabilities, it works better for everyone
- At any point in our lives, personal self-esteem, identity, and well-being are deeply affected by our ability to function in our physical surroundings with a sense of comfort, independence and control (Leslie Kanes Weisman, 4/99)
- Usability and aesthetics are mutually compatible"

23. Scotch and Schriner, "Disability as Human Variation," 152, 154–55.

24. Prior to this invention, of course, visually impaired and blind travelers solved this problem by asking the bus driver to announce the stops or asking fellow passengers if they did not memorize the routes and know the stops from frequent use.

25. Bill Long, "Smart Buses: Solving the Problem of Calling Bus Stops" (paper presented at the 60th Convention of the National Federation of the Blind, July 7, 2000).

26. Peter Singer, *Practical Ethics*, 2nd ed. (New York: Cambridge University Press, 1993), 184. ("[T]he main point is clear: killing a disabled infant is not morally equivalent to killing a person. Very often it is not wrong at all.") Idem., 191. Peter Singer reiterated his views in two public presentations in 1999: Address at Princeton University (October 12, 1999) and Address at the 2nd Annual Meeting of the American Society for Bioethics and Humanities, Philadelphia, Pa. (October 29, 1999).

27. Susan Daniels, Address at the Conference of the Association for Higher Education and Disability, Atlanta, Ga. (July 14, 1999).

28. 42 U.S.C. §§ 12101–12213 (1994).

29. William G. Johnson, Preface to *Annals of the American Academy of Political and Social Science* 549, 8 (1997).

30. Nancy R. Mudrick and Adrienne Asch, "Investigation and Enforcement of a Disability Discrimination Statue: Complaints of Employment Discrimination Filed in New York State," *Journal of Disability Policy Studies* 7 (1996): 21, 27.

31. See Feldblum, "Definition of Disability."

32. 401 U.S. 424 (1971).

33. I recognize that persons filing complaints alleging that employers regard them as im-

paired when they believe they are not impaired will not be claiming a need for employer-provided "reasonable accommodation." They may be claiming that the glasses they wear or the medications they take to control blood pressure are their accommodations to their physical characteristics but that employers believe those employee-provided accommodations are inadequate or ineffective measures for successful job performance.

If the nation adopted the "regard as" formulation of disability I suggest and analyzed whether a person had been "regarded as" disabled because of an inability to perform in an existing environment, it would then have to recognize that the "reasonable accommodations" employers may be asked to pay for are necessary only because the existing environment does not permit all potential employees to function effectively. It is an accommodation to the interactions of their biology with the existing, hitherto unaccommodating and impairing environment.

34. Ian F. Haney López addresses the social construction of racial categories in "The Social Construction of Race," in Delgado, *CRT: The Cutting Edge*, 191, and "White by Law," in Delgado, *CRT: The Cutting Edge*, 542.

35. Not all of these factors have been systematically explored to determine which factors are more important at different times, or whether there is a pattern of responses that makes shortened lifespan more disturbing, for example, than visibility, either to people who live with the conditions themselves or to their associates. For discussions of attitudes toward people with disabilities, see generally, Harold E. Yuker ed., *Attitudes toward Persons with Disabilities* (New York: Springer, 1988); Richard F. Antonak and Hanoch Livneh, *The Measurement of Attitudes toward People with Disabilities* (Springfield, Ill.: C.C. Thomas, 1988); Elaine Makas, "Positive Attitudes toward Disabled People: Disabled and Nondisabled Persons' Perspectives," *Journal of Social Issues* 49 (1988): 44. For discussions of the psychological impact of disability upon individuals and families, see John S. Rolland, *Families, Illness, and Disability: An Integrative Treatment Model* (New York: Basic Books, 1994); Rosalyn Benjamin Darling, "Parental Entrepreneurship: A Consumerist Response to Professional Dominance," *Journal of Social Issues* 44 (1988): 141; Philip M. Ferguson et al., "The Experience of Disability in Families: A Synthesis of Research and Parent Narratives," in *Prenatal Testing and Disability Rights*, edited by Erik Parens and Adrienne Asch (Washington, D.C.: Georgetown University Press, 2000), 72. For classic material on living as a person with a disability, see Beatrice A. Wright, *Physical Disability—A Psychosocial Approach*, 2d ed. (New York: Harper, 1983).

36. Harlan Hahn, "The Politics of Physical Differences: Disability and Discrimination," *Journal of Social Issues* 44 (1988): 39.

37. Brief of Amici Curiae.

38. Nora E. Groce, *Everyone Here Spoke Sign Language: Hereditary Deafness on Martha's Vineyard* (Cambridge, Mass.: Harvard University Press, 1985).

39. See *PGA Tour, Inc. v. Martin*, 204 F.3d 994 (9th Cir. 2000), cert. granted, 121 S. Ct. 30 (September 26, 2000) (No. 00–24).

40. *Sutton v. United Air Lines, Inc., 527 U.S. 471 (1999).*

41. *Murphy v. United Parcel Serv., Inc.*, 527 U.S. 516 (1999).

42. Although I have not litigated or investigated cases filed under the Americans with Disabilities Act, I base the comments in the foregoing section partly on my years of work dealing with cases of employer-devised medical standards under the New York State Human Rights Law. From 1974 to 1977 and then from 1980 to 1985, I worked

with the New York State Division of Human Rights in several professional capacities, examining the legitimacy of employers' vision, blood pressure, and other medical requirements as they applied to positions of truck driver, nurse, lifeguard, and other positions. New York's Human Rights law contained no "reasonable accommodation" provision, yet that law was successfully used by complainants to show that many employer medical standards were, in fact, not job related.

43. Peller, "Race Consciousness."
44. Ibid., 128.
45. Ibid., 130
46. Ibid., 135.
47. Ibid., 150.
48. Ibid., 151.
49. For a discussion of the cites of and barriers to self-organization among people with disabilities, see generally Richard K. Scotch, *From Good Will to Civil Rights: Transforming Federal Disability Policy* (Philadelphia: Temple University Press, 1984); Richard K. Scotch, "Disability as the Basis for a Social Movement: Advocacy and the Politics of Definition," *Journal of Social Issues* 44 (1988): 159.
50. I write about a part of my own development in Adrienne Asch, "Personal Reflections," *American Psychologist* 39 (1984): 551; and in Philip M. Ferguson and Adrienne Asch, "Lessons from Life: Personal and Parental Perspectives on School, Childhood, and Disability," in *Schooling and Disability 108*, edited by Douglas Biklen et al. (Chicago: University of Chicago Press, 1989).
51. *Individuals with Disabilities in Education Act*, 20 U.S.C. § 1415 (1994).
52. *Olmstead v. L.C.*, 527 U.S. 581 (1999) (holding that the ADA requires states to provide community-based treatment for individuals with mental disabilities when treatment professionals determine that the placement is appropriate, the treatment is not opposed by the affected parties, and placement can be reasonably accommodated).
53. The mother of a seventh-grade girl who is blind reported this story to me on September 23, 2000.
54. *Board of Education v. Rowley*, 458 U.S. 176 (1982).
55. For well-worked-out discussions of exemplary programs that incorporate a wide range of students thought "too disabled" to be in the public schools, see Gail McGregor and R. Timm Vogelsberg, *Inclusive Schooling Practices: Pedagogical and Research Foundations: A Synthesis of the Literature that Informs Best Practices about Inclusive Schooling* (Baltimore: Philips H. Brookes Publishing, 1998); and Dorothy K. Lipsky and Alan Gartner, "Taking Inclusion into the Future," *Education Leadership*, 56, 2, October 1998, 78.
56. Duncan Kennedy, "A Cultural Pluralist Case for Affirmative Action in Legal Academia," in Crenshaw et al., *CRT: The Key Writings*, 159, 162 (expressing statements made by Randall Kennedy).
57. Ibid., 167–168.
58. Iris Marion Young, *Justice and the Politics of Difference* (Princeton, N.J.: Princeton University Press, 1990), 40.
59. I recognize that members of the Deaf community join together based on a shared language, ASL, that gives them a status of both a linguistic and a disability community. Even the statement of including Deaf people as members of the disability community is controversial, since many reject the label of disability when it is applied to them. However, because people who are Deaf, as well as deaf people who do not

identify with the Deaf cultural world, avail themselves of the provisions of the Americans with Disabilities Act to obtain telephone relay services and the right to ASL interpreters or real-time captioners, I believe it is not inappropriate to consider them, for some purposes, members of the large population of people impaired in environments without provisions for communicating in a means other than spoken language.

60. For discussions of "disability culture," see Mary Johnson, "Emotion and Pride: The Search for a Disability Culture," *Disability Rag* 7 (January/February 1987): 7; Paul K. Longmore, "The Second Phase: From Disability Rights to Disability Culture," *Disability Rag* 16 (September/October 1995), 4; and *Vital Signs: Crip Culture Talks Back* (Marquette, Miss.: Brace Yourself Productions, 1995).

61. H. Taylor, M. R. Kagan, and S. Leichenko, *The ICD Survey of Disabled Americans: Bringing Disabled Americans into the Mainstream* (New York: Louis Harris and Associates, 1986), 9–10; "New Harris Survey Marks Strong Approval for ADA Nine Years After Passage," available at http://www.nod.org/press.html#poll; retrieved April 15, 1999.

62. Personal communication with Carol Gill (June 1999).

63. Anthony Appiah, "'But Would That Still Be Me?' Notes on Gender, 'Race' Ethnicity, as Sources of 'Identity,'" *Journal of Philosophy* 87, 10 (1990): 493, 497; reprinted in *Race, Sex: Their Sameness, Difference and Interplay*, edited by Naomi Zack (New York: Routledge, 1997), 75–81

64. Stubblefield, "Racial Identity," 368; Wasserstrom, as cited in Stubblefield, "Racial Identity," 368.

65. Jeffrey R. Botkin, "Fetal Privacy and Confidentiality," *Hastings Center Report* 25 (September–October 1995): 32.

66. For discussions of disability as inimical to at least some parents' hopes, see William Ruddick, "Ways to Limit Prenatal Testing," in *Prenatal Testing and Disability Rights*, edited by Erik Parens and Adrienne Asch (Washington, D.C.: Georgetown University Press, 2000), 95.

67. Philip M. Ferguson et al., "The Experience of Disability in Families," 72.

68. See Letter from Professor Ruth Colker, supra note 4.

69. Illustrative books about motherhood that neglect mothers with disability, although they carefully include many other "marginalized" mothers are: Faye Ginsburg and Rayna Rapp, eds., *Conceiving the New World Order: The Global Politics of Reproduction* (Berkeley: University of California Press, 1995); Julia E. Hanigsberg and Sara Ruddick, eds., *Mother Troubles: Rethinking Contemporary Maternal Dilemmas* (Boston: Beacon, 1999); Cynthia Garcia Coll, Janet L. Surrey, and Kathy Weingarten, eds., *Mothering against the Odds: Diverse Voices of Contemporary Mothers* (New York: Guilford Press, 1998); and Evelyn Nakano Glenn, Grace Chang, and Linda Rennie Forcey, eds., *Mothering: Ideology, Experience, and Agency* (New York: Routledge, 1994).

70. Christopher Nolan, *Under the Eye of the Clock: A Memoir* (New York: St. Martin's Press, 2000).

71. Young, "Justice and Politics of Difference," 46–47.

72. Longmore, "The Second Phase," 9.

73. Martha Minow, *Not Only for Myself: Identity, Politics and the Law* (New York: New Press, 1997), 56–57.

74. For discussions of the social construction of disability from within the field of bioethics, see Erik Parens and Adrienne Asch, "The Disability Rights Critique of Prenatal

Genetic Testing: Reflections and Recommendations," *Hastings Center Report* 29 (September–October 1999), 51; Adrienne Asch, "Why I Haven't Changed My Mind about Prenatal Diagnosis: Reflections and Refinements," in *Prenatal Testing and Disability Rights* 234, edited by Erik Parens and Adrienne Asch (Washington, D.C.: Georgetown University Press, 2000); Margaret Olivia Little, "Cosmetic Surgery, Suspect Norms, and the Ethics of Complicity," in *Enhancing Human Traits*, edited by Erik Parens (Washington, D.C.: Georgetown University Press, 1998), 162; and Tom Shakespeare, "Arguing About Disability and Genetics," *Interaction* 13 (2000):11–14.

75. Gregory H. Williams, "Reflections on the ADA: Rethinking the Past, and Looking toward the Future," *Ohio State Law Journal* 62 (2000), 1, 9.

76. Peter Putnam, "If You Had a Choice," *Jewish Braille Review* (October 1963) 25, 30.

77. Ibid., 32.

78. See Gregory H. Williams, *Life on the Color Line: The True Story of a White Boy Who Discovered He Was Black* (New York: Dutton, 1995), which according to Williams details his "personal transition from a white American to a black American."

79. Williams, "Reflections on the ADA," 9.

Bibliography

Adaptive Environments Center, Inc. "Universal Design." Available at http://www.adaptenv.org/universal; retrieved February 27, 2001.

Americans with Disabilities Act, 42 U.S.C. § 12111(a)(7) (1994).

Antonak, Richard F., and Hanoch Livneh. *The Measurement of Attitudes toward People with Disabilities: Methods, Psychometrics, and Scales.* Springfield, Ill.: C.C. Thomas, 1988.

Appiah, Anthony. "'But Would That Still Be Me?' Notes on Gender, 'Race,' Ethnicity, as Sources of 'Identity.'" *The Journal of Philosophy* 87, 10 (October 1990): 493–499. Reprinted in *Race, Sex: Their Sameness, Difference and Interplay*, edited by Naomi Zack. New York: Routledge, 1997, 75–81.

Asch, Adrienne. "Personal Reflections," *American Psychologist* 39 (1984).

———. "Why I Haven't Changed My Mind about Prenatal Diagnosis: Reflections and Refinements." In *Prenatal Testing and Disability Rights*, edited by Erik Parens and Adrienne Asch. Washington, D.C.: Georgetown University Press, 2000.

Bd. of Educ. v. Rowley, 458 U.S. 176 (1982).

Bell, Derrick A., Jr. "*Brown v. Board of Education* and the Interest Convergence Dilemma." In *Critical Race Theory: The Key Writings that Formed the Movement*, edited by Kimberlé Crenshaw, Neil Gotanda, Garry Peller, and Kendall Thomas. New York: New Press, 1995.

———. "The Civil Rights Chronicles: The Chronicle of the DeVine Gift." In *Critical Race Theory: The Cutting Edge*, edited by Richard Delgado. Philadelphia: Temple University Press, 1995.

———. "Racial Realism." In *Critical Race Theory: The Key Writings that Formed the Movement*, edited by Kimberlé Crenshaw, Neil Gotanda, Garry Peller, and Kendall Thomas. New York: New Press, 1995.

Berkeley Journal of Employment & Labor Law. ADA Symposium Issue 21, 1 (2000). [No editor]

Bickenbach, Jerome E. *Physical Disability and Social Policy*. Buffalo, N.Y.: University of Toronto Press, 1993.

Bickenbach, Jerome E., Somnath Chatterji, E. M. Badley, and T. B. Üstün. "Models of Disablement, Universalism and the International Classification of Impairments, Disabilities and Handicaps." *Society, Science and Medicine* 48 (1999).

Board of Education v. Rowley, 458 U.S. 176 (1982).

Botkin, Jeffrey R. "Fetal Privacy and Confidentiality." *Hastings Center Report* 25 (September–October 1995).

Bowe, Frank. *Handicapping America: Barriers to Disabled People.* New York: Harper & Row, 1978.

————. *Rehabilitating America: Toward Independence for Disabled and Elderly People.* New York: Harper & Row, 1980.

Brief of Amici Curiae in Support of Respondents, *Univ. of Ala. at Birmingham Bd. of Trs. v. Garrett*, 193 F.3d 1214 (11th Cir.) (No. 99–1240).

Brightman, Alan J., ed. *Ordinary Moments: The Disabled Experience.* Rockville, Md.: Aspen Publishers, Inc, 1984.

Coll, Cynthia Garcia, Janet L. Surrey, and Kathy Weingarten, eds. *Mothering against the Odds: Diverse Voices of Contemporary Mothers.* New York: Guilford Press, 1998.

Crenshaw, Kimberlé, Neil Gotanda, Garry Peller, and Kendall Thomas, eds. *Critical Race Theory: The Key Writings that Formed the Movement.* New York: New Press, 1995.

Daniels, Susan. Address at the Conference of the Association for Higher Education and Disability, Atlanta, Ga. (July 14, 1999).

Darling, Rosalyn Benjamin. "Parental Entrepreneurship: A Consumerist Response to Professional Dominance." *Journal of Social Issues* 44 (1988).

Delgado, Richard, ed. *Critical Race Theory: The Cutting Edge.* Philadelphia: Temple University Press, 1995.

Feldblum, Chai R. "Definition of Disability Under Federal Anti-Discrimination Law: What Happened? Why? And What Can We Do About It?" *Berkeley Journal of Employment and Labor Law* 22 (2000).

Ferguson, Philip M., and Adrienne Asch. "Lessons from Life: Personal and Parental Perspectives on School, Childhood, and Disability." In *Schooling and Disability*. Eighty-eighth Yearbook of the National Society for the Study of Education, edited by Douglas Biklen, Dianne L. Ferguson, Alison Ford, and Kenneth J. Rehage. Chicago: University of Chicago Press, 1989.

Ferguson, Philip M., Alan Gartner, and Dorothy K. Lipsky. "The Experience of Disability in Families: A Synthesis of Research and Parent Narratives." In *Prenatal Testing and Disability Rights*, edited by Erik Parens & Adrienne Asch. Washington, D.C.: Georgetown University Press, 2000.

Fine, Michelle, and Adrienne Asch. "Disability beyond Stigma: Social Interaction, Discrimination, and Activism." *Journal of Social Issues* 44 (1988).

Francis, Leslie Pickering, and Anita Silvers, eds. *Americans with Disabilities: Exploring Implications of the Law for Individuals and Institutions.* New York: Routledge, 2000.

Freeman, Alan David. "Derrick Bell—Race and Class: The Dilemma of Liberal Reform." In *Critical Race Theory: The Key Writings that Formed the Movement*, edited by Kimberlé Crenshaw, Neil Gotanda, Garry Peller, and Kendall Thomas. New York: New Press, 1995.

————. "Legitimizing Racial Discrimination through Antidiscrimination Law: A Critical Review of Supreme Court Doctrine." In *Critical Race Theory: The Key Writings that Formed the Movement*, edited by Kimberlé Crenshaw, Neil Gotanda, Garry Peller, and Kendall Thomas. New York: New Press, 1995.

Ginsburg, Faye, and Rayna Rapp eds. *Conceiving the New World Order: The Global Politics of Reproduction*. Berkeley: University of California Press, 1995.

Glenn, Evelyn Nakano, Grace Chang, and Linda Rennie Forcey. *Mothering: Ideology, Experience, and Agency*. New York: Routledge, 1994.

Gliedman, John, and William Roth. *The Unexpected Minority: Handicapped Children in America*. New York: Harcourt Brace Jovanovich, 1980.

Goffman, Erving. *Stigma: Notes on the Management of Spoiled Identity*. Englewood Cliffs, N.J., Prentice-Hall, 1963.

Greenhouse, Linda. "Justices Give the States Immunity from Suits by Disabled Workers." *New York Times*, February 22, 2001, A1.

Griggs v. Duke Power Co., 401 U.S. 424 (1971)4.

Groce, Nora E. *Everyone Here Spoke Sign Language: Hereditary Deafness on Martha's Vineyard*. Cambridge, Mass.: Harvard University Press, 1985.

Hahn, Harlan. "Paternalism and Public Policy." *Society* 20 (March–April 1983).

————. "The Politics of Physical Differences: Disability and Discrimination." *Journal of Social Issues* 44 (1988).

Hanigsberg, Julia E., and Sara Ruddick, eds. *Mother Troubles: Rethinking Contemporary Maternal Dilemmas*. Boston: Beacon, 1999.

Hockenberry, John. *Moving Violations: War Zones, Wheelchairs, and Declarations of Independence*. New York: Hyperion, 1995.

Individuals with Disabilities in Education Act, 20 U.S.C. § 1415 (1994).

Johnson, Mary. "Emotion and Pride: The Search for a Disability Culture." *Disability Rag* 7 (January–February 1987).

Johnson, William G. Preface to *Annals of the American Academy of Political and Social Science*. "The Americans with Disabilities Act: Social Contract or Special Privilege?" Series: The Annals of the American Academy of Political and Social Science 549, 1997.

Katz, Irwin, R. G. Hass, and J. Bailey, J. "Attitudinal Ambivalence and Behavior toward People with Disabilities." In *Attitudes toward Persons with Disabilities*, edited by Harold E. Yuker. New York: Springer, 1988.

Kennedy, Duncan. "A Cultural Pluralist Case for Affirmative Action in Legal Academia." In *Critical Race Theory: The Key Writings that Formed the Movement*, edited by Kimberlé Crenshaw, Neil Gotanda, Garry Peller, and Kendall Thomas. New York: New Press, 1995.

Lawrence, Charles R., III. "The Id, the Ego, and Equal Protection: Reckoning with Unconscious Racism." In *Critical Race Theory: The Key Writings that Formed the Movement*, edited by Kimberlé Crenshaw, Neil Gotanda, Garry Peller, and Kendall Thomas. New York: New Press, 1995.

Lipsky, Dorothy K., and Alan Gartner. "Taking Inclusion into the Future." *Educational Leadership* 56 (October 1998).

Little, Margaret Olivia. "Cosmetic Surgery, Suspect Norms, and the Ethics of Complicity." In *Enhancing Human Traits: Ethical and Social Implications*, edited by Erik Parens. Washington, D.C.: Georgetown University Press, 1988.

Long, Bill. "Smart Buses: Solving the Problem of Calling Bus Stops." Paper presented at the 60th Convention of the National Federation of the Blind, July 7, 2000.

Longmore, Paul K. "The Second Phase: From Disability Rights to Disability Culture." *Disability Rag* 16 (September–October, 1995).

López, Ian F. Haney. "The Social Construction of Race." In *Critical Race Theory: The Cutting Edge*, edited by Richard Delgado. Philadelphia: Temple University Press, 1995.

———. "White by Law." In *Critical Race Theory: The Cutting Edge*, edited by Richard Delgado. Philadelphia: Temple University Press, 1995.

Makas, Elaine. "Positive Attitudes toward Disabled People: Disabled and Nondisabled Persons' Perspectives." *Journal of Social Issues* 44 (1988).

Matson, Floyd W. *Walking Alone and Marching Together: A History of the Organized Blind Movement in the United States, 1940–1990*. Baltimore, Md.: National Federation of the Blind, 1990.

Matsuda, Mari. "Looking to the Bottom: Critical Legal Studies and Reparations." In *Critical Race Theory: The Key Writings that Formed the Movement*, edited by Kimberlé Crenshaw, Neil Gotanda, Garry Peller, and Kendall Thomas. New York: New Press, 1995.

McGregor, Gail, and R. Timm Vogelsberg. *Inclusive Schooling Practices: Pedagogical and Research Foundations: A Synthesis of the Literature that Informs Best Practices about Inclusive Schooling*. Allegheny University of Health Sciences; Baltimore: Paul H. Brookes Publishing, 1998.

Minow, Martha. *Not Only for Myself: Identity, Politics and the Law*. New York: New Press, 1997.

Mudrick, Nancy R., and Adrienne Asch. "Investigation and Enforcement of a Disability Discrimination Statute: Complaints of Employment Discrimination Filed in New York State." *Journal of Disability Policy Studies* 7 (1996).

Murphy v. United Parcel Serv., Inc., 527 U.S. 516 (1999).

National Council on Disability. *Promises to Keep: A Decade of Federal Enforcement of the Americans with Disabilities Act*. Washington, DC: US GPO, 2000.

"New Harris Survey Marks Strong Approval for ADA Nine Years After Passage." Available at http://www.nod.org/press.html#poll; retrieved April 15, 1999.

Nolan, Christopher. *Under the Eye of the Clock: A Memoir*. New York: St. Martin's Press, 2000.

Olmstead v. L.C., 527 U.S. 581 (1999)

Parens, Erik, and Adrienne Asch. 1999. "The Disability Rights Critique of Prenatal Genetic Testing: Reflections and Recommendations." *Hastings Center Report* 29 (September–October 1999).

Peller, Gary. "Race-Consciousness." In *Critical Race Theory: The Key Writings that Formed the Movement*, edited by Kimberlé Crenshaw, Neil Gotanda, Garry Peller, and Kendall Thomas. New York: New Press, 1995.

PGA Tour, Inc. v. Martin, 204 F.3d 994 (9th Cir. 2000), cert. granted, 121 S. Ct. 30 (September 26, 2000) (No. 00–24).

Phillips, Marilyn J. "Damaged Goods: Oral Narratives of the Experience of Disability in American Culture." *Social Science and Medicine* 30 (2000).

Putnam, Peter. "If You Had a Choice." *Jewish Braille Review* (October 1963)

Rolland, John S. *Families, Illness, and Disability: An Integrative Treatment Model*. New York: BasicBooks, 1994.

Ruddick, William. "Ways to Limit Prenatal Testing." In *Prenatal Testing and Disability Rights*, edited by Erik Parens and Adrienne Asch. Washington, D.C.: Georgetown University Press, 2000.

Scotch, Richard K. "Disability as the Basis for a Social Movement: Advocacy and the Politics of Definition." *Journal of Social Issues* 44 (1988).

———— *From Good Will to Civil Rights: Transforming Federal Disability Policy.* Philadelphia: Temple University Press, 1984.

Scotch, Richard K., and Kay Schriner. "Disability as Human Variation: Implications for Policy." *Annals of the American Academy of Political and Social Science*, 549 (1977).

Shakespeare, Tom. "Arguing About Disability and Genetics." *Interaction*, 13 (2000).

Shapiro, Joseph P. *No Pity: People with Disabilities Forging a New Civil Rights Movement.* New York: Times Books, 1994.

Silvers, Anita. "Formal Justice." In *Disability, Difference, Discrimination: Perspectives on Justice in Bioethics and Public Policy*, edited by Anita Silvers, David Wasserman, and Mary B. Mahowald. Lanham, Md.: Rowman & Littlefield Publishers, 1998.

Singer, Peter M. *Practical Ethics.* 2d ed. New York: Cambridge University Press, 1993.

Stroman, Duane F. *The Awakening Minorities: The Physically Handicapped.* Lanham, Md: University Press of America, 1982.

Stubblefield, Anna. "Racial Identity and Non-Essentialism about Race." *Social Theory & Practice* 21 (1995).

Sutton v. United Air Lines, Inc., 527 U.S. 471 (1999).

Taylor, H., M. R. Kagan, and S. Leichenko. *The ICD Survey of Disabled Americans: Bringing Disabled Americans into the Mainstream.* New York: Louis Harris and Associates, 1986.

tenBroek, Jacobus. "The Right to Live in the World: The Disabled in the Law of Torts." *California Law Review* 54 (1966).

Univ. of Ala. at Birmingham Bd. of Trs. v. Garrett, No. 99–1240, 2001 U.S. LEXIS 1700 (February 21, 2001).

Vital Signs: Crip Culture Talks Back. Color video. 48 minutes. Directed by David T. Mitchell, and Sharon Snyder. Marquette, Miss.: Brace Yourselves Productions, 1997.

Williams, Gregory Howard. *Life on the Color Line: The True Story of a White Boy Who Discovered He Was Black.* New York: Dutton, 1995.

————. "Reflections on the ADA: Rethinking the Past, and Looking toward the Future." *Ohio State Law Journal* 62, 1 (2000).

Williams, Patricia J. *The Alchemy of Race and Rights.* Cambridge, Mass.: Harvard University Press, 1991.

Wright, Beatrice A. *Physical Disability—A Psychosocial Approach.* 2d ed. New York: Harper, 1983.

Young, Iris Marion. *Justice and the Politics of Difference.* Princeton, N.J.: Princeton University Press, 1990.

Yuker, Harold E., ed. *Attitudes toward Persons with Disabilities.* New York: Springer, 1988.

Zola, Irving Kenneth. "Toward the Necessary Universalizing of a Disability Policy." *Milbank Quarterly* 67 (1989).

Why the Intersexed Shouldn't Be Fixed

Insights from Queer Theory and Disability Studies

ঐ৯

Sumi Colligan

The initiatives the Intersex Society of North America (ISNA) promoted to prevent "corrective" surgery for genitals not clearly identifiable as male or female have recently come to my attention.[1] This discovery has stimulated my own reflections on the parallels between American cultural representations and the everyday struggles of the intersexed and those of people with disabilities. Both groups are subjected to anomalous classification, medical management, silencing, and shame; both groups titillate the projected, and often repressed, fantasies of outsiders; and both intersexed and disabled individuals and organizations are challenging the assumptions that underlie these negative images to reclaim their own impassioned, desirable, and desirous bodies. These activists seek to assert the value of their own presence in the world and to raise questions about a system of cultural ordering that renders them symbolically, if not literally, neutered or "fixed."

David Mitchell and Sharon Snyder (1997) point out that while there is an abundance of critical theory on the body, disability remains largely untheorized, often appearing as a natural backdrop for the exploration of already established social issues and themes. They explain: "Within this common critical methodology physical difference exemplifies the evidence of social deviance even as the constructed nature of physicality itself fades from view" (5). Yet opportunities to explore the cultural construction of physicality and its intersections with race, class, gender, and sexuality are abundant, appearing both within the realms of popular and medical culture. These references are often quite explicit and should not require the sensitized lens of disability studies for quick detection. For example, apropos of disability and the trans and/or nebulously gendered, talk show host Jerry Springer is quoted as saying:

When you think of all the things that could go wrong at birth or at least not be as they ought to be, from blindness to mental retardation to cystic fibrosis to, indeed, the entire litany of possible birth defects, why do we assume that the one thing that can never be out of sync is our gender identity? And yet, while we are quick to heap our love and compassion and charity on any of these disabilities, if it has something to do with sex suddenly we don't want to hear about it. . . . And so with the same compassion that we are offering to those who are trying to fix other parts of their body that perhaps aren't working as they should, why not a word of understanding to those whose gender seems to be out of whack? (cited in Gamson 1998, 106)

A number of issues here go unquestioned: Why are charity and compassion considered to be a desirable and automatic response to certain kinds of physical variation? Why is there an assumption that disability has nothing to do with sex? Why do genitals and gender identity have to match? Why is being fixed a moral imperative?

It is instructive to begin to explore these intersections and parallels by interrogating the meaning of *fixed*. The dictionary definition of the verb indicates "to set in order," "to repair," "to attach or fasten immovably"; even the noun, *fix*, is defined as "an embarrassing or uncomfortable position."[2] Through the lens of *fixed*, I consider how and why Western cultures have come to disable the intersexed and neuter the disabled, subjecting them to similar disciplines of normalization. Then I evaluate postmodern responses (drawing primarily from disability studies and queer theory) to the normalization of varyingly disabled and gendered bodies, weighing lessons that emerge from the situated perspectives and lived experiences of individuals with these bodies. My overall argument is that, whereas flexible categories may be an antidote to the pressures and techniques of normalization, our imagining of these categories should not become too malleable and disengaged from the real bodies and lives who occupy the categories. With ever more powerful tools of normalization emerging, often more difficult to locate, identify, and contain than those that came before them, we must remain vigilant of the forces of erasure and remain anchored to our bodies and our right to occupy the world as we are or want to be.

Intersexuality and Disability as Cultural Spectacle

During the sixteenth and seventeenth centuries in Western Europe, prior to the advent of modern medical hegemony, a humanist revival of the classics rekindled an interest in aberrant bodies and their possible meanings. The lines between religion, science, and pornography were not clearly drawn. In post-Reformation England especially, "monsters were to be read as God's advertisements" (Gilbert 2000, 147), revealing the misdeeds of the onlookers. More specifically, "to view the monstrous body was, in these terms, to view the inner self. In this context, the hermaphrodite or disabled body was read as a materialization of social, political or moral corruption" (148). Such bodies also became objects of intense scrutiny because they disrupted established patterns of policing bodies, challenging the boundaries of what it meant to be human.

The late seventeenth century saw a transition from a more religiously infused view of variant corporealities to one focusing more on commercialization and classification. This transition took the form of popular entertainment, marked by freak shows that enjoyed their heyday from the mid-nineteenth century into the early decades of the twentieth century. Disability studies theorist Rosemarie Garland-Thomson (1997) avers that "freak shows framed and choreographed bodily differences that we now call 'race,' 'ethnicity,' and 'disability'" (64). Bodies that were put on display were objectified and stripped of all their humanity, frequently viewed as samples of inferior evolutionary forms.

This ritual staging of freakdom also entailed an underscoring of lack and excess, in which malformations of bodies and sexuality became significantly entwined. Conjoined twins and hermaphrodites were often displayed in close association, representing a blurring of bodies that defied common assumptions about gender and personhood (Garland-Thomson 2001b, 14). Additionally, race, sexuality, and disability mutually informed one another, as in the case of depictions of female Hottentot genitals that linked large clitorises with a penchant for lesbianism (Garland-Thomson 1997, 76). Of course, the female body, in whatever guise, has generally been viewed as unable to achieve ideal form, revealing ways in which cultural constructions of all forms of physicality are intimately interconnected.

As spectacle gave way to the hegemonic inroads of allopathic medicine and ushered in the age of charity and medical reformation, "freaks" became increasingly removed from public view and instead subjected to probing medical techniques and inquisitions, confined to sequestered spaces and to the expert eye. The privileges and routines of normalization were to become universally available (at least, that was the "promise"), with "freaks" no longer publicly present to offer reassurance or unmask the mythology of normalcy.

Medicalizing Intersexed/Disabled Bodies: Retrofitting and Reform

Michel Foucault has documented the forces that have converged in the last two centuries in Western Europe and the United States that contribute to the medical scrutiny of the flesh and its moral attributes. For example, in *The Birth of a Clinic* (1973), Foucault describes processes by which the bodies of individuals undergoing medical treatment came to be viewed as discrete and docile entities whose hidden recesses contained the secrets to their ailments. Likewise, in *The History of Sexuality* (1978), he addresses a range of professions (demography, pedagogy, medicine, and psychiatry among them) that emerged during this period to shape the contours of modernity. These fields used their professional powers to name, locate, regulate, punish, and remold individuals associated with aberrant corporealities. Foucault referred to these approaches as "bio-power," as they are "techniques that make possible a special alliance between specialized knowledge and institutionalized power in the state's management of life" (Halperin 1995, 41).

However, whereas Foucault draws out the implications of the deployment of these forms of power/knowledge to define and contain illness, madness, and sexuality, historian Henri-Jacques Stiker (1997) notes that disability is lacking from Foucault's analysis. I contend that such an analysis should be broadened to include the role that the development of statistics played in turning disability into deviance, a process that included upholding a statistical norm against which all else was rendered abnormal (Davis 1997, 11).[3] Moreover, the analysis should consider the manner in which the growth of the rehabilitation industry was cata-lyzed by a drive to remove the "lack" and restore the disabled body to its "as-sumed, prior normal state" (Stiker 1997, 122). As we shall see, all these powers collided and collaborated to refashion, retrofit, and reform intersexed and dis-abled bodies to eradicate their "abnormalities" from our social presence and/or to render them invisible.[4]

In Foucault's introduction to *Herculine Barbin: Being the Recently Dis-covered Diary of a Nineteenth Century French Hermaphrodite* (1980), he states that by the mid–1800s, medical doctors had concluded that everyone had a "true" sex, which even when masked, could be discerned by the penetrating eye of science. This conviction was also corroborated by Alice Dreger (1998), a re-searcher of French and British physicians between 1860 and 1915, who remarks that "the history of hermaphroditism is largely the history of struggles over the 'realities' of sex—the nature of 'true' sex, the proper role of the sexes, the ques-tion of what sex can, should, or must mean" (15). The medical examination of hermaphrodites rested on the assumption of sexual dimorphism such that one's true sex could only be read as male or female. The sorting out of the sexes was conducted by navigating one's way through "genital geography" (89), decipher-ing anatomical excesses and deficiencies, and distinguishing "veritable" from "pseudo vulvas" (119). If anatomy alone wasn't quick to release its secrets, doc-tors would also seek clues in behaviors and aptitudes because of an assumed linear correlation between genitals and gendered attractions and performances (ergo, testicles and ovaries are us). Additionally, parents were interrogated for recollections of maternal impressions and "hereditary antecedents" (70), physi-cal indicators of past parental transgressions.[5] Overall, if bodies and actions didn't conform to medical expectations and social conventions, they were forced to comply to nature's imagined calling by medical declaration and legal protocol.

In the past fifty years, surgery and hormonal therapy have become rou-tine, technical solutions for individuals whose genitals are deemed medically problematic. That normative physicality is being constructed here should be readily apparent and is captured humorously by intersex ("intersex" is in com-mon use now because it doesn't carry the mythical connotations of "hermaph-rodite") writer Raphael Carter (1998) who defines ambiguous genitalia as "genitalia that refuse to declare their sex to doctors—no doubt on the principle that under interrogation by the enemy you should give only name, rank and serial number" (10). This queering of medical authority serves to underscore the invasive consequences of accepted medical definitions and procedures. Intersex reporter Martha Coventry (2000) reveals that according to scientific standards, "girls, if they perceive themselves, or want to be perceived as fully 'feminine,' should have clitorises no longer than $3/8$ inch at birth. Boys, if they hope to grow up 'masculine,' should have penises that are about one inch in stretched length at birth. Girls should have vaginas fit for future intercourse, and boys should have urethra openings at the tip of the penis (55) in order to be able to urinate standing up.

Of course, the irony here is that self-identity has nothing to do with this medical intervention because surgeons now generally perform these reconstructive feats on the intersexed in infancy. Biologist Anne Fausto-Sterling (1998) argues that the intersexed excite discomfort in medical professionals because "they possess the irritating ability to live sometimes as one sex and sometimes as the other, and they raise the specter of homosexuality" (46). It is clear, then, that intersexed babies are being fixed, at least in part, as a form of rehabilitation that facilitates their bodily deployment into society according to heteronormative measures. In keeping with the body's truth, doctors, however, contend that their medical tampering is simply a means of restoring the infants to their naturally gendered state, denying the role that culture plays in enforcing this imperative (Kessler 1998).

In parallel fashion, in the last several centuries, people with disabilities have been subjected to pacification through the medical gaze's fixation on essentialized and internalized bodily truths and to reform through the disciplined practices of sheltered workshops, special education, and physical rehabilitation. The benevolence and charity that have been extended to these individuals rest on their willingness, through medical treatment, physical retraining, and mental acquiescence, to strive to achieve normative standards of bodily appearance and physical, linguistic, and cognitive use. By means of these institutional practices, "the disabled are to be 'raised up,' restored" (Stiker 1997, 108). Indeed, historian Stiker concludes: "rehabilitation marks the appearance of a culture that attempts to complete the act of identification, of making identical" (128).

Alternatively, for those who can't be medically disappeared as with the intersexed, there remains the role of desexualized, childlike, dependents who are destined to institutionalization as they await the promise of cure. As historian Paul Longmore (1997, 136) notes, these individuals are extended the benevolent hand of charity because, particularly in the United States, their images help reaffirm the virtue and moral fitness of its nondisabled citizens. Stiker asserts that cure suggests removal and that rehabilitation suggests assimilation (1997). Regardless of an emphasis on cure or rehabilitation, "compassion tends to be channeled into normalizing" (Dreger 1998, 198). And either way, intersexed and disabled persons, viewed as destabilizing physical, sexual, gendered, and classificatory presences, have clearly been the targets of coercive regimes of routinization which have nearly, but not so successfully, extinguished their bodily knowledge and their desires.

Fixing Bodies, Extinguishing Desires: Constructing Asexuality

The aforementioned regulatory discourses and practices have played a significant role in constructing the asexuality of the intersexed and of people with disabilities. Both intersexed and disabled bodies have been construed as threatening, with their imagined excesses and deficiencies. Consequently, these bodies have been stripped of their ability to pleasure and be pleasured through the mechanism of denial, the social erasure of sexuality. From this standpoint, both intersexed and disabled bodies are lurking in the social margins, fluctuating between the overly intrusive and the wispy. In this vein, James Porter (1997) notes:

> viewed in itself (an essentializing perspective—but that is part of the point), a disabled body seems somehow too much a body, too real, too corporeal: it is a body that, so to speak, stands in its own way. From another angle, which is no less reductive, a disabled body seems to be lacking something essential, something to make it identifiable and something to identify with; a body that is deficiently itself, not quite a body in the full sense of the word, not real enough. (xii)

And as Foucault has aptly demonstrated, societal regulatory regimes have been deployed not only to survey these excesses and deficiencies but to contain them as well.

Medicalization of the intersexed and disabled has profoundly shaped their cultural representations and interpersonal relationships, as well as their phenomenological experiences of and with their own bodies. Whereas historically, the intersexed conjured up erotic associations, more recently, repeated medical diagnosis and intervention and medical jargon bantered about in exclusionary or hushed tones have contributed to shrouding disabled/intersexed bodies with an aura of taboo, secrecy, and shame (Kessler 1998). Overall, medical and cultural assumptions about sex being reserved for heterosexed, symmetrical, and genitally specific bodies tend to promote the expectation that sex and sexuality are privileges awarded to the "normate"[6] only (Saxton 1984; Atkins and Martson 1999).

The rigid molding of bodies to conform to conventional standards and allowances clearly exacts a toll in conceiving of alternative means of desiring. For the intersexed, "to grow up in a world in which there is no name, at least no spoken name, for what you are" is frightening and confusing (Holmes 1998, 221). Fear of rejection undermines sexual choices. For instance, Morgan Holmes (1998), an intersexed bisexual, explains: "I learned then that my desire wasn't necessarily linked to my physical difference. However, even that knowledge could not assuage the fear that my lovers of whatever sex, but particularly female, would know I had a fake 'cunt' and would abandon me" (224). In this way, the expectation that our bodies should be strictly products of nature and not culture (as if any human body occupies space outside of culture), awards sexual gratification and relationships to those whose bodies pass the test of normative authenticity.

The story of a person called Toby who was brought up as a girl, then lived as a boy, eventually adopted the label of neuter, and in 1987, endeavored to form a self-help group for others who similarly self-identified, further illustrates the psychic cost of growing up with a body that the surrounding culture denies is possible. "As Toby conceived it, the group's purpose was to provide a forum for people who think of themselves as neuter and/or asexual to make (nonsexual) connections with others" (Kessler 1998, 77). Toby's hope was that such a group would provide "'a setting free of pressure to define ourselves in terms of maleness or femaleness'" (77). While asexuality should be respected as a chosen identity and practice, the fact that abstinence is the only acceptable alternative in our society for the unmarried, disabled, or nonheteronormative leaves me wondering why neuter was the one option to fill the interspace. Is this yet one more instance of a presence concealed as an absence because Western binary categories disallow more creative possibilities?

What is perhaps most remarkable in the testimonies of intersex though, particularly those individuals whose bodies have escaped medical tampering, is the sense of contentedness with their own bodies. In the video ISNA produced, "Hermaphrodites Speak" (1996), Angela Moreno describes the delight she received from her large clitoris at the age of twelve before doctors insisted on performing a "clitoral reduction" as "time in the pleasure garden before the fall." She asserts that what has been most profoundly removed from the intersexed through medical intervention is a uniquely "hermaphroditic eroticism."

Unfortunately, the idea that our bodies harbor our deepest truths tends to obscure the part that our culture and its naturalizing agents play in imposing these so-called truths upon us. Instead we are cast in the role of deceivers if we don't wear our bodies on our sleeves, for we are said to deprive others of their ability to manage us, anchor us, and fix our meaning. Joshua Gamson (1998) suggests that on television talk shows, for example, "any dissonance between genital status and genital identity [is taken] as a sign of inauthenticity" (97). Foucault would, in fact, argue that this compulsion to speak incessantly of our sexualities is a manifestation of modern surveillance techniques rather than an expression of our innermost thoughts. This point would indicate that, as much as discourse may attempt to contain the truth of our bodies, there will inevitably be discontinuities between the stories we tell and our bodies themselves. From this vantage point, there can never be a complete correlation between our genital status and our gender identities, no matter who we are. Moreover, David Halperin (1995) further complicates this issue of truth telling by stating that "coming out" has the advantage of "claiming back . . . a certain interpretive authority" (13), but never effectively eliminates the "superior and knowing gaze" (35) of the outside viewer.

On the other hand, those of us who have visible disabilities are often neutralized by external fixations that rob us of the opportunity to speak our own pleasures and desires. Part of the problem is that the larger society simply assumes that sexuality and disability are so antithetical to one another that there is no discussion to be had. Certain British disability theorists assert: "In modern Western societies, sexual agency (that is, potential or actual independent sexual activity) is considered the essential element of full adult personhood, replacing the role formerly taken by paid work: because disabled people are infantalized, and denied the status of active subjects, so consequently their sexuality is undermined" (Shakespeare, Gillespie-Sells, and Davies 1996, 9–10).[7] Eli Clare (1999) argues further that, because disabled bodies are equated so thoroughly with medical pathology, they are generally denied even the distorted and magnified sexuality attributed to many marginalized people (109).

The tendency to deny any recognition to the sexuality of people with disabilities also contributes to a blurring of their gender identification such that they share a gender ambiguity not so dissimilar from the intersexed. Disability and queer writer Eli Clare (1999) explains: "The construction of gender depends not only on the male and female body, but also on the nondisabled body" (112). This refusal to read disabled bodies correctly may even pose a problem for entry and acceptance into gay, lesbian, bisexual, and transgender subcultures as they, too, rely upon visible markers to signify group membership (Atkins 1998). Attention to the more culturally loaded, but misunderstood qualities of disabled bodies may cause "their less visible identity to be neglected" (xxxix). More generally, visuality and visibility produce complex and contradictory effects for those whose bodies are deemed unnatural because the impulse to stabilize our identities and to mold us into singular subjects is there regardless of the source of our visibility (i.e., by our appearance, our actions, and/or our words). The fact that all of us, in some way, participate in this dynamic suggests that these misreadings are powerful cultural scripts to resist and transform.

Destablizing Fixation and Containment

Significant challenges to the paradigms of deviance and cure are contributing to a flourishing body of normalcy studies. Fitting into the larger domain of critical theory, this line of inquiry probes the assumptions that underlie the unmarked categories in a society, exposing the constructed character of normalcy and revealing the institutional practices that create aberrations from the norm. Queer theorists have been particularly vocal about demonstrating the inherent instability of the concept of normal and unmasking the inequalities such a concept preserves. Indeed in its most liberatory sense, "queer" is not so much an embodied state or a sexual orientation as a proclivity to disclose, loosen up, and reshape the ties that bind us (see McRuer 1997).

Although the potential for breaking out of the mold of normal is always present, queer theorists Michael Warner (1999) and Alexandra Chasin (2000) offer compelling analyses concerning how and why the magnet of normalcy has functioned to undermine the more progressive agendas of the gay and lesbian movements, promoting gay marriage and being co-opted by capitalism. The broader point here is that normalcy is seductive, often beckoning us with social legitimacy and material rewards or tempting us in unexamined guises. However, its lure can limit public knowledge concerning the varieties of bodies and sexual expressions and further marginalize those who can't or won't be fixed. Both intersex and disability rights movements would benefit from heeding these concerns, avoiding containment as niche movements, lest we be the ones to be left permanently on the fringe.

Clearly, then, the struggle between normalization and transgression is a constant, with no clear victor emerging. Disability theorist Rosemarie Garland-Thomson (2001a, 348) suggests that disabled bodies offer testimony to the inherent instability of all bodies, making them a particular target for fixation and containment. Photography has been a favorite technique for such containment because it sanctions the stare, a common, but disfavored approach to relating to disability. As with the rise of the gay and lesbian movements, capitalism has been very much at the heart of these images, whether the images are used to solicit charity or encourage consumerism. Also, as with these movements, the emphasis on a commodified visuality limits public knowledge of disability and narrows the scope of a disability rights agenda because this focus simply reinforces previously scripted ways both of seeing and market-based routes to inclusion. On the other hand, Thomson asserts that some more recent forms of photography, such as advertising that promotes disability fashions, does have a certain radical potential. She clarifies: "In other words, the conjunction of the visual discourse of high fashion, which has traditionally trafficked exclusively in standardized, stylized bodies, with the visual discourse of disability, which has traditionally traded in the pathetic, earnest, or sensational creates a visual disjuncture that calls previous images of disability into question" (368–369).

In all these cases then, rupture rarely marks unconditional openings for progressive social change. At the same time, the promise and benefits of normalization are, at best, partial, and at worst, downright deceptive and contradictory, leaving room to articulate ongoing cultural critiques and oppositional strategies. Moreover, because normal does not always successfully parade as authentic, its incomplete replication sometimes creates a space for subversion and transgression.

Overlapping Coalitions and Demedicalization

Although power is often deployed in order to fix and contain unruly bodies, Halperin (1995) points out: "Power is also positive and productive. It produces possibilities of action, of choice, and, ultimately, it produces the conditions for the exercise of freedom" (17). For the intersexed, the disjuncture between medical definitions and protocol, on one hand, and self-definition, on the other, has contributed to simple instances of medical noncompliance as well as more collective efforts to disavow, subvert or transform both accepted medical treatment and the binary rigidity of conventional gender classification.

In the past decade, intersexed individuals have formed a group called the Intersex Society of North America (ISNA) to take umbrage with the assumption that they require fixing as well as to seek out alliances with other activist groups who are likely to be supportive of their cause. In fact, it was actually the disenchantment of ISNA recruits with their surgical outcomes that served as the initial catalyst for group identification (Kessler 1998). Members of ISNA now question the medical assertion that genitals are natural signifiers of gender. Apropos this point, Cheryl Chase, the organization's founder, retorts, "What are genitals for? It is my position that my genitals are for my pleasure" (cited in Nussbaum 1999, 43).

Although ISNA's original mission was to establish a forum for intersexed individuals to network and share their stories, it quickly assumed a more politicized agenda, demanding that medical and allied personnel assume a more proactive role in preparing the intersexed infant's parents to facilitate the infant's entry into the social world (Chase 1998, 197). Nonetheless, their efforts at social transformation are tempered by an acknowledgment of the rigidity of our current gender system. Chase states in this regard:

> While it is fascinating to think about the potential development of new genders or subject positions grounded in forms of embodiment that fall outside the familiar male/female dichotomy, we recognize that the two-sex gender model is currently hegemonic and therefore advocate that children be raised as boys or girls, according to which designation seems most likely to offer the child the greatest future sense of comfort. (198)

In fact, in a recent conversation I had with Chase, she further explained that ISNA's overarching mission is to ensure the bodily integrity and informed consent of intersex children. Gender issues are often the preoccupation of outsiders who think about and rally behind intersex agendas. However, while Chase supports a greater flexibility in gender role socialization, she states that such a flexibility is not an accommodation for the intersexed but an openness that would benefit everyone.

ISNA's campaign to halt genital surgery on infants has also extended to efforts to publicly affiliate their cause with U.S. government initiatives to curtail the practice of female genital mutilation. By referring to "intersex surgeries as 'IGM' to heighten the association with 'FGM'" (Kessler 1998, 81), ISNA members have hoped to garner wider support for their cause from first-world feminists. However, Chase (1998, 205) reports that this campaign has not been particularly successful because many first-world feminists have refused to see these surgeries as anything but medical, rejecting the claim that these operations are human and gender rights violations. Just recently (July 2001), the National Organization for Women (NOW) did pass a resolution supporting ISNA in their fight for informed consent. Yet, interestingly NOW insisted on using the term *intersex girls* instead of *intersex children* (which was what ISNA wanted), again essentializing categories of gender and reinscribing intersexuality as a matter of gender.

Despite the strategic concessions ISNA has made to gender binaries, it aligns itself most visibly with queer activism. In this regard, Chase contends that most intersexuals share a sense of queer identity, even when they self-identify as heterosexual, because their bodies have been made to feel queer (Dreger 1998, 178). It was, in fact, Chase's (1998, 196) exposure to groups such as Transgender Nation that helped to form her own critical consciousness concerning the damaging effects of normalizing categories and to imagine her own concerns in terms of broader struggles for social justice. Her realization that "the body I was born with was not diseased, just different" (195) moved her to build alliances with individuals and organizations whose experiences either in some way paralleled hers or who would be likely to promote the demedicalization of atypical sexual anatomy.

On a somewhat parallel course, disability rights activists have argued that while medical treatment may be necessary or desirable in order to save lives or reduce physical discomfort, fatigue, and frustration, the ideology of cure suggests that individuals with disease or disability are unwelcome members of society, to be eliminated rather than accommodated (Kemp 1981). Although disability studies theorists and activists have loudly critiqued this ideology, the fact remains that it continues to refashion itself in new guises as evidenced most recently by the Human Genome Project. Feminist philosopher Susan Wendell (1996) warns: "The desire for perfection and control of the body, or for the elimination of differences that are feared, poorly understood, and widely considered to be marks of inferiority, easily masquerades as the compassionate desire to prevent or stop suffering" (156). Additionally, Kessler (1998, 124) asserts that scientists see themselves as "creating technology, not culture" and so, too, with the intersexed, physicians foresee a day when intersexuality will be addressed by genetic screening and altered in utero.

Because queer is about coalition building, it seems worthwhile to consider why ISNA has appeared more obviously aligned with the queer movement than with the disability rights movement. My first impetus might be to conclude that the gay and lesbian movements have had more apparent successes. After all, homosexuality hasn't been considered a mental disorder since 1973. However, new categories such as "gender dysphoria" and "gender identity disorder" have been installed in its stead (Clare 1999, 96). Perhaps even more disturbing is the search for the gay gene, a quest that even some gay scientists endorse. As McRuer (1997) warns: "If a gay gene is secured, there is no reason to assume that homophobia will suddenly end. Indeed, in a culture already primed to see difference as a regrettable biological fact, there is nothing to keep heterosexuals from seeing homosexuality similarly as a natural but regrettable biological destiny, all the while doing nothing to change the institutions that secure heterosexual dominance" (210). Hence, success rarely achieves finality.

Alternatively, clues to the disidentification of some ISNA members with disability may rest with common sense understandings of the term *disability* itself. Chase herself has confided in me that many intersexed people reject this label because of its association with pathology. Mitchell and Snyder (2000) characterize this disassociation as "methodological distancing," a process by which other identity-based inquiries (such as race, feminist, and sexuality studies) have "positioned disability as the 'real' limitation from which they must escape" (3). As these disability theorists indicate, such a move may be understandable inasmuch as these inquiries are attempting to refute the culturally constructed foundation of these allegations of inferiority for their own groups. Nonetheless, such positioning only serves to reinforce the stigma already attached to disability, a stigma that will never be fully eroded unless all equations of physical difference with inferiority are challenged.

On the other hand, Chase asserts that she has learned a lot from the disability rights movement, citing as evidence the story of a Japanese woman, who, after repeated painful surgeries to be taller, decided that it was better to be short and became a disability activist in Japan. Further, intersex, transgender, and disability rights activists Diana Courvant and Emi Koyama argue that intersexuality and disability are significantly intertwined, describing them as a "confluence of rivers" merging into "one larger river." [8] "Methodological distancing" then is simply one more manifestation of the seduction of normality, a stance which members of all groups are sometimes complicit in holding.[9] Nevertheless, there are always individuals present to remind us of our broader common agenda of eliminating the notion that some human bodies aren't good enough to make their rightful claim to human dignity and sociality. Clearly, until we dismantle the authenticity of disability as the ultimate measure of inferiority, the inclination in Western cultures to pathologize and seek to limit any form of bodily difference will remain.

A Call for Fluidity and Longevity

It is at this intersection of my own disabled, feminist, and queer identification, that I would like to address my own thoughts on the real and ongoing threat of physical erasure. The anthropological record amply demonstrates that, whereas the cultural salience of particular body parts may be historically and culturally specific, the body has always served as a cultural template for social order and disorder. Moreover, the body is likely to continue to do so, albeit in potentially novel and historically contingent ways. Given this caveat, although an insistence on bodily control, autonomy, and integrity can be an effective response to bodily incursion, too great an emphasis on discrete and wholesome bodies may undermine the value of individuals, who for various reasons lack control of their own bodies, have bodies that are surgically scarred or don't conform to "normate" concepts of wholeness, or whose lives are explicitly interwoven with others who help sustain them. Likewise, the notion that the general significance that Western cultures attach to bodies can be minimized by performative and/or surgical play may be valuable inasmuch as this play blurs bodily categories and reveals their constructed and fluid character (Kessler 1998, 118). Nonetheless, such free play may not be accessible to all and may inadvertently give license to scientific free play over which we have little or no censure.

Challenging conventional categories and culturally entrenched modes of thought concerning the body is a crucial step in creating a space for all bodies, but we must do so from an embodied perspective, lest we become not only blurred, but literally and physically effaced. This is not an argument for an essentialized embodiment because any such argument may be used to obscure the role of culture in molding all our bodies or may be deployed to further mark the boundaries for inclusion and exclusion into the realm of civility and humanity. Indeed, it seems particularly ironic that we confidently exoticize and barbarize the practice of clitorectomy in some African societies even as we engage in self-starvation and full body makeovers (and as Chase [1998, 205] points out, even as we overlook the ongoing practice of clitorectomies in the West). Rather, it is from the positionality of our embodied differences, falling as they might on the continuum of cultural/natural physical variance, that we should insist on a recognition of our embodied dignity and cultural integrity at the center of a culturally imagined human community. After all, "it is from the eccentric positionality occupied by the queer subject that it may become possible to envision . . . [the means] for restructuring . . . the relations among power, truth, and desire" (Halperin 1995, 64), a restructuring that has the potential for releasing us all from these cumbersome fixations.

I believe that Will Roscoe's (1998) research on multiple genders in Native North America may offer some clue to routes to embodiment which grant us both flexibility as well as social recognition and respect because it challenges the assumption "that the fluidity of human desire and the ambiguities of human categories make stable identities and cultural continuity impossible" (5). Indeed, he asserts that beliefs about human categories may be avowedly constructionist and still experience longevity. In other words, a call for embodiment need not "shore up identities" nor be divisive.[10] We need not be fixed to be anchored. Along these same lines, anthropologist Esther Newton (2000) posits, while keeping in mind that history is neither static nor spun from a single narrative, that some claim to identity is necessary for survival, allowing us to place ourselves "in a narrative of history" (209). Arriving at similar conclusions, "disability theory provides a recognition of the social construction of labeling terms, without falling into the bind of postmodern plasticity by continually grounding itself in the "messiness" of bodily variety" (Atkins and Martson 1999, 20). It is from this grounded lens of bodily messiness that we should and must insist on speaking our bodies, our names, and our desires. Clearly, one of the most salient lessons both the queer and the disability rights movements provide is that from this human spectrum of bodily messiness has arisen and will arise cultural precedents, knowledge, and innovation which enhance the survival of us all.

Notes

1. ISNA founder Cheryl Chase (1998, 189) reports that one in two thousand births results in genital anomalies that call into question the gender status of the newborn.
2. These definitions are taken from *Webster's New Universal Unabridged Dictionary*, 2nd ed. (1979, 694).
3. The French statistician Adolphe Quetelet (1796–1847) was the first to express the power of the norm to set standards for desirable behavior and bodies (Davis 1997, 11).
4. The line of inquiry I am taking here, comparing the medical disciplining of intersexed and impaired bodies, has also been recommended by Shelly Tremain (1999, 122).
5. Similar explanations were put forward for disability during the Victorian era (Stiker 1997, 93).
6. *Normate* is a term used by Rosemarie Garland-Thomson (1997, 8) to refer to all those who conform to cultural constructions of normality in a particular society.
7. In fact, Tom Shakespeare et al. (1996, 6) argue that disability rights activists themselves have played a part in rendering the sexuality of individuals with disabilities invisible by placing civil rights agendas at the forefront of their activism.
8. The comments by Cheryl Chase, Diana Courvant, and Emi Koyama included here were made at the First International Queer Disability Conference held at San Francisco State University on June 2, 2002.
9. For example, disability rights activists have also engaged in "methodological distancing" as evidenced by the resistance of some activists to include AIDS as a disability under the Americans with Disabilities Act (Fleisher and Zames 2001, 90).
10. Here Will Roscoe is disagreeing somewhat with queer theorists who contend: "Even as the categories that mark us as different are necessary for claiming rights and benefits, it is only when they are unworkable that we are really safe. From this angle, muddying the categories rather than shoring them up, pointing out their instability and fluidity, along with their social roots, is the key to liberation" (Gamson 1998, 222).

Works Cited

Atkins, Dawn. 1998. Introduction: Looking queer. In *Looking queer: Body image and identity in lesbian, bisexual, gay, and transgendered communities*, edited by Dawn Atkins. New York: Harrington Park Press.

Atkins, Dawn, and C. Martson. 1999. Creating accessible queer community: Intersections and fractures with dis/ability praxis. *Journal of Gay, Lesbian, and Bisexual Identity* 4 (1): 3–22.

Carter, Raphael. 1998. The murk manual: How to understand medical writing on intersex. *Chrysalis: The Journal of Transgressive Gender Identities* 2 (5): 10, 30.

Chase, Cheryl. 1998. Hermaphrodites with attitude: Mapping the emergence of intersex activism. *Gay and Lesbian Quarterly* 4: 189–211.

Chasin, Alexandra. 2000. *Selling out: The gay and lesbian movement goes to market.* New York: St. Martin's Press.

Clare, Eli. 1999. *Exile and pride: Disability, queerness, and liberation.* Cambridge, Mass.: South End Press.

Coventry, Martha. 2000. Making the cut. *Ms.* 10 (6), 52–60.

Davis, Lennard. 1997. Constructing normalcy: The bell curve, the novel, and the invention of the disabled body in the nineteenth century. In *The Disability Studies Reader,* edited by Lennard Davis. New York: Routledge.

Dreger, Alice Domurat. 1998. *Hermaphrodites and the medical invention of sex.* Cambridge, Mass.: Harvard University Press.

Fausto-Sterling, Anne. 1998. The five sexes: Why male and female are not enough. In *Women's lives: Multicultural perspectives,* edited by Gwyn Kirk and Margo Okaza-Rey. Mountain View, Calif.: Mayfield.

Fleisher, Doris Zames, and Frieda Zames. 2001. *The disability rights movement: From charity to confrontation.* Philadelphia: Temple University Press.

Foucault, Michel. 1973. *The birth of a clinic.* London: Tavistock.

———. 1978. *The history of sexuality.* New York: Vintage.

———. 1980. *Herculine Barbin: Being the recently discovered diary of a nineteenth century French hermaphrodite.* New York: Pantheon.

Gamson, Joshua. 1998. *Freaks talk back: Tabloid talk shows and sexual nonconformity.* Chicago: University of Chicago Press.

Garland-Thomson, Rosemarie. 1997. *Extraordinary bodies: Figuring physical disability in American culture and literature.* New York: Columbia University Press.

———. 2001a. Seeing the disabled: Visual rhetorics of disability in popular photography. In *The new disability history: American perspectives,* edited by Paul Longmore and Lauri Umansky. New York: New York University Press.

———. 2001b. Toward a feminist disability theory. Paper presented at the Gender and Disability Conference, Institute for Research on Women, Rutgers University, New Brunswick, N.J., March 2–3, 2001.

Gilbert, Ruth. 2000. "Strange notions": Treatments of Early Modern hermaphrodites. In *Madness, disability, and social exclusion: The archaeology and anthropology of "difference,"* edited by June Hubert. London: Routledge.

Halperin, David. 1995. *Saint Foucault: Toward a gay hagiography.* New York: Oxford University Press.

Hermaphrodites speak (Film). 1996. Produced by ISNA.

Holmes, Morgan. 1998. In(to)visibility: Intersexuality in the field of queer. In *Looking queer: Body image and identity in lesbian, bisexual, gay, and transgender communities,* edited by Dawn Atkins. New York: Harrington Park Press.

Kemp, Evan. 1981. Aiding the disabled, no pity please. *New York Times,* September 3, p. 3.

Kessler, Suzanne. 1998. *Lessons from the intersexed.* New Brunswick, N.J.: Rutgers University Press.

Longmore, Paul. 1997. Conspicuous contribution and American cultural dilemmas: Telethon rituals of cleansing and renewal. In *The body and physical difference: Discourses of disability,* edited by David Mitchell and Sharon Snyder. Ann Arbor: University of Michigan Press.

McRuer, Robert. 1997. *The queer renaissance: Contemporary American literature and the reinvention of lesbian and gay identities.* New York: New York University Press.

Mitchell, David, and Sharon Snyder. 1997. Introduction: Disability studies and the double bind of representation. In *The body and physical difference: Discourses of disability,* edited by D. Mitchell and S. Snyder. Ann Arbor: University of Michigan Press.

————. 2000. *Narrative prosthesis: Disability and the dependencies of discourse*. Ann Arbor: University of Michigan Press.

Newton, Esther. 2000. *Margaret Mead Made Me gay: Personal essays, public ideas*. Durham, N.C.: Duke University Press.

Nussbaum, Emily. 1999. The sex that dare not speak its name. *Lingua Franca*. May/June: 42–51.

Porter, James. 1997. Foreword to *The body and physical difference: Discourses of disability*, edited by D. Mitchell and S. Snyder. Ann Arbor: University of Michigan Press.

Roscoe, Will. 1998. *Changing ones: Third and fourth genders in Native North America*. New York: St. Martin's Griffin.

Saxton, Martha. 1984. Born and unborn: The implications of reproductive technologies for people with disabilities. In *Test-tube women: What future motherhood*, edited by Rita Arditti, R. D. Klein, and S. Minden. London: Pandora Press.

Shakespeare, Tom, Kath Gillespie-Sells, and Dominic Davies. 1996. *The sexual politics of disability: Untold desires*. London: Cassell.

Stiker, Henri-Jacques. 1997. *A history of disability*. Ann Arbor: University of Michigan Press.

Tremain, Shelly. 1999. Book review. *Journal of Gay, Lesbian, and Bisexual Identity* 4: 119–123.

Warner, Michael. 1999. *The trouble with normal: Sex, politics, and the ethics of queer life*. Cambridge, Mass.: Harvard University Press.

Wendell, Susan. 1996. *The rejected body: Feminist philosophical reflections on disability*. New York: Routledge.

Interpreting Women

ℐℒℴ

BRENDA JO BRUEGGEMANN

Sign language interpreters fascinate me. They are predominantly women (and white women at that)—almost 85 percent so—and their work in what Mary Louise Pratt and others have called the "contact zone"—right here in our own country as it occurs between deaf and hearing worlds and cognitions and between the radically different modalities and languages of visual-spatial, embodied American Sign Language (ASL) and print-centered, often disembodied contemporary English—strikes me as even more fraught with tensions about who "speaks" (Roof and Weigman 1995); the problems of speaking for others (Alcoff 1994); the politics of translation (Spivak 1992); and the ethics of care, justice, and representation (Robinson 1999), than just about any other translating, interpreting, scene—literally or metaphorically—that I can imagine. Sign language interpreters fascinate me because their cultural space, "working the hyphens" as Michelle Fine (1994) would call it, and performing in the kind of hybrid third space that Homi Bhabha (1994) has written about resonates often with my own "hard-of-hearing" doubly hyphenated existence in both deaf and hearing worlds.

Two of my closest friends and colleagues in both my personal and professional life are interpreters—and my entry and return points into the Gallaudet d/Deaf community over the past twelve years have come at their hands. Outside the Gallaudet academic community, I have often, although not always, used two different long-standing interpreter-friends as my contact points at academic conferences and some academic social gatherings—helping me to work the hyphens between the hearing academic world and my own hard-of-hearing capabilities. Their bodies and interpretations often become my third space.

And it is a remarkably fluid space, yet fraught with ethical choices at every turn. Let me present three scenes with one interpreter to illustrate. First, a few years ago, at a College of Humanities faculty meeting on my campus some one hundred of us were treated to a sneak preview of a sophisticated video made about the College of Humanities' sophisticated new "World Media and Culture

61

Center" and its soon-to-be-open cyber-café that promised to "bridge cross-cultural communication and send Ohio State well ahead into the twenty-first century." The video was slated to be shown at numerous halftimes of upcoming OSU basketball games, piquing the curiosity—and prying open the pocketbooks, it was hoped—of wealthy alumni and parents of potential future Buckeyes.

While the video preview played on a giant auditorium screen in the Wexner Center Film and Video Theater, it was my interpreter and I who sat, together, kindred and frustrated—in the dark both literally and figuratively—while the wonders of cross-cultural communication and shared knowledge unfolded on the screen. Without the addition of either open or closed captions on the video clip and with the Wexner Center auditorium darkened enough that sign language interpretation of what was being said on the video was impossible to see as well, we both felt alternatively embarrassed and angry at the abundant ironies. Even more abundantly ironic was the fact that I was currently then serving on the College of Humanities' Diversity Committee; the Dean had appointed me to this committee, in fact, because of the disability perspective I could bring to the committee and its work. And further, I was slated to stand and speak for five minutes at this specific faculty meeting about a new Diversity Enhancement Award we would be putting in place that year. Thus, I had made sure I had my longest-standing and favorite interpreter there (we have known each other now at OSU for nine years), principally to be sure I could field questions well from the faculty audience after I spoke. When the clip ended and the lights went back up, my interpreter immediately signed, "Do you want me to say something?" "No," I asserted, "I will." And then I did.

The entanglement of her advocacy, her ability and willingness to speak (again, literally and figuratively) for me, and her shared space in the darkened moment of frustration with me plays in numerous corners of the ethical room that sign language interpreters almost always occupy. This recounted scene and its moment of advocacy on the part of the interpreter—an example of the politics of interpretation and representation in full action—and the personal and professional shared intimacy of an awkward moment with an interpreter happens daily in the life of many deaf people. Melanie Metzger's book, *Sign Language Interpreting: Deconstructing the Myth of Neutrality* (1999) makes some of these politic and ethical situations of sign language interpretation quite evident.

At another College of Humanities faculty meeting two years later—with a new Dean who now had me chairing the Diversity Committee and who was also helping me secure an American Sign Language program for language credits at Ohio State as well as developing an undergraduate and graduate minor in Disability Studies—the same interpreter is with me again. At this particular meeting, we were voting on whether a unit that had existed, and flourished, in the College for over a decade as a division (one notch below a department) could, at long last, become a full-fledged department, with the budget and tenure-initiating status that comes along with departmenthood at OSU. The discussion period before the vote was marked as twenty minutes on the official agenda.

One senior member of the College faculty stood, the moment that discussion was called, and read from a prepared speech/letter for the full twenty minutes. Thus, no one else was given the floor to speak. He was, of course, speaking against the granting of department status to this unit (as he had apparently also done some years earlier when a similar vote had been made on granting the Women's Studies Center the title of department as well).

As his letter/speech went on and on, my interpreter increasingly became the subject of increasing scrutiny herself. Although I couldn't see this from the audience behind me, I could in fact see and sense it playing out on her own body and expressions. Suddenly we were both very sorry that we had decided she should be up on the stage in the auditorium where this meeting was held, alongside the table occupied by the Dean, Associate Dean, and Assistant Dean (so that she could hear them best). For when the speaker kept speaking, and the faculty-audience became increasingly impatient, their eyes and attention, naturally, began to cast about. And sign language interpreters always make a good focal point in almost any predominantly hearing-world environment. Thus, there she was, stuck on the stage, the center of the shifting attention.

To complicate things even more, good interpreters are trained to register the tone and "voice" of the speech and speaker largely through body position and pronounced facial expressions (quite pronounced, that is, for the hearing world's sense of propriety but actually quite reserved often in terms of Deaf culture's facial and body expressions while signing). And I could tell that my interpreter was suddenly, but profoundly, struggling with a significant ethical choice: should she register, with accuracy, the "tone" of this speaker so that I could "hear" it myself (as she was mostly trained to do), or should she protect the chance that her interpretation would be viewed as mockery of his speech and possibly too, in extension or collaboration (since deaf people are sadly and so often perceived as somehow only extensions or composites of their interpreters) of my own views—as if I judged his speech in mockery.

No easy scene. No small dilemma. What was created was a communicative triangle that was surely restrictive to all engaged in it. In the end, she chose to go deadpan and to interpret only with hand signs and virtually no facial expression or body movement; in other words, she chose to violate one part of her training (about accurate representation of tone and register) to not violate another (misrepresenting herself or her client's intent). This scene and all her choices—damned if she did, damned if she didn't—have played in my mind many times since.

They've played so because only four months before that she was interpreting for me at a very different kind of scene and her engagement there was also dramatically different. I had organized a literary event called "A Triple Blind Reading" on my campus; three of my treasured friends and colleagues, all with sight loss ("call it blindness," one of them, Georgina Kleege, would say) who also happened to be very accomplished writers, would be reading from their poetry and prose. One would read from an essay, one from poetry, and one from a piece of short fiction. Each of these three authors employs different kinds of technology to accomplish a public reading like this (and to complete their own writing and research); considering these differences was also to be a part of the discussion afterwards with the audience, to explore (and exploit) the idea of "blind reading."

I had asked my favorite OSU interpreter to work the event if she could, not only because I knew and trusted her interpreting but also because she had been gaining great skills over the last couple of years at artistic interpreting. I didn't necessarily need an interpreter myself—I would be sitting front row and center for the event (I was to introduce each reader) and I had read all of their texts, in print, beforehand. But I had also just requested her in case a person, especially an OSU student, with hearing loss showed up on the scene at the last minute; this way, I could ensure quality interpreting from the outset.

What happened that night was very very memorable for me—as it was for many in the audience. The reading took place in the Wexner Center Film and Video Theater (ominously, in the same place as the bad College faculty meeting with the uncaptioned World Media Center video some two years before). And Carolyn, the interpreter (not her real name), rose to the occasion. By the last reader, she was in total artistic performance mode. (Some interpreters gain advanced skills in certain kinds of interpreting—academic, public schools, legal and medical, artistic, e.g.) The last "reader" more or less performed orally a short story he had written (with only a small tape recorder ear-prompting him on his own text and this device, quite uncannily, was virtually unseen by the audience)—and Carolyn, more or less performed (not just interpreted) in sign language about two feet from him. It was mesmerizing.

Afterwards—in fact, for weeks afterwards—those who had attended this event continued to remark to me how deeply engaged they had been with both performances at the same time and how, too, they felt that this deep engagement couldn't have happened with any kind of "regular" artistic reading. (These kinds of comments, by the way, always leave me both beaming with pride and yet squirming uncomfortably since the disabled body has always been this kind of double-sided spectacle—inspirational pride and look-away-quickly discomfort—for our culture at large.) Carolyn, the interpreter, was truly lost in her own performance. So much so that at the end, before she darted out, she approached me and apologized since she had only just then realized that "I forgot to check with you, to register if the interpretation was working for you [it was, and how!] . . . I just got so caught up in performing it."

When I put those two events, just four months apart, beside each other, I am amazed. In both of them stand the same interpreter and the same "client" (that's me). Yet in one, the communicative and rhetorical situation seems to demand defying her training and removing all self and expression from the event—in order, in large part, to protect me. While in the other, the situation called for a kind of transcendence of her training and a total self-immersion and overt expressiveness—in large part, abandoning me. And yet in both, the Other audience outside our two-part dialogue plays a significant role. In short, interpreters are not, in fact are never (I'd wager), interpreting only for their designated (deaf) clients. Strange but true.

My examples here still only skim the surface of an incredibly complex set of issues around ethics, caring, and representation in the profession of sign language interpreting. The particular points of my own use of interpreters, only on certain occasions, both adds to and yet simplifies some of this potential complexity. Because, for example, I myself do speak and write well enough in English, because I have been successfully mainstreamed, because I lipread quite well and do use, with some success, numerous kinds of assistive listening technologies in my job, and because, finally, I now occupy a position of relative authority in "the hearing world"—all of these particulars make interpreting for me far less an unbalanced communication dynamic to begin with. That is, my interpreters don't usually find themselves in the uncomfortable situation of assisting communication for someone they often feel is not being regarded as (let's just be forthright here) intelligent, equal, communicatively capable on par with the one speaking, literally, in the dominant tongue. (Still, this "deaf-downgrading" factor does happen to me from time to time too.)

Interpreters do indeed throw their voices a lot. In helping them deal with the murkier issues around matters of "voice" and representation, to assist in navigating their way through what Melanie Metzger has called their long-standing "myth of neutrality" (1999), they have a field-wide code of ethics. It attempts, I would argue, to wrestle with and tame some of the more powerful sides of their latent authority, to contextualize their "caring" for their clients, and to attempt fashioning more clearly their representations of both their selves and their clients. I see and hear this code referred to often—hardly neutral, I sense its mythical sleeping dragon-like power in their lives and work.

To illustrate, I have reconstructed here a bit of dialogue from a three and a half-hour-long interview I conducted with five interpreters in the Washington D.C. area. All five of these interpreters were trained by Gallaudet University's own interpreter program, all were recommended to me as "the best in the business," and all five also promised me they were more than willing to talk about issues of authority and representation in their profession. And they held true to that promise, running me through three audiotapes and two sets of batteries and driving my transcriber nearly crazy with their animated, often overlapping, discussion. There are five women (counting myself) in on this discussion and one man, who also happens to be regarded as "the best interpreter in the D.C. area." Later, I will have more to say about him in particular. At this particular juncture, they are discussing the interpreters' code of ethics and sharing their interpretations of it; they are also imagining various scenes that test their authority and representative roles within the frame of this code:

Jack: What I get into trouble with is when there are certain moral issues
that are coming into play that have nothing to do with the code. Like

my favorite example: I'm interpreting for a deaf person who I know is taking medication already. I've interpreted for them in another situation. They go to see a different doctor. I'm interpreting for the same person. The doctor says, "Are you taking any medication because this medication I'm giving you really doesn't go well with many drugs." The deaf person says, "No, I'm not on anything else." The doctor is not going to prescribe them otherwise. If I follow the letter of the code, I'm not supposed to say anything. You can be damned sure, before I'm out of there, I'm gonna be saying to the person, "you are taking something." Or, "Doctor, she is on something. You better ask again." Because I'm not going to go to bed thinking somebody could kill them. Just because the code says you don't say anything—I tell them, "Are you sure about the medicine you're taking?"

Kate: Yeah, you go to the deaf person first.

June: That's what I do.

Jack: Yes, of course.

June: I say, "Remember?" And they go, "Oh yes! Thank you."

Jack: Unless the deaf person really refuses to remember, or can't remember.

June: Then I'll leave it alone, of course.

Jack: No, then I tell the doctor.

June: You do?

Jack: Yes! If they're going to be taking another medication.

June: But, if they consciously—

Elaine: Yeah, what if they make that decision?

Jack: If you're sure they understood your question. But what if they forgot? What if there is something about what they got that they can't remember they're taking something else?

June: Dementia? Okay. Different story, but—

Elaine: If they consciously decide not to tell the doctor—

June: If it's clear they're just siding—

Jack: Yeah, yeah. I would leave it.

June: But if they forgot, like elderly people. . . . All right, thank you.

Jack: What if the reason is because they want to kill themselves? Am I going to participate in their suicide?

Carla: Yes! Because it's their right to make that decision. I mean, because you know what: if they weren't there, and it was a hearing person, they could make that decision for themselves. I mean that's sometimes the place I have to go—even though I may not agree with it. Sometimes I say, "Okay. If there were no need for an interpreter here, this person has that right to make that decision." I may not agree with it. I may for the rest of my life hate myself for going along with it, but it's not my right to make that decision. Another example of what would be considered a break in the code of ethics. Early on, when I first started interpreting, I was in a situation. And, you know, the deaf community in general is extremely small, and in D.C., it's even smaller. And there was a situation where a deaf person had a situation that was very emotional, shall we say. And I had to interpret in this particular situation. And there's supposedly a clause in the code of ethics that everything is confidential. You aren't supposed to talk about what happens with regard to your work.

June: To anyone. This is my favorite: you're not even supposed to tell anyone you're interpreting. You're supposed to tell them you're going out for ice cream.

Jack: That's not in the code.

June: That's what I was taught.

Carla: That's some people's interpretation of it still. One of my teachers still abides by it. Confidentiality. Doesn't talk about anything. This situation was so incredibly emotional. It was so unfair. Everything about it was just garbage. And here I am a brand new—I mean I had probably been out of school six months. It was a situation I was qualified for, but I had all of this stuff. It's like a therapist who has all of this stuff that's passed through them. And then you're with it, and what do you do with it? It took me a while to find a way to be with that and to go process it because I wasn't gonna sit and hold that. But there are people that say that an interpreter's confidentiality is it. And that the number one tenet of the code of ethics is confidentiality. We're not supposed to talk about it. There are some people that say, like she said, that you're not even supposed to admit that you interpret, much less where it is or what you do or any of that.

Elaine: Yeah, like if you were in a therapy session yourself, and it [an interpreting situation] really hits home for you, you're not supposed to go back to your own therapist and tell them what happened.

Carla: Right, right. Or you're sitting in an interpreting situation and something really affects you—or whatever kind of session—and you're sitting there, and the thing is really getting to you and you're crying. Well, you aren't supposed to have any feelings because then you're being partial. Hellllloooo!

Brenda (me): That makes me think, though . . . again, about the authority undercurrent—this notion that you do carry a lot of authority.

I have been interviewing interpreters (as well as audiologists, deaf educators, and deaf women authors/performers) and studying deaf women's autobiography for several years now; I have also been attending their professional conferences and gatherings, reading their textbooks and training materials, and just generally watching them at what they do every chance I get. I have been exploring the nature of female authority in relation to deafness. Each of these three fields—audiology, sign language interpreting, and deaf education—is composed of over 85 percent women, and I am convinced that these women construct and carry out a unique kind of authority in relation to the speech-centered, male-dominant modes of communication in our culture. I am particularly interested in the rhetorical appeal of *ethos*—the construction of moral character— because as a relational concept, *ethos* will help me analyze the fluid, flexible, ethically fraught third space that these professional women occupy between deaf and hearing worlds.

For theoretical and analytical lenses, I am attending to work on feminist ethics of care and representation, the dynamics of caring and speaking for others, and various frameworks for cross-cultural communication. In considering the stances and scenes of interpreting women, I have observed at least six key elements and issues around representation and the construction of their authority that they frequently encounter and embody.

First, there is the way that an ethics of care and ethics of justice occur in often-entangled operations with each other. The scene the five interpreters are playing out above is one they might ethically practice on as part of their ethical training. But too, they tell me, these are actually the kinds of large but small decisions they make almost every day they interpret. The dimensions of, and boundaries around, their service to and representation of their d/Deaf clients governs their collective and individual views of care and justice and impacts their way of doing their job both in a general philosophical position they take but also in reacting to any individualized situation of interpretation dynamics. They must respond, for example, to the Deaf community's charge that they gain profit off the weakness of the deaf person's literacy skills in our culture and that they should do more to address this potential exploitation of power and literacy imbalance.

One illustration of justice and care ethically entangled with each other occurred at a recent conference held in Washington D.C.—the first-ever international conference on Disability Studies sponsored by the National Institutes for Disability Research and Rehabilitation. An entire contingent from Gallaudet University occupied the better part of one large table near the front of the room and proceeded, increasingly as the conference wore on, to alienate the two interpreters who were supposed to be working for them on the stage and who were clearly not quite qualified to interpret the level of international academic discourse going on in that room. Although they continued to interpret, the interpreters' expressions, in response, became deadpan and their bodies registered their own mental, emotional absence from the scene and their job. They became, that is, the very picture of empty rhetoric as the table of Deaf scholars from Gallaudet University began to ignore them, just sign-chatting among themselves and glancing occasionally at the real-time captioning screen, clearly dissatisfied with the interpreting they had been provided with.

A second key issue or element in interpretive authority dynamics, as is obvious from this alienating scene, is how complex representation issues are encountered repeatedly by sign language interpreters. The interpreters at this

NIDRR convention, for example, were clearly encountering some thick and tough representational dilemmas. What to do when the code of your profession suggests that you continue to interpret for those who have clearly discounted you? What to do when you find yourself quite unqualified for the discussion at hand (and this happens to them more often than I think they want to admit)? And yet, if you withdraw, there will likely be no communication path for or potential involvement by your deaf client in this current interaction. Thus, you are damned if you do (stay and attempt an interpretation) but also damned if you don't (withdraw yourself, take your disqualifications and flee). Which representation to choose?

Ethically co-constructed situations where an interpreter might know or sense that the deaf person is already in a power-under situation—as in a medical scene like the one played out by the group discussion earlier—are microcosms of the way power plays out at large in our culture. And again, it is primarily women negotiating these scenes. The complex of representational issues that sign language interpreters encounter in their authoritative "speaking" space need to be even more carefully coded, catalogued, and categorized so that interpreters in training and practice might have better frames within which to understand their own authority.

Such frames might help deal with the third key issue—their particular/situational and general/cultural gender-based constructions of authority. It is Jack (the single male in the group) who makes the definitive pronouncement about what is in the code of ethics and what is not there. Note how much Jack centers and even drives this conversation, even in the three-minute clip I have pulled from a three-hour exchange. In three other group-arranged discussions with other sets of interpreters that I've conducted in other locations, this has been the pattern: the single male authorizes more often and more forcibly, often making what seems to be far clearer and more definitive pronouncements on ethical dilemmas. Jack's female cohorts all tease him—both affectionately but quite seriously—about "getting away with murder" and "having a lot of authority" because he is a man, they say. (Not because, for example, he is just naturally more talented at what he does.) For the most part, he agrees with them.

Why, I wonder, have all those interpreters who have been deemed the "best of the best" that I've encountered in interviewing three sets of interpreters now—one group in D.C. area (here), one in Boston, and one in Columbus—why do they always give the guy in the group the "best of the best" crown? Why at Gallaudet University Press Editorial Board meetings I've attended—six of them now—has there always been a male interpreter (and only a single male) on hand? Why are male interpreters almost always CODA (Children of Deaf Adults) or gay, as more than one person has quipped to me? What patterns of gender-based communication, as explored by sociolinguistic scholars such as Deborah Tannen, apply to male and female interpretive strategies and their negotiation of authority in between speech and sign?

In these interrogative frames I might further explore, for example, how

Carla waits a while to enter the dialogue; yet when she does find her way in, she enters quite fully and forcibly, taking a friendly but firm position that complicates Jack's considerably. This holding back but then heavy-handed authoritative positioning by a female interpreter has happened more than once in the data I have.

Finally, in looking more closely at situational and cultural conversational norms as they influence and play upon gender-based dynamics in an interpreting situation, I want to consider the quite varied ways that interpreters I have used at my university and at professional meetings and national conferences around the country have responded to, served, interacted with me. The range is quite astonishing, sometimes enlightening and sometimes, yes, disturbing, and it is always, I think, an ethical co-construction of our mutual, sometimes complementary and sometimes competing, authorities.

A fourth set of representational dilemmas that sign language interpreters often encounter, that are also often complementary and competing at the same time, are their ethical conflicts about their own positions as mere instruments or powerful advocates. Sign language interpreters' individual and collective ethical and authoritative positionings have swung heavily on a historical pendulum—from an early view of interpreters as heavy advocates for their deaf clients, interfering and speaking for them often, to a later equally problematic view that marked them as mere objective instruments, as only tools of communication (not communicative subjective individuals themselves). And now there is some attempt to swing between those poles, as one interpreter tells me—to keep shifting their locus of authority for each situation in a sort of interpretive standpoint epistemology. This still-in-process historical swing over the advocate (or not) role that interpreters can play in relation to the clients they work for and with occupies their field and training discussions quite a bit: Is an interpreter merely a kind of communicative conduit? Are they a unique form of access technology? And (or?) are they real people and an active, engaged part of the dia– no, make that tria-logue?

In trying to answer these questions for themselves—to figure ways to represent their own part in the conversations and communication they interpret— we (and they) must also imagine the way they go about imagining the "others" they serve. This is the fifth key representational and authority-constructing element of their work. In exploring the way that a (deaf) Other is a reflection of their own (hearing) selves, the audience analysis emphasis in much of rhetorical history and theory—from at least Aristotle forward—might come in handy as in considering the way that an interpreter is a twice-over kind of third space between her deaf client (curious, see, that the hearing person in the communicative exchange is never the client) and those who are hearing.

Who exactly is the audience in an interpreting scene, we might have to begin by asking here. Is it the interpreter herself—as audience to both parties, conduit between them? Or is it the deaf client—for whose benefit the interpreter is supposed to exist? But what about, too, the hearing person/people in the exchange—who are obviously receiving/listening/attending as well? Aren't they clients and audience too? Who speaks (and how) in this triangulated communication space? Who listens (and why?) Who authorizes (and what makes their authority so?) What kind of rhetorical triangle is this?

In working to answer the audience and authority dynamics framed in these kinds of questions, interpreters also engage in a sixth and final representational act: they are deeply involved in the politics of translation. In exploring the always-shifting standpoint of an interpretive triangle, they must turn to issues of translation, transliteration, and communicative and crosscultural (mis)understandings in general. Sign language interpreters by and large have a discomforting awareness that too much depends upon them, that hearing people often only have conversations with them (not with the deaf person they are interpreting for), that their authority is simply too great, that the balance of communication is off-kilter to begin with and the triangle askew, near to collapsing. In our country, for example, they fret over how much—too much—authority they occupy politically and interpersonally when they translate back and forth between visual-spatial, embodied, nonprint versions of sign language (clearly the nondominant language in the exchange, no matter who begins or authorizes it) and the dominant, empowered spoken/written and disembodied English.

But then too, these interpreters often express discomfort over their lack of authority. They often express dissatisfaction over: how often they are neglected by both of the other parties in the triangular exchange; how easily they are made into nothing but an almost nonhuman instrument; how often they are put in situations they have no business being in, aren't qualified for, haven't been trained for, don't have a way out of; and how, too, they don't much like being "replaced" with things such as real-time captioning and other assistive listening technologies where the human component (seems to) disappear.

Mostly, however, in considering the politics of translation that they often engage, I am riveted by the quite strong discomfort most of them express when the situation demands that they must "voice" for a deaf person. While they often don't mind turning a hearing voice into sign language, most confess that they feel awkward—even fearful and disgusted by—the communication dynamics that occur when they must become a deaf person's "voice."

What strikes me here then, and finally, is how the power of *willing speech*—of speech that is one's own will, of speech that is easy and willing, of the ability to will speech to occur—is no authority to be ignored. The way our entire rhetorical, cultural imperative to *will* speech, to create willing speech, lies in the hands, literally and figuratively, of women as interpreters (and audiologists and educators too) when they work to construct the literate and rhetorical life of their deaf and hard-of-hearing "subjects" is an issue we've long "skirted" as one "just about deafness." But, I believe, it is far, far more. The authority of these women, as interpreters, represents perhaps one of the keenest examples we could imagine of rhetoric's long-standing educational, political, and personal power—the endowment of willing speech. Interpreting women is not only about understanding (interpreting) these women who interpret with the authority of willing speech, but it is also about how women are themselves interpreted in (and occupy) such fluid and ethically complex roles in relation to the will of speech in our culture at large.

Works Cited

Alcoff, Linda. 1994. The problem of speaking for others. In *Feminist nightmares: Women at odds: Feminism and the problem of sisterhood*, edited by Susan Ostrov Weisser and Jennifer Fleischner. New York: New York University Press.

Bhabha, Homi K. 1994. *The location of culture*. London: Routledge.

Fine, Michelle. 1994. Working the hyphens: Reinventing self and other in qualitative research. In *Handbook of qualitative research*, edited by Norman K. Denzin and Yvonna S. Lincoln. Thousand Oaks, Calif.: Sage.

Metzger, Melanie. 1999. *Sign language interpreting: Deconstructing the myth of neutrality*. Washington D.C.: Gallaudet University Press.

Robinson, Fiona. 1999. *Globalizing care: Ethics, feminist theory, and international relations*. Boulder, Colo.: Westview Press.

Roof, Judith and Robyn Wiegman, eds. 1995. *Who can speak?: Authority and critical identity*. Urbana: University of Illinois Press.

Spivak, Gayatri Chakravorty. 1992. The politics of translation. In *Destabilizing theory: Contemporary feminist debates*, edited by Michèle Barrett and Anne Phillips. Stanford, Calif.: Stanford University Press.

Integrating Disability, Transforming Feminist Theory

☙❧

ROSEMARIE GARLAND-THOMSON

Over the last several years, disability studies has moved out of the applied fields of medicine, social work, and rehabilitation to become a vibrant new field of inquiry within the critical genre of identity studies. Charged with the residual fervor of the civil rights movement, Women's Studies and race studies established a model in the academy for identity-based critical enterprises that followed, such as gender studies, queer studies, disability studies, and a proliferation of ethnic studies, all of which have enriched and complicated our understandings of social justice, subject formation, subjugated knowledges, and collective action.

Even though disability studies is now flourishing in disciplines such as history, literature, religion, theater, and philosophy in precisely the same way feminist studies did twenty-five years ago, many of its practitioners do not recognize that disability studies is part of this larger undertaking that can be called identity studies. Indeed, I must wearily conclude that much of current disability studies does a great deal of wheel reinventing. This is largely because many disability studies scholars simply do not know either feminist theory or the institutional history of Women's Studies. All too often, the pronouncements in disability studies of what we need to start addressing are precisely issues that feminist theory has been grappling with for years. This is not to say that feminist theory can be transferred wholly and intact over to the study of disability studies, but it is to suggest that feminist theory can offer profound insights, methods, and perspectives that would deepen disability studies.

Conversely, feminist theories all too often do not recognize disability in their litanies of identities that inflect the category of woman. Repeatedly, feminist issues that are intricately entangled with disability—such as reproductive technology, the place of bodily differences, the particularities of oppression, the ethics of care, the construction of the subject—are discussed without any reference to disability. Like disability studies practitioners who are unaware of feminism, feminist scholars are often simply unacquainted with disability studies' perspectives. The most sophisticated and nuanced analyses of disability, in my view, come from scholars conversant with feminist theory. And the most compelling and complex analyses of gender intersectionality take into consideration what I call the ability/disability system—along with race, ethnicity, sexuality, and class.

I want to give the omissions I am describing here the most generous interpretation I can. The archive, Foucault has shown us, determines what we can know. There has been no archive, no template for understanding disability as a category of analysis and knowledge, as a cultural trope, and an historical community. So just as the now widely recognized centrality of gender and race analyses to all knowledge was unthinkable thirty years ago, disability is still not an icon on many critical desktops. I think, however, that feminist theory's omission of disability differs from disability studies' ignorance of feminist theory. I find feminist theory and those familiar with it quick to grasp the broad outlines of disability theory and eager to consider its implications. This, of course, is because feminist theory itself has undertaken internal critiques and proved to be porous and flexible. Disability studies is news, but feminist theory is not. Nevertheless, feminist theory is still resisted for exactly the same reasons that scholars might resist disability studies: the assumption that it is narrow, particular, and has little to do with the mainstream of academic practice and knowledge (or with themselves). This reductive notion that identity studies are intellectual ghettos limited to a narrow constituency demanding special pleading is the persistent obstacle that both feminist theory and disability studies must surmount.

Disability studies can benefit from feminist theory and feminist theory can benefit from disability studies. Both feminism and disability studies are comparative and concurrent academic enterprises. Just as feminism has expanded the lexicon of what we imagine as womanly, has sought to understand and destigmatize what we call the subject position of woman, so has disability studies examined the identity *disabled* in the service of integrating people with disabilities more fully into our society. As such, both are insurgencies that are becoming institutionalized, underpinning inquiries outside and inside the academy. A feminist disability theory builds on the strengths of both.

Feminist Disability Theory

My title here, "Integrating Disability, Transforming Feminist Theory," invokes and links two notions, integration and transformation, both of which are fundamental to the feminist project and to the larger civil rights movement that informed it. Integration suggests achieving parity by fully including that which has been excluded and subordinated. Transformation suggests reimagining established knowledge and the order of things. By alluding to integration and transformation, I set my own modest project of integrating disability into feminist theory in the politicized context of the civil rights movement to gesture toward the explicit relation that feminism supposes between intellectual work and a commitment to creating a more just, equitable, and integrated society.

This chapter aims to amplify feminist theory by articulating and fostering feminist disability theory. In naming feminist disability studies here as an academic field of inquiry, I am sometimes describing work that is already underway, some of which explicitly addresses disability, and some of which gestures implicitly to the topic. At other times, I am calling for study that needs to be done to better illuminate feminist thought. In other words, this chapter, in part, sets an agenda for future work in feminist disability theory. Most fundamentally, though, the goal of feminist disability studies, as I lay it out in this chapter, is to augment the terms and confront the limits of the ways we understand human diversity, the materiality of the body, multiculturalism, and the social formations that interpret bodily differences. The fundamental point I will make here is that integrating disability as a category of analysis and a system of representation deepens, expands, and challenges feminist theory.

Academic feminism is a complex and contradictory matrix of theories, strategies, pedagogies, and practices. One way to think about feminist theory is to say that it investigates how culture saturates the particularities of bodies with meanings and probes the consequences of those meanings. Feminist theory is a collaborative, interdisciplinary inquiry and a self-conscious cultural critique that interrogates how subjects are multiply interpellated: in other words, how the representational systems of gender, race, ethnicity, ability, sexuality, and class mutually construct, inflect, and contradict one another. These systems intersect to produce and sustain ascribed, achieved, and acquired identities—both those that claim us and those that we claim for ourselves. A feminist disability theory introduces the ability/disability system as a category of analysis into this diverse and diffuse enterprise. It aims to extend current notions of cultural diversity and to more fully integrate the academy and the larger world it helps shape.

A feminist disability approach fosters complex understandings of the cultural history of the body. By considering the ability/disability system, feminist disability theory goes beyond explicit disability topics such as illness, health, beauty, genetics, eugenics, aging, reproductive technologies, prosthetics, and access issues. Feminist disability theory addresses such broad feminist concerns as the unity of the category *woman*, the status of the lived body, the politics of appearance, the medicalization of the body, the privilege of normalcy, multiculturalism, sexuality, the social construction of identity, and the commitment to integration. To borrow Toni Morrison's (1992) notion that blackness is an idea that permeates American culture, disability too is a pervasive, often unarticulated, ideology informing our cultural notions of self and other. Disability—like gender—is a concept that pervades all aspects of culture: its structuring institutions, social identities, cultural practices, political positions, historical communities, and the shared human experience of embodiment.

Integrating disability into feminist theory is generative, broadening our collective inquiries, questioning our assumptions, and contributing to feminism's intersectionality. Introducing a disability analysis does not narrow the inquiry, limit the focus to only women with disabilities, or preclude engaging other manifestations of feminisms. Indeed, the multiplicity of foci we now call feminisms is not a group of fragmented, competing subfields but rather a vibrant, complex conversation. In talking about feminist disability theory, I am not proposing yet another discrete feminism but suggesting instead some ways that thinking about disability transforms feminist theory. Integrating disability does not obscure our critical focus on the registers of race, sexuality, ethnicity, or gender, nor is it additive. Rather, considering disability shifts the conceptual framework to strengthen our understanding of how these multiple systems intertwine, redefine, and mutually constitute one another. Integrating disability clarifies how this aggregate of systems operates together, yet distinctly, to support an imaginary norm and structure of the relations that grant power, privilege, and status to that norm. Indeed, the cultural function of the disabled figure is to act as a synecdoche for all forms that culture deems nonnormative.

We need to study disability in a feminist context to direct our highly honed critical skills toward the dual scholarly tasks of unmasking and reimagining disability, not only for people with disabilities, but for everyone. As Simi Linton (1998) puts it, studying disability is "a prism through which one can gain a broader understanding of society and human experience" (118). It deepens our understanding of gender and sexuality, individualism and equality, minority group definitions, autonomy, wholeness, independence, dependence, health, physical appearance, aesthetics, the integrity of the body, community, and ideas of progress and perfection in every aspect of cultures. A feminist disability theory introduces what Eve Sedgwick (1990) has called a "universalizing view" of disability that will replace an often persisting "minoritizing view." Such a view will cast disability as "an issue of continuing, determinative importance in the lives of people across the spectrum" (1). In other words, understanding how disability operates as an identity category and cultural concept will enhance how we understand what it is to be human, our relationships with one another, and the experience of embodiment. The constituency for feminist disability studies is all of us, not only women with disabilities: disability is the most human of experiences, touching every family and—if we live long enough—touching us all.

The Ability/Disability System

Feminist disability theory's radical critique hinges on a broad understanding of disability as a pervasive cultural system that stigmatizes certain kinds of bodily variations. At the same time, this system has the potential to incite a critical politics. The informing premise of feminist disability theory is that disability, like femaleness, is not a natural state of corporeal inferiority, inadequacy, excess, or a stroke of misfortune. Rather, disability is a culturally fabricated narrative of the body, similar to what we understand as the fictions of race and gender. The disability/ability system produces subjects by differentiating and marking bodies. Although this comparison of bodies is ideological rather than biological, it nevertheless penetrates into the formation of culture, legitimating an unequal distribution of resources, status, and power within a biased social and architectural environment. As such, disability has four aspects: first, it is a system for interpreting and disciplining bodily variations; second, it is a relationship between bodies and their environments; third, it is a set of practices that produce both the able-bodied and the disabled; fourth, it is a way of describing the inherent instability of the embodied self. The disability system excludes the kinds of bodily forms, functions, impairments, changes, or ambiguities that call into question our cultural fantasy of the body as a neutral, compliant instrument of some transcendent will. Moreover, disability is a broad term within which cluster ideological categories as varied as sick, deformed, crazy, ugly, old, maimed, afflicted, mad, abnormal, or debilitated—all of which disadvantage people by devaluing bodies that do not conform to cultural standards. Thus, the disability system functions to preserve and validate such privileged designations as beautiful, healthy, normal, fit, competent, intelligent—all of which provide cultural capital to those who can claim such status, who can reside within these subject positions. It is, then, the various interactions between bodies and world that materialize disability from the stuff of human variation and precariousness.

A feminist disability theory denaturalizes disability by unseating the dominant assumption that disability is something that is wrong with someone. By this I mean, of course, that it mobilizes feminism's highly developed and complex critique of gender, class, race, ethnicity, and sexuality as exclusionary and oppressive systems rather than as the natural and appropriate order of things. To do this, feminist disability theory engages several of the fundamental premises of critical theory: (*a*) that representation structures reality, (*b*) that the margins define the center, (*c*) that gender (or disability) is a way of signifying relationships of power, (*d*) that human identity is multiple and unstable, (*e*) that all analysis and evaluation have political implications.

To elaborate on these premises, I discuss here four fundamental and interpenetrating domains of feminist theory and suggest some of the kinds of critical inquiries that considering disability can generate within these theoretical arenas. These domains are: (*a*) representation, (*b*) the body, (*c*) identity, and (*d*) activism. While I have disentangled these domains here for the purposes of setting up a schematic organization for my analysis, these domains are, of course, not discrete in either concept or practice, but rather tend to be synchronic.

Representation

The first domain of feminist theory that can be deepened by a disability analysis is representation. Western thought has long conflated femaleness and disability, understanding both as defective departures from a valued standard. Aristotle, for example, defined women as "mutilated males." Women, for Aristotle, have "improper form"; we are "monstrosit[ies]" (1944, 27–8, 8–9). As what Nancy Tuana (1994) calls "misbegotten men" (18), women thus become the primal freaks in Western history, envisioned as what we might now call congenitally deformed as a result of what we might now term genetic disability. More recently, feminist theorists have argued that female embodiment is a disabling condition in sexist culture. Iris Marion Young (1990b), for instance, examines how enforced feminine comportment delimits women's sense of embodied agency, restricting them to "throwing like a girl" (141). Young concludes that, "Women in a sexist society are physically handicapped" (153). Even the general American public associates femininity with disability. A recent study on stereotyping showed that housewives, disabled people, blind people, so-called retarded people, and the elderly were all judged as being similarly incompetent. Such a study suggests that intensely normatively feminine positions—such as a housewife—are aligned with negative attitudes about people with disabilities (Fiske, Cuddy, and Glick 2001).[1]

Recognizing how the concept of disability has been used to cast the form and functioning of female bodies as nonnormative can extend feminist critiques. Take, for example, the exploitation of Saartje Bartmann, the African woman exhibited as a freak in nineteenth-century Europe (Gilman 1985; Fausto Sterling 1995). Known as the Hottentot Venus, Bartmann's treatment has come to represent the most egregious form of racial and gendered degradation. What goes unremarked in studies of Bartmann's display, however, are the ways that the language and assumptions of the ability/disability system were implemented to pathologize and exoticize Bartmann. Her display invoked disability by presenting as deformities or abnormalities the characteristics that marked her as raced and gendered. I am not suggesting that Bartmann was disabled but rather that the concepts of disability discourse framed her presentation to the Western eye. Using disability as a category of analysis allows us to see that what was normative embodiment in her native context became abnormal to the Western mind. More important, rather than simply supposing that being labeled as a freak is a slander, a disability analysis presses our critique further by challenging the premise that unusual embodiment is inherently inferior. The feminist interrogation of gender since Simone de Beauvoir (1952/1974) has revealed how women are assigned a cluster of ascriptions, like Aristotle's, that mark us as other. What is less widely recognized, however, is that this collection of interrelated characterizations is precisely the same set of supposed attributes affixed to people with disabilities.

The gender, race, and ability systems intertwine further in representing subjugated people as being pure body, unredeemed by mind or spirit. This sentence of embodiment is conceived of as either a lack or an excess. Women, for example, are considered castrated, or to use Marge Piercy's (1969) wonderful term, "penis-poor." They are thought to be hysterical or have overactive hormones. Women have been cast as alternately having insatiable appetites in some eras and as pathologically self-denying in other times. Similarly, disabled people have supposedly extra chromosomes or limb deficiencies. The differences of disability are cast as atrophy, meaning degeneration, or hypertrophy, meaning enlargement. People with disabilities are described as having aplasia, meaning absence or failure of formation, or hypoplasia, meaning underdevelopment. All these terms police variation and reference a hidden norm from which the bodies of people with disabilities and women are imagined to depart.

Female, disabled, and dark bodies are supposed to be dependent, incomplete, vulnerable, and incompetent bodies. Femininity and race are performances of disability. Women and the disabled are portrayed as helpless, dependent, weak, vulnerable, and incapable bodies. Women, the disabled, and people of color are always ready occasions for the aggrandizement of benevolent rescuers, whether strong males, distinguished doctors, abolitionists, or Jerry Lewis hosting his telethons. For example, an 1885 medical illustration of a pathologically "love deficient" woman, that is, the cultural stereotype of the ugly woman or perhaps the lesbian, suggests how sexuality and appearance slide into the terms of disability (fig. 1). This illustration shows that the language of deficiency and abnormality is used simultaneously to devalue women who depart from the mandates of femininity by equating them with disabled bodies. Such an interpretive move economically invokes the subjugating effect of one oppressive system to deprecate people marked by another system of representation.

Subjugated bodies are pictured as either deficient or as profligate. For instance, what Susan Bordo (1993) describes as the too-muchness of women also haunts disability and racial discourses, marking subjugated bodies as ungovernable, intemperate, or threatening. The historical figure of the monster, as well, invokes disability, often to serve racism and sexism. Although the term has expanded to encompass all forms of social and corporeal aberration, *monster* originally described people with congenital impairments. As departures from the normatively human, monsters were seen as category violations or grotesque hybrids. The semantics of monstrosity are recruited to explain gender violations such as Julia Pastrana, for example, the Mexican Indian "bearded woman," whose body was displayed in nineteenth-century freak shows both during her lifetime and after her death. Pastrana's live and later her embalmed body spectacularly confused and transgressed established cultural categories. Race, gender, disability, and sexuality augmented one another in Pastrana's display to produce a spectacle of embodied otherness that is simultaneously sensational, sentimental, and pathological (Garland-Thomson 1999). Furthermore, much current feminist work theorizes figures of hybridity and excess such as monsters, grotesques, and cyborgs to suggest their transgressive potential for a feminist politics (Haraway 1991; Braidotti 1994; Russo 1994). However, this metaphorical invocation

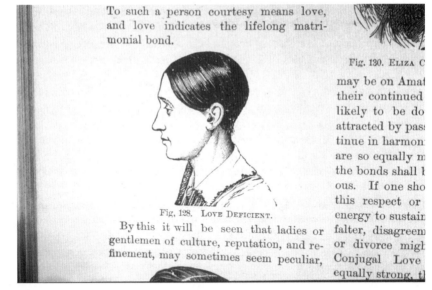

To such a person courtesy means love, and love indicates the lifelong matrimonial bond.

Fig. 130. ELIZA C

may be on Amai
their continued
likely to be do
attracted by pas:
tinue in harmon
are so equally m
the bonds shall I
ous. If one sho
this respect or
energy to sustain
falter, disagreem
or divorce migl
Conjugal Love
equally strong, tl

Fig. 128. LOVE DEFICIENT.

By this it will be seen that ladies or gentlemen of culture, reputation, and refinement, may sometimes seem peculiar,

FIGURE 1. An 1885 physiognometric drawing of a supposedly pathologically "Love Deficient" woman

seldom acknowledges that these figures often refer to the actual bodies of people with disabilities. Erasing real disabled bodies from the history of these terms compromises the very critique they intend to launch and misses an opportunity to use disability as a feminist critical category.

Such representations ultimately portray subjugated bodies not only as inadequate or unrestrained but also at the same time as redundant and expendable. Bodies marked and selected by such systems are targeted for elimination by varying historical and crosscultural practices. Women, people with disabilities or appearance impairments, ethnic Others, gays and lesbians, and people of color are variously the objects of infanticide, selective abortion, eugenic programs, hate crimes, mercy killing, assisted suicide, lynching, bride burning, honor killings, forced conversion, coercive rehabilitation, domestic violence, genocide, normalizing surgical procedures, racial profiling, and neglect. All these discriminatory practices are legitimated by systems of representation, by collective cultural stories that shape the material world, underwrite exclusionary attitudes, inform human relations, and mold our senses of who we are. Understanding how disability functions along with other systems of representation clarifies how all the systems intersect and mutually constitute one another.

The Body

The second domain of feminist theory that a disability analysis can illuminate is the investigation of the body: its materiality, its politics, its lived experience, and its relation to subjectivity and identity. Confronting issues of representation is certainly crucial to the cultural critique of feminist disability theory. But we should not focus exclusively on the discursive realm. What distinguishes a feminist disability theory from other critical paradigms is that it scrutinizes a wide range of material practices involving the lived body. Perhaps because women and the disabled are cultural signifiers for the body, their actual bodies have been subjected relentlessly to what Michel Foucault calls "discipline" (1979). Together, the gender, race, ethnicity, sexuality, class, and ability systems exert tremendous social pressures to shape, regulate, and normalize subjugated bodies. Such disciplining is enacted primarily through the two interrelated cultural discourses of medicine and appearance.

Feminist disability theory offers a particularly trenchant analysis of the ways that the female body has been medicalized in modernity. As I have already suggested, both women and the disabled have been imagined as medically abnormal—as the quintessential sick ones. Sickness is gendered feminine. This gendering of illness has entailed distinct consequences in everything from epidemiology and diagnosis to prophylaxis and therapeutics.

Perhaps feminist disability theory's most incisive critique is revealing the intersections between the politics of appearance and the medicalization of subjugated bodies. Appearance norms have a long history in Western culture, as is witnessed by the anthropometric composite figures of ideal male and female bodies made by Dudley Sargent in 1893 (fig. 2). The classical ideal was to be worshiped rather than imitated, but increasingly, in modernity, the ideal has migrated to become the paradigm that is to be attained. As many feminist critics have pointed out, the beauty system's mandated standard of the female body has become a goal to be achieved through self-regulation and consumerism (Wolf 1991; Haiken 1997). Feminist disability theory suggests that appearance and health norms often have similar disciplinary goals. For example, the body braces developed in the 1930s to ostensibly correct scoliosis, discipline the body to conform to dictates of both the gender and the ability systems by enforcing standardized female form similarly to the nineteenth-century corset, which, ironically, often disabled female bodies. Although both devices normalize bodies, the brace is part of medical discourse while the corset is cast as a fashion practice.

Similarly, a feminist disability theory calls into question the separation of reconstructive and cosmetic surgery, recognizing their essentially normalizing function as what Sander L. Gilman (1998) calls "aesthetic surgery." Cosmetic surgery, driven by gender ideology and market demand, now enforces feminine body standards and standardizes female bodies toward what I have called the "normate"—the corporeal incarnation of culture's collective, unmarked, normative characteristics (Garland-Thomson 1997, 8). Cosmetic surgery's twin, reconstructive surgery, eliminates disability and enforces the ideals of what might be thought of as the normalcy system. Both cosmetic and reconstructive procedures commodify the body and parade mutilations as enhancements that correct flaws to improve the psychological well being of the patient. The conception of the

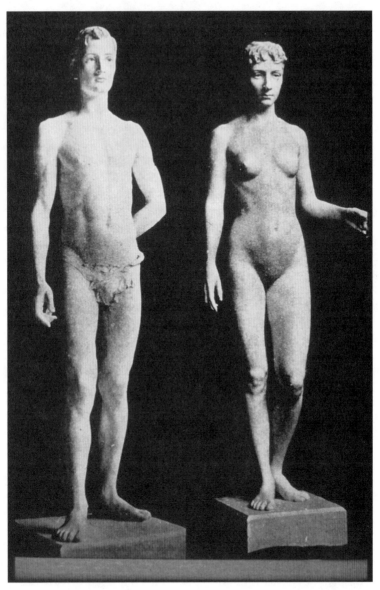

FIGURE 2. 1893 anthropometric composite figures by Dudley Sargent of normative man and woman in European culture

body as what Susan Bordo (1993, 246) terms "cultural plastic" through surgical and medical interventions increasingly pressures people with disabilities or appearance impairments to become what Michel Foucault (1975, 135) calls "docile bodies." The twin ideologies of normalcy and beauty posit female and disabled bodies, particularly, as not only spectacles to be looked at, but as pliable bodies to be shaped infinitely so as to conform to a set of standards called *normal* and *beautiful*.

Normal has inflected beautiful in modernity. What is imagined as excess body fat, the effects of aging, marks of ethnicity such as supposedly Jewish noses, bodily particularities thought of as blemishes or deformities, and marks of history such as scarring and impairments are now expected to be surgically erased to produce an unmarked body. This visually unobtrusive body may then pass unnoticed within the milieu of anonymity that is the hallmark of social relations beyond the personal in modernity. The purpose of aesthetic surgery, as well as the costuming of power, is not to appear unique—or to "be yourself," as the ads endlessly promise—but rather not to be conspicuous, not to look different. This flight from the nonconforming body translates into individual efforts to look normal, neutral, unmarked, to *not* look disabled, queer, ugly, fat, ethnic, or raced. Beauty, then, dictates corporeal standards that create not distinction but utter conformity to a bland look that is at the same time unachievable so as to leash us to consumer practices that promise to deliver such sameness. In the language of contemporary cosmetic surgery, the unreconstructed female body is persistently cast as having abnormalities that can be corrected by surgical procedures that supposedly improve one's appearance by producing ostensibly natural-looking noses, thighs, breasts, chins, and so on. Thus, our unmodified bodies are presented as unnatural and abnormal while the surgically altered bodies are portrayed as normal and natural. The beautiful woman of the twenty-first century is sculpted surgically from top to bottom, generically neutral, all irregularities regularized, all particularities expunged. She is thus nondisabled, deracialized, and de-ethnicized.

In addition, the politics of prosthetics enters the purview of feminism when we consider the contested use of breast implants and prostheses for breast cancer survivors. The famous 1993 *New York Times* cover photo of the fashion model, Matushka, baring her mastectomy scar or Audre Lorde's account of breast cancer in *The Cancer Journals* (1980) challenge the sexist assumption that the amputated breast must always pass for the normative, sexualized one either through concealment or prosthetics. A vibrant feminist conversation has emerged about the politics of the surgically altered, the disabled breast. Diane Price Herndl (2002) challenges Audre Lorde's refusal of a breast prosthesis after mastectomy and Iris Marion Young's classic essay "Breasted Experience" (1990a) queries the cultural meanings of breasts under the knife.

Another entanglement of appearance and medicine involves the spectacle of the female breast, both normative and disabled. In January 2000, the San Francisco-based The Breast Cancer Fund mounted a public awareness poster campaign, called Obsessed with Breasts, which showed women boldly displaying mastectomy scars. The posters parodied familiar commercial media sites—a Calvin Klein perfume ad, a *Cosmopolitan* magazine cover, and a Victoria Secret catalog cover—that routinely represent women's breasts as only sexual in nature. The posters replace the now unremarkable eroticized breast with the

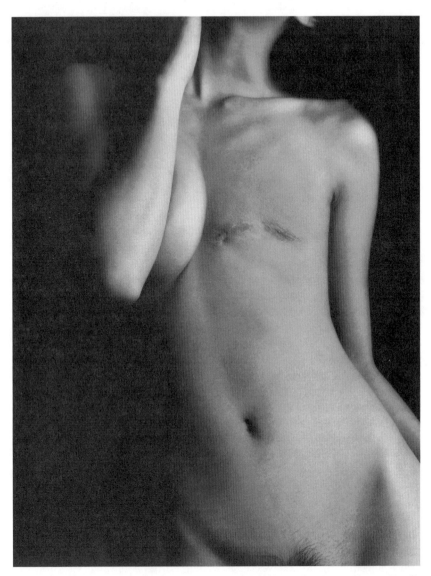

FIGURE 3. Obsessed with Breasts poster. Image taken from The Breast Cancer Fund's *Obsessed with Breasts* campaign, *www.breastcancerfund.org*. Photographer: Henard Jue

forbidden image of the amputated breast (fig. 3). In doing so, they disrupt the visual convention of the female breast as sexualized object for male appropriation and pleasure. The posters thus produce a powerful visual violation by exchanging the spectacle of the eroticized breast, which has been desensationalized by its endless circulation, with the medicalized image of the scarred breast, which has been concealed from public view. The Breast Cancer Fund used these remarkable images to challenge both sexism in medical research and treatment for breast cancer as well as the oppressive representational practices that make everyday erotic spectacles of women's breasts while erasing the fact of the amputated breast.

Feminist disability theory can press far its critique of the pervasive will-to-normalize the nonstandard body. Take two related examples: first, the surgical separation of conjoined twins and, second, the surgical assignment of gender for the intersexed, people with ambiguous genitalia and gender characteristics. Both forms of embodiment are regularly—if infrequently—occurring, congenital bodily variations that spectacularly violate sacred ideologies of Western culture. Conjoined twins contradict our notion of the individual as discrete and autonomous quite similarly to the way pregnancy does. Intersexed infants challenge our insistence that biological gender is unequivocally binary. So threatening to the order of things is the natural embodiment of conjoined twins and intersexed people that they are almost always surgically normalized through amputation and mutilation immediately after birth (Clark and Myser 1996; Dreger 1998a; Kessler 1990; Fausto-Sterling 2000). Not infrequently, one conjoined twin is sacrificed to save the other from the supposed abnormality of their embodiment. Such mutilations are justified as preventing suffering and creating well-adjusted individuals. So intolerable is their insult to dominant ideologies about who patriarchal culture insists that we are, that the testimonies of adults with these forms of embodiment who say that they do not want to be separated is routinely ignored in establishing the rationale for medical treatment (Dreger 1998b). In truth, these procedures benefit not the affected individuals, but rather they expunge the kinds of corporeal human variations that contradict the ideologies the dominant order depends upon to anchor truths it insists are unequivocally encoded in bodies.

I do not want to oversimplify here by suggesting that women and disabled people should not use modern medicine to improve their lives or help their bodies function more fully. But the critical issues are complex and provocative. A feminist disability theory should illuminate and explain, not become ideological policing or set orthodoxy. The kinds of critical analyses I am discussing offer a counterlogic to the overdetermined cultural mandates to comply with normal and beautiful at any cost. The medical commitment to healing, when coupled with modernity's faith in technology and interventions that control outcomes, has increasingly shifted toward an aggressive intent to fix, regulate, or eradicate ostensibly deviant bodies. Such a program of elimination has often been at the expense of creating a more accessible environment or providing better support services for people with disabilities. The privileging of medical technology over less ambitious programs such as rehabilitation has encouraged the cultural conviction that disability can be extirpated; inviting the belief that life with a disability is intolerable. As charity campaigns and telethons repeatedly affirm, cure rather than adjustment or accommodation is the overdetermined cultural response to disability (Longmore 1997). For instance, a 1949 March of Dimes poster

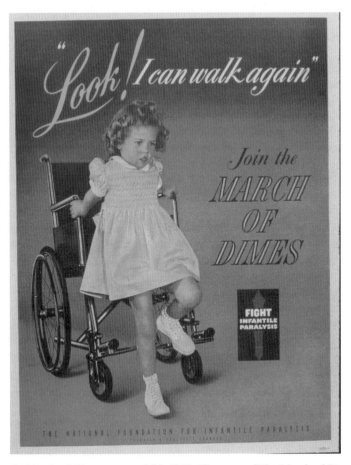

FIGURE 4. March of Dimes poster child, 1949 *(Courtesy of The March of Dimes Birth Defects Foundation)*

shows an appealing little girl stepping out of her wheelchair into the supposed redemption of walking: "Look, I Can Walk Again!" the text proclaims, while at once charging the viewers with the responsibility of assuring her future ambulation (fig. 4). Nowhere do we find posters suggesting that life as a wheelchair user might be full and satisfying, as many people who actually use them find their lives to be. This ideology of cure is not isolated in medical texts or charity campaigns but in fact permeates the entire cultural conversation about disability and illness. Take, for example, the discourse of cure in get well cards. A 1950 card, for instance, urges its recipient to "snap out of it." Fusing racist, sexist, and ableist discourses, the card recruits the Mammy figure to insist on cure. The stereotypical racist figure asks, "Is you sick, Honey?" and then exhorts the recipient of her care to "jes hoodoo all dat illness out o you."

The ideology of cure directed at disabled people focuses on changing bodies imagined as abnormal and dysfunctional rather than on exclusionary attitudinal, environmental, and economic barriers. The emphasis on cure reduces the cultural tolerance for human variation and vulnerability by locating disability in bodies imagined as flawed rather than social systems in need of fixing. A feminist disability studies would draw an important distinction between prevention and elimination. Preventing illness, suffering, and injury is a humane social objective. Eliminating the range of unacceptable and devalued bodily forms and functions the dominant order calls disability is, on the other hand, a eugenic undertaking. The ostensibly progressive sociomedical project of eradicating disability all too often is enacted as a program to eliminate people with disabilities through such practices as forced sterilization, so-called physician-assisted suicide and mercy killing, selective abortion, institutionalization, and segregation policies.

A feminist disability theory extends its critique of the normalization of bodies and the medicalization of appearance to challenge some widely held assumptions about reproductive issues as well. The cultural mandate to eliminate the variations in form and function that we think of as disabilities has undergirded the reproductive practices of genetic testing and selective abortion (Saxton 1998; Rapp 1999; Parens and Asch 2000). Some disability activists argue that the "choice" to abort fetuses with disabilities is a coercive form of genocide against the disabled (Hubbard 1990). A more nuanced argument against selective abortion comes from Adrienne Asch and Gail Geller (1996), who wish to preserve a woman's right to choose whether to bear a child, but who at the same time object to the ethics of selectively aborting a wanted fetus because it will become a person with a disability. Asch and Geller counter the quality-of-life and prevention-of-suffering arguments so readily invoked to justify selective abortion, as well as physician-assisted suicide, by pointing out that we cannot predict or, more precisely, control in advance such equivocal human states as happiness, suffering, or success. Neither is any amount of prenatal engineering going to produce the life that any of us desire and value. Indeed, both hubris and a lack of imagination characterize the prejudicial and reductive assumption that having a disability ruins lives. A vague notion of suffering and its potential deterrence drives much of the logic of elimination that rationalizes selective abortion (Kittay 2000). Life chances and quality are simply far too contingent to justify prenatal prediction.

Similarly, genetic testing and applications of the Human Genome Project as the key to expunging disability are often critiqued as enactments of eugenic ideology, what the feminist biologist Evelyn Fox Keller (1992) calls a "eugenics of normalcy." The popular utopian belief that all forms of disability can be eliminated through prophylactic manipulation of genetics will only serve to intensify the prejudice against those who inevitably will acquire disabilities through aging and encounters with the environment. In the popular celebrations of the Human Genome Project as the quixotic pinnacle of technological progress, seldom do we hear a cautionary logic about the eugenic implications of this drive toward what Priscilla Wald (2000, 1) calls "future perfect." Disability scholars have entered the debate over so-called physician-assisted suicide as well, by arguing that oppressive attitudes toward disability distort the possibility of un-biased free choice (Battin, Rhodes, and Silvers 1998). The practices of genetic and prenatal testing as well as physician-administered euthanasia, then, become potentially eugenic practices within the context of a culture deeply intolerant of disability. Both the rhetoric and the enactment of this kind of disability discrimi-nation create a hostile and exclusionary environment for people with disabili-ties that perhaps exceeds the less virulent architectural barriers that keep them out of the workforce and the public sphere.

Integrating disability into feminism's conversation about the place of the body in the equality and difference debates produces fresh insights as well. Whereas liberal feminism emphasizes sameness, choice, and autonomy, cultural feminism critiques the premises of liberalism. Out of cultural feminism's insis-tence on difference and its positive interpretation of feminine culture comes the affirmation of a feminist ethic of care. This ethic of care contends that care giv-ing is a moral benefit for its practitioners and for humankind. A feminist dis-ability studies complicates both the feminist ethic of care and liberal feminism in regard to the politics of care and dependency.

A disability perspective nuances feminist theory's consideration of the eth-ics of care by examining the power relations between the givers and receivers of care. Anita Silvers (1995) has argued strongly that being the object of care precludes the equality that a liberal democracy depends upon, and undermines the claim to justice as equality that undergirds a civil rights approach used to counter discrimination (1995). Eva Kittay (1999, 4), on the other hand, formu-lates a "dependency critique of equality," which asserts that the ideal of equal-ity under liberalism repudiates the fact of human dependency, the need for mutual care, and the asymmetries of care relations. Similarly, Barbara Hillyer (1993) has called attention to dependency in order to critique a liberal tendency in the rhetoric of disability rights. Disability itself demands that human interdepen-dence and the universal need for assistance be figured into our dialogues about rights and subjectivity.

Identity

The third domain of feminist theory that a disability analysis complicates is identity. Feminist theory has productively and rigorously critiqued the iden-tity category of woman, on which the entire feminist enterprise seemed to rest. Feminism increasingly recognizes that no woman is ever *only* a woman, that she occupies multiple subject positions and is claimed by several cultural identity categories (Spelman 1988). This complication of *woman* compelled feminist theory to turn from an exclusively male/female focus to look more fully at the exclusionary, essentialist, oppressive, and binary aspects of the category woman itself. Disability is one such identity vector that disrupts the unity of the classi-fication woman and challenges the primacy of gender as a monolithic category.

Disabled women are, of course, a marked and excluded—albeit quite varied—group within the larger social class of women. The relative privileges of normative femininity are often denied to disabled women (Fine and Asch 1988). Cultural stereotypes imagine disabled women as asexual, unfit to reproduce, overly dependent, unattractive—as generally removed from the sphere of true womanhood and feminine beauty. Women with disabilities often must struggle to have their sexuality and rights to bear children recognized (Finger 1990). Disability thus both intensifies and attenuates the cultural scripts of femininity. Aging is a form of disablement that disqualifies older women from the limited power allotted females who are young and meet the criteria for attracting men. Depression, anorexia, and agoraphobia are female-dominant, psychophysical disabilities that exaggerate normative gendered roles. Feminine cultural practices such as footbinding, clitorectomies, and corseting, as well as their less hyperbolic costuming rituals such as stiletto high heels, girdles, and chastity belts— impair women's bodies and restrict their physical agency, imposing disability on them.

Banishment from femininity can be both a liability and a benefit. Let me offer—with some irony—an instructive example from popular culture. Barbie, that cultural icon of femininity, offers a disability analysis that clarifies both how multiple identity and diversity is commodified and how the commercial realm might offer politically useful feminist counterimages. Perhaps the measure of a group's arrival into the mainstream of multiculturalism is to be represented in the Barbie pantheon. While Barbie herself still identifies as able-bodied—despite her severely deformed body—we now have several incarnations of Barbie's "friend," Share-A-Smile Becky. One Becky uses a cool hot pink wheelchair; another is Paralympic Champion Becky, brought out for the 2000 Sydney Olympics in a chic red-white-and-blue warm-up suit with matching chair. Most interesting however is Becky, the school photographer, clad in a preppy outfit, complete with camera and red high-top sneakers (fig. 5). As she perkily gazes at an alluring Barbie in her camera's viewfinder, this Becky may be the incarnation of what Erica Rand (1995) has called "Barbie's queer accessories."

A disabled, queer Becky is certainly a provocative and subversive fusion of stigmatized identities, but more important is that Becky challenges notions of normalcy in feminist ways. The disabled Becky, for example, wears comfortable clothes: pants with elastic-waists no doubt, sensible shoes, and roomy shirts. Becky is also one of the few dolls with flat feet and legs that bend at the knee. The disabled Becky is dressed and poised for agency, action, and creative engagement with the world. In contrast, the prototypical Barbie performs excessive femininity in her restrictive sequined gowns, crowns, and push-up bras. So while Becky implies on the one hand that disabled girls are purged from the feminine economy, on the other hand, Becky also suggests that disabled girls might be liberated from those oppressive and debilitating scripts. The last word on Barbies comes from a disability activist who quipped that he would like to outfit a disabled doll with a power wheelchair and a briefcase to make her a

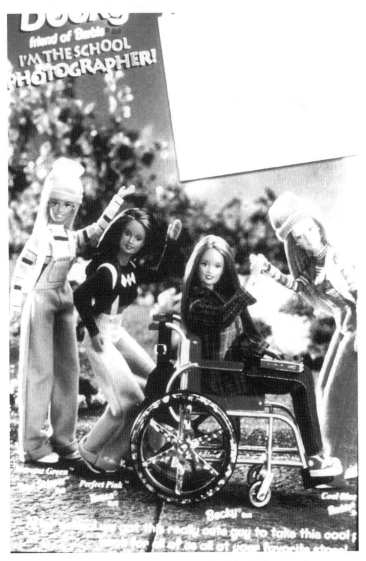

FIGURE 5. Barbie's friend Becky, the School Photographer

civil rights lawyer who enforces the *Americans with Disabilities Act* (1990). He wants to call her "Sue-Your-Ass-Becky."[2] I think she would make a very good role model.

The paradox of Barbie and Becky, of course, is that the ultra-feminized Barbie is a target for sexual appropriation both by men and beauty practices while the disabled Becky escapes such sexual objectification at the potential cost of losing her sense of identity as a feminine sexual being. Some disabled women negotiate this possible identity crisis by developing alternate sexualities, such as lesbianism (Brownworth and Raffo 1999). However, what Harlan Hahn (1988) calls the "asexual objectification" of people with disabilities complicates the feminist critique of normative sexual objectification. Consider the 1987 *Playboy* magazine photos of the paraplegic actress Ellen Stohl. After becoming disabled, Stohl wrote to editor Hugh Hefner that she wanted to pose nude for *Playboy* because "sexuality is the hardest thing for disabled persons to hold onto" ("Meet Ellen Stohl" 1987, 68). For Stohl, it would seem that the performance of excessive feminine sexuality was necessary to counter the social interpretation that disability cancels out sexuality. This confirmation of normative heterosexuality was then for Stohl no Butlerian parody but rather the affirmation she needed as a disabled woman to be sexual at all.

Ellen Stohl's presentation by way of the sexist conventions of the porn magazine illuminates the relation between identity and the body, an aspect of subject formation that disability analysis can offer. Although binary identities are conferred from outside through social relations, these identities are nevertheless inscribed on the body as either manifest or incipient visual traces. Identity's social meaning turns on this play of visibility. The photos of Stohl in *Playboy* both refuse and insist on marking her impairment. The centerfold spread—so to speak—of Stohl nude and masturbating erases her impairment to conform to the sexualized conventions of the centerfold. This photo expunges her wheelchair and any other visual clues to her impairment. In other words, to avoid the cultural contradiction of a sexual, disabled woman, the pornographic photos must offer up Stohl as visually nondisabled. But to appeal to the cultural narrative of overcoming disability that sells so well seems novel and capitalizes on sentimental interest; Stohl must be visually dramatized as disabled at the same time. So *Playboy* includes several shots of Stohl that mark her as disabled by picturing her in her wheelchair, entirely without the typical porn conventions. In fact, the photos of her using her wheelchair invoke the asexual poster child. Thus, the affirmation of sexuality that Stohl sought by posing nude in the porn magazine came at the expense of denying, through the powerful visual register, her identity as a woman with a disability, even while she attempted to claim that identity textually.

Another aspect of subject formation that disability confirms is that identity is always in transition. Disability reminds us that the body is, as Denise Riley (1999, 224) asserts, "an unsteady mark, scarred in its long decay." As Caroline Walker Bynum's (1999) intriguing work on werewolf narratives suggests, the body is in a perpetual state of transformation. Caring for her father for over twenty years of Alzheimer's disease prompted Bynum to investigate how we can understand individual identity as continuous even though both body and mind can and do change dramatically, certainly over a lifetime and sometimes quite suddenly. Disability invites us to query what the continuity of the self might depend upon if the body perpetually metamorphoses. We envision our racial, gender, or ethnic identities as tethered to bodily traits that are relatively secure.

Disability and sexual identity, however, seem more fluid, although sexual mutability is imagined as elective where disability is seldom conceived of as a choice. Disability is an identity category that anyone can enter at any time, and we will all join it if we live long enough. As such, disability reveals the essential dynamism of identity. Thus, disability attenuates the cherished cultural belief that the body is the unchanging anchor of identity. Moreover, it undermines our fantasies of stable, enduring identities in ways that may illuminate the fluidity of all identity.

Disability's clarification of the body's corporeal truths also suggests that the body/self materializes—in Judith Butler's (1993) sense—not so much through discourse, but through history. The self materializes in response to an embodied engagement with its environment, both social and concrete. The disabled body is a body whose variations or transformations have rendered it out of sync with its environment, both the physical and the attitudinal environments. In other words, the body becomes disabled when it is incongruent both in space and in the milieu of expectations. Furthermore, a feminist disability theory presses us to ask what kinds of knowledge might be produced through having a body radically marked by its own particularity, a body that materializes at the ends of the curve of human variation. For example, an alternative epistemology that emerges from the lived experience of disability is nicely summed up in Nancy Mairs's book title, *Waist High in the World* (1996), which she irreverently considered calling "cock high in the world."[3] What perspectives or politics arise from encountering the world from such an atypical position? Perhaps Mairs's epistemology can offer us a critical positionality called *sitpoint theory*, a neologism I can offer that interrogates the ableist assumptions underlying the notion of standpoint theory (Hartsock 1983).

Our collective cultural consciousness emphatically denies the knowledge of vulnerability, contingency, and mortality. Disability insists otherwise, contradicting such phallic ideology. I would argue that disability is perhaps the essential characteristic of being human. The body is dynamic, constantly interactive with history and environment. We evolve into disability. Our bodies need care; we all need assistance to live. An equality model of feminist theory sometimes prizes individualistic autonomy as the key to women's liberation. A feminist disability theory, however, suggests that we are better off learning to individually and collectively accommodate bodily limits and evolutions than trying to eliminate or deny them.

Identity formation is at the center of feminist theory. Disability can complicate feminist theory often quite succinctly by invoking established theoretical paradigms. This kind of theoretical intertextuality inflects familiar feminist concepts with new resonance. Let me offer several examples: the idea of "compulsory ablebodiedness," which Robert McRuer (1999) has coined, extends Adrienne Rich's (1986) famous analysis of "compulsory heterosexuality." Joan Wallach Scott's (1988, 1) germinal work on gender is recruited when we discuss disability as "a useful category of analysis." The feminist elaboration of the gender system informs my use of the term *disability system*. Lennard Davis

(1995) suggests that the term *normalcy studies* supplant the name *disability studies* in the way that *gender studies* sometimes succeeds *feminism*. The oft-invoked distinction between sex and gender clarifies a differentiation between impairment and disability, even though both binaries are fraught. The concept of performing disability cites (as it were) Judith Butler's (1990) vigorous critique of essentialism. Reading disabled bodies as exemplary instances of "docile bodies" invokes Foucault (1979). To suggest that identity is lodged in the body, I propose that the body haunts the subject, alluding to Susan Bordo's (1994, 1) notion regarding masculinity that "the penis haunts the phallus." My own work has complicated the familiar discourse of the gaze to theorize what I call the stare, which I argue produces disability identity. Such theoretical shorthand impels us to reconsider the ways that identity categories cut across and redefine one another, pressuring both the terms *woman* and *disabled.*

A feminist disability theory can also highlight intersections and convergences with other identity-based critical perspectives such as queer and ethnic studies. Disability coming-out stories, for example, borrow from gay and lesbian identity narratives to expose what previously was hidden, privatized, and medicalized in order to enter into a political community. The politicized sphere into which many scholars come out is feminist disability studies, which enables critique, claims disability identity, and creates affirming counternarratives. Disability coming-out narratives raise questions about the body's role in identity by asking how markers so conspicuous as crutches, wheelchairs, hearing aids, guide dogs, white canes, or empty sleeves can be closeted.

Passing as nondisabled complicates ethnic and queer studies' analyses of how this seductive but psychically estranging access to privilege operates. Some of my friends, for example, have measured their regard for me by saying, "But I don't think of you as disabled." What they point to in such a compliment is the contradiction they find between their perception of me as a valuable, capable, lovable person and the cultural figure of the disabled person whom they take to be precisely my opposite: worthless, incapable, and unlovable. People with disabilities routinely announce that they do not consider themselves as disabled. Although they are often repudiating the literal meaning of the word *disabled*, their words nevertheless serve to disassociate them from the identity group of the disabled. Our culture offers profound disincentives and few rewards to identifying as disabled. The trouble with such statements is that they leave intact, without challenge, the oppressive stereotypes that permit, among other things, the unexamined use of disability terms such as *crippled, lame, dumb, idiot, moron* as verbal gestures of derision. The refusal to claim disability identity is in part due to a lack of ways to understand or talk about disability that are not oppressive. People with disabilities and those who care about them flee from the language of *crippled* or *deformed* and have no other alternatives. Yet, the Civil Rights Movement and the accompanying black-is-beautiful identity politics have generally shown white culture what is problematic with saying to black friends, "I don't think of you as black." Nonetheless, by disavowing disability identity, many of us learned to save ourselves from devaluation by a complicity that perpetuates oppressive notions about ostensibly real disabled people. Thus, together we help make the alternately menacing and pathetic cultural figures who rattle tin cups or rave on street corners, ones we with impairments often flee from more surely than those who imagine themselves as nondisabled.

Activism

The final domain of feminist theory that a disability analysis expands is activism. There are many arenas of what can be seen as feminist disability activism: marches; protests; The Breast Cancer Fund poster campaign I discussed earlier; action groups such as the Intersex Society of North America (ISNA); and Not Dead Yet, which opposes physician-assisted suicide; or the American Disabled for Accessible Public Transit (ADAPT). What counts as activism cuts a wide swath through U.S. society and the academy. I want to suggest here two unlikely, even quirky, cultural practices that function in activist ways but are seldom considered as potentially transformative. One practice is disabled fashion modeling and the other is academic tolerance. Both are different genres of activism from the more traditional marching-on-Washington or chaining-your-self-to-a-bus modes. Both are less theatrical but perhaps fresher and more interestingly controversial ways to change the social landscape and to promote equality, which I take to be the goal of activism.

The theologian and sociologist, Nancy Eiesland (1994, 98), has argued that in addition to legislative, economic, and social changes, achieving equality for people with disabilities depends upon cultural "resymbolization." Eiesland asserts that the way we imagine disability and disabled people must shift for real social change to occur. Whereas Eiesland's work resymbolizes our conceptions of disability in religious iconography, my own examinations of disabled fashion models do similar cultural work in the popular sphere, introducing some interesting complications into her notion of resymbolization.

Images of disabled fashion models in the media can shake up established categories and expectations. Because commercial visual media are the most widespread and commanding source of images in modern, image-saturated culture, they have great potential for shaping public consciousness—as feminist cultural critics are well aware. Fashion imagery is the visual distillation of the normative, gilded with the chic and the luxurious to render it desirable. The commercial sphere is completely amoral, driven as it is by the single logic of the bottom line. As we know, it sweeps through culture seizing with alarming neutrality anything it senses will sell. This value-free aspect of advertising produces a kind of pliable potency that sometimes can yield unexpected results.

Take, for example, a shot from the monthly fashion feature in *WE Magazine*, a *Cosmopolitan* knock-off targeted toward the disabled consumer market (fig. 6). In this conventional, stylized, high fashion shot, a typical female model—slender, white, blonde, clad in a black evening gown—is accompanied by her

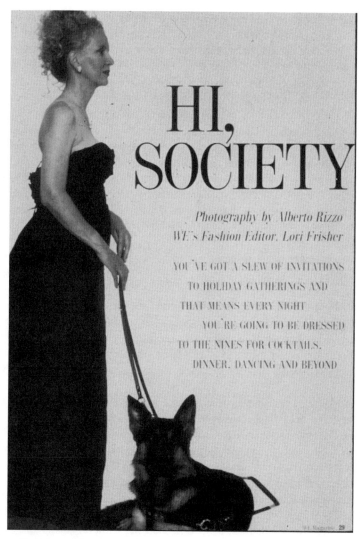

FIGURE 6. Blind model with service dog *(Photographer: Alberto Rizzo)*

service dog. My argument is that public images such as this are radical because they fuse two previously antithetical visual discourses, the chic high fashion shot and the earnest charity campaign. Public representations of disability have traditionally been contained within the conventions of sentimental charity images, exotic freak show portraits, medical illustrations, or sensational and forbidden pictures. Indeed, people with disabilities have been excluded most fully from the dominant, public world of the marketplace. Before the civil rights initiatives of the mid-twentieth century began to transform the public architectural and institutional environment, disabled people were segregated to the private and the medical spheres. Until recently, the only available public image of a woman with a service dog that shaped the public imagination was a street-corner beggar or a charity poster. By juxtaposing the elite body of a visually normative fashion model with the mark of disability, this image shakes up our assumptions about the normal and the abnormal, the public and the private, the chic and the desolate, the compelling and the repelling. Introducing a service dog—a standard prop of indigents and poster children—into the conventional composition of an upscale fashion photo forces the viewer to reconfigure assumptions about what constitutes the attractive and the desirable.

I am arguing that the emergence of disabled fashion models is inadvertent activism without any legitimate agent for positive social change. Their appearance is simply a result of market forces. This both troubling and empowering form of entry into democratic capitalism produces a kind of instrumental form of equality: the freedom to be appropriated by consumer culture. In a democracy, to reject this paradoxical liberty is one thing; not to be granted it is another. Ever straining for novelty and capitalizing on titillation, the fashion-advertising world promptly appropriated the power of disabled figures to provoke responses. Diversity appeals to an upscale liberal sensibility these days, making consumers feel good about buying from companies that are charitable toward the traditionally disadvantaged. More important, the disability market is burgeoning. At 54 million people and growing fast as the baby boomers age, their spending power was estimated to have reached the trillion-dollar mark in 2000 (Williams 1999).

For the most part, commercial advertising presents disabled models in the same way as nondisabled models, simply because all models look essentially the same. The physical markings of gender, race, ethnicity, and disability are muted to the level of gesture, subordinated to the overall normativity of the models' appearance. Thus, commercial visual media cast disabled consumers as simply one of many variations that compose the market to which they appeal. Such routinization of disability imagery—however stylized and unrealistic it may be— nevertheless brings disability as a human experience out of the closet and into the normative public sphere. Images of disabled fashion models enable people with disabilities, especially those who acquire impairments as adults, to imagine themselves as a part of the ordinary, albeit consumerist, world rather than as a special class of excluded untouchables and unviewables. Images of impairment as a familiar, even mundane, experience in the lives of seemingly successful, happy, well-adjusted people can reduce the identifying against oneself that is the overwhelming effect of oppressive and discriminatory attitudes toward people with disabilities. Such images, then, are at once liberatory and oppressive. They do the cultural work of integrating a previously excluded group into the dominant order—for better or worse—much like the inclusion of women in the military.

This form of popular resymbolization produces counterimages that have activist potential. A clearer example of disability activism might be Aimee Mullins, who is a fashion model, celebrity, champion runner, a Georgetown University student, and double amputee. Mullins was also one of *People Magazine's* 50 Most Beautiful People of 1999. An icon of disability pride and equality, Mullins exposes—in fact calls attention to—the mark of her disability in most photos, refusing to normalize or hide her disability in order to pass for nondisabled. Indeed, the public version of her career is that her disability has been a benefit: she has several sets of legs, both cosmetic and functional, and so is able to choose how tall she wants to be. Photographed in her prosthetic legs, she embodies the sexualized jock look that demands women be both slender and fit (fig. 7). In her cosmetic legs, she captures the look of the high fashion beauty in the controversial shoot by Nick Knight called Accessible, showcasing outfits created by designers such as Alexander McQueen (fig. 8). But this is high fashion with a difference. In the jock shot, her functional legs are brazenly displayed, and even in the voguishly costumed shot, the knee joints of her artificial legs are exposed. Never is there an attempt to disguise her prosthetic legs; rather all of the photos thematically echo her prostheses and render the whole image chic. Mullins's prosthetic legs—whether cosmetic or functional—parody, indeed proudly mock, the fantasy of the perfect body that is the mark of fashion, even while the rest of her body conforms precisely to fashion's impossible standards. So rather than concealing, normalizing, or erasing disability, these photos use the hyperbole and stigmata traditionally associated with disability to quench postmodernity's perpetual search for the new and arresting image. Such a narrative of advantage works against oppressive narratives and practices usually invoked about disabilities. First, Mullins counters the insistent narrative that one must overcome an impairment rather than incorporating it into one's life and self, even perhaps as a benefit. Second, Mullins counters the practice of passing for nondisabled that people with disabilities are often obliged to enact in the public sphere. Mullins uses her conformity with beauty standards to assert her disability's violation of those very standards. As legless and beautiful, she is an embodied paradox, asserting an inherently disruptive potential.

What my analysis of these images reveals is that feminist cultural critiques are complex. On the one hand, feminists have rightly unmasked consumer capitalism's appropriation of women as sexual objects for male gratification. On the other hand, these images imply that the same capitalist system in its drive to harvest new markets can produce politically progressive counterimages and counternarratives, however fraught they may be in their entanglement with consumer culture. Images of disabled fashion models are both complicit and critical of the beauty system that oppresses all women. Nevertheless, they suggest that consumer culture can provide the raw material for its own critique.

The concluding version of activism I offer is less controversial and subtler than glitzy fashion spreads. It is what I call academic activism, the activism of integrating education, in the very broadest sense of that term. The academy is no ivory tower but rather it is the grass roots of the educational enterprise.

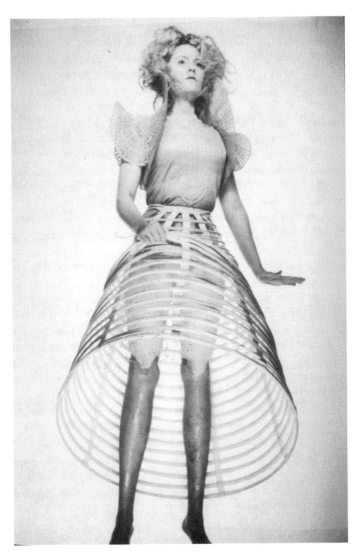

FIGURE 7. Aimee Mullins using functional legs *(Photo by Nick Knight)*

Scholars and teachers shape the communal knowledge and the pedagogical archive that is disseminated from kindergarten to the university. Academic activism is most self-consciously vibrant in the aggregate of interdisciplinary identity studies—of which Women's Studies is exemplary—that strive to expose the workings of oppression, examine subject formation, and offer counternarratives for subjugated groups. Their cultural work is building an archive through historical and textual retrieval, canon reformation, role modeling, mentoring, curricular reform, and course and program development.

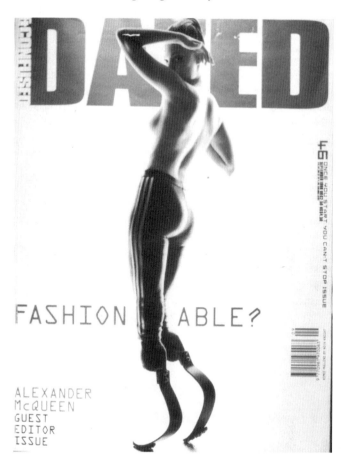

FIGURE 8. Aimee Mullins using cosmetic legs *(Photo by Nick Knight)*

A specific form of feminist academic activism can be deepened through the complication of a disability analysis. I call this academic activism the methodology of intellectual tolerance. By this I do not mean tolerance in the more usual sense of tolerating each other—although that would be useful as well. What I mean is the intellectual position of tolerating what has been thought of as incoherence. As feminism has embraced the paradoxes that have emerged from its challenge to the gender system, it has not collapsed into chaos, but rather it developed a methodology that tolerates internal conflict and contradiction. This method asks difficult questions, but accepts provisional answers. This method recognizes the power of identity, at the same time that it reveals identity as a fiction. This method both seeks equality and it claims difference. This method allows us to teach with authority at the same time that we reject notions of pedagogical mastery. This method establishes institutional presences even while it acknowledges the limitations of institutions. This method validates the personal but implements disinterested inquiry. This method both writes new stories and recovers traditional ones. Considering disability as a vector of identity that intersects gender is one more internal challenge that threatens the coherence of woman, of course. But feminism can accommodate such complication and the contradictions it cultivates. Indeed the intellectual tolerance I am arguing for espouses the partial, the provisional, the particular. Disability experience and acceptance can inform such an intellectual habit. To embrace the supposedly flawed body of disability is to critique the normalizing phallic fantasies of wholeness, unity, coherence, and completeness. The disabled body is contradiction, ambiguity, and partiality incarnate.

My claim here has been that integrating disability as a category of analysis, an historical community, a set of material practices, a social identity, a political position, and a representational system into the content of feminist—indeed into all inquiry—can strengthen the critique that is feminism. Disability, like gender and race, is everywhere, once we know how to look for it. Integrating disability analyses will enrich and deepen all our teaching and scholarship. Moreover, such critical intellectual work facilitates a fuller integration of the sociopolitical world—for the benefit of everyone. As with gender, race, sexuality, and class: to understand how disability operates is to understand what it is to be fully human.

Notes

This chapter was originally printed in *NWSA Journal*, volume 14(3), published by Indiana University Press. Used by permission of the publisher.

1 Interestingly, in Fiske's study, feminists, businesswomen, Asians, Northerners, and black professionals were stereotyped as highly competent, thus envied. In addition to having very low competence, housewives, disabled people, blind people, so-called retarded people, and the elderly were rated as warm, thus pitied.

2. Personal conversation with Paul Longmore, San Francisco, California, June 2000.

3. Personal conversation with Nancy Mairs, Columbus, Ohio, April 17, 1998.

Works Cited

Americans with Disabilities Act of 1990. [cited August 15, 2002]. Available at http://www.usdoj.gov/crt/ada/pubs/ada.txt.

Aristotle. 1944. *Generation of animals.* Translated by A. L. Peck. Cambridge, Mass.: Harvard University Press.

Asch, Adrienne, and Gail Geller. 1996. Feminism, bioethics and genetics. In *Feminism, bioethics: Beyond reproduction*, edited by S. M. Wolf, 318–350. Oxford, U.K.: Oxford University Press.

Battin, Margaret P., Rosamond Rhodes, and Anita Silvers, eds. 1998. *Physician assisted suicide: Expanding the debate.* New York: Routledge.

Bordo, Susan. 1993. *Unbearable weight: Feminism, Western culture and the body.* Berkeley: University of California Press.

———. 1994. Reading the male body. In *The male body*, edited by Laurence Goldstein, 265–306. Ann Arbor: University of Michigan Press.

Braidotti, Rosi. 1994. *Nomadic subjects: Embodiment and sexual difference in contemporary feminist thought.* New York: Columbia University Press.

Brownworth, Victoria A., and Susan Raffo, eds. 1999. *Restricted access: Lesbians on disability.* Seattle, Wash.: Seal Press.

Butler, Judith. 1993. *Bodies that matter.* New York: Routledge.

———. 1990. *Gender trouble.* New York: Routledge.

Bynum, Caroline Walker. 1999. Shape and story: Metamorphosis in the Western tradition. Paper presented at the NEH Jefferson Lecture, Washington, D.C., March 22.

Clark, David L., and Catherine Myser. 1996. Being humaned: Medical documentaries and the hyperrealization of conjoined twins. In *Freakery: Cultural spectacles of the extraordinary body*, edited by Rosemarie Garland-Thomson, 338–355. New York: New York University Press.

Davis, Lennard. 1995. *Enforcing normalcy: Disability, deafness, and the body.* New York: Verso.

de Beauvoir, Simone. (1952/1974). *The second sex.* Translated by H. M. Parshley. New York: Vintage Press.

Dreger, Alice Domurat. 1998a. *Hermaphrodites and the medical invention of sex.* Cambridge, Mass.: Harvard University Press.

———. 1998b. The limits of individuality: Ritual and sacrifice in the lives and medical treatment of conjoined twins. In *Freakery: Cultural spectacles of the extraordinary body*, edited by Rosemarie Garland-Thomson, 338–355. New York: New York University Press.

Eiesland, Nancy. 1994. *The disabled God: Toward a liberatory theology of disability.* Nashville, Tenn.: Abingdon Press.

Fausto Sterling, Anne. 1995. Gender, race, and nation: The comparative anatomy of Hottentot women in Europe, 1815–1817. In *Deviant bodies: Cultural perspectives in science and popular culture*, edited by Jennifer Terry and Jacqueline Urla, 19–48. Bloomington: Indiana University Press.

———. 2000. *Sexing the body: Gender politics and the construction of sexuality.* New York: Basic Books.

Fine, Michelle, and Adrienne Asch, eds. 1988. *Women with disabilities: Essays in psychology, culture, and politics.* Philadelphia: Temple University Press.

Finger, Anne. 1990. *Past due: A story of disability, pregnancy, and birth.* Seattle, Wash.: Seal Press.

Fiske, Susan T., Amy J. C. Cuddy, and Peter Glick. 2001. A model of (often mixed) stereotype content: Competence and warmth respectively follow from perceived status and competition. Unpublished study.

Foucault, Michel. 1979. *Discipline and punish: The birth of the prison.* Translated by Alan M. Sheridan-Smith. New York: Vintage Books.

Garland-Thomson, Rosemarie. 1997. *Extraordinary bodies: Figuring physical disability in American culture and literature.* New York: Columbia University Press

———. 1999. Narratives of deviance and delight: Staring at Julia Pastrana, "The extraordinary Lady." In *Beyond the binary*, edited by Timothy Powell, 81–106. New Brunswick, N.J.: Rutgers University Press.

Gilman, Sander L. 1985. *Difference and pathology: Stereotypes of sexuality, race, and madness.* Ithaca, N.Y.: Cornell University Press.

————. 1998. *Creating beauty to cure the soul*. Durham, N.C.: Duke University Press.

————. 1999. *Making the body beautiful*. Princeton, N.J.: Princeton University Press.

Hahn, Harlan. 1988. Can disability be beautiful? *Social Policy* 18 (winter): 26–31.

Haiken, Elizabeth. 1997. *Venus envy: A history of cosmetic surgery*. Baltimore, Md.: Johns Hopkins University Press.

Haraway, Donna. 1991. *Simians, cyborgs, and women*. New York: Routledge.

Hartsock, Nancy. 1983. The feminist standpoint: Developing their ground for a specifically feminist historical materialism. In *Discovering reality*, edited by Sandra Harding and Merrell Hintikka, 283–305. Dortrecht, Holland: Reidel Publishing.

Herndl, Diane Price. 2002. Reconstructing the posthuman feminist body: Twenty years after Audre Lorde's *Cancer Journals*. In *Disability studies: Enabling the humanities*, edited by Brenda Brueggemann, Rosemarie Garland-Thomson, and Sharon Snyder, 144–155. New York: MLA Press.

Hillyer, Barbara. 1993. *Feminism and disability*. Norman: University of Oklahoma Press.

Hubbard, Ruth. 1990. Who should and who should not inhabit the world? In her *The politics of women's biology*, 179–198. New Brunswick, N.J.: Rutgers University Press.

Keller, Evelyn Fox. 1992. Nature, nurture and the Human Genome Project. In *The code of codes: Scientific and social issues in the Human Genome Project*, edited by Daniel J. Kevles and Leroy Hood, 281–299. Cambridge, Mass.: Harvard University Press.

Kessler, Suzanne J. 1990. *Lessons from the intersexed*. New Brunswick, N.J.: Rutgers University Press.

Kittay, Eva Feder. 1999. *Love's labor: Essays on women, equality, and dependency*. New York: Routledge.

Kittay, Eva, with Leo Kittay. 2000. On the expressivity and ethics of selective abortion for disability: Conversations with my son. In *Prenatal testing and disability rights*, edited by Erik Parens and Adrienne Asch, 165–195. Georgetown, Md.: Georgetown University Press.

Linton, Simi. 1998. *Claiming disability: Knowledge and identity*. New York: New York University Press.

Longmore, Paul K. 1997. Conspicuous contribution and American cultural dilemmas: Telethon rituals of cleansing and renewal. In *The body and physical difference: Discourses of disability*, edited by David Mitchell and Sharon Snyder, 134–158. Ann Arbor: University of Michigan Press.

Lorde, Audre. 1980. *The cancer journals*. San Francisco, Calif.: Spinsters Ink.

Mairs, Nancy. 1996. *Waist high in the world: A life among the nondisabled*. Boston, Mass.: Beacon Press.

McRuer, Robert. 1999. Compulsory able-bodiedness and queer/disabled existence. Paper presented at the Modern Language Association Convention, Chicago, Ill., December 28.

Meet Ellen Stohl. 1987. *Playboy*, July, 68–74.

Morrison, Toni. 1992. *Playing in the dark: Whiteness and the literary imagination*. Cambridge, Mass.: Harvard University Press.

Parens, Erik, and Adrienne Asch. 2000. *Prenatal testing and disability rights*. Georgetown, Md.: Georgetown University Press.

Piercy, Marge. 1969. Unlearning not to speak. In her *Circles on water*, 97. New York: Doubleday.

Rand, Erica. 1995. *Barbie's queer accessories*. Durham, N.C.: Duke University Press.

Rapp, Rayna. 1999. *Testing women, testing the fetus: The social impact of amniocentesis in America.* New York: Routledge.

Rich, Adrienne. 1986. Compulsory heterosexuality and lesbian existence. In her *Blood, bread, and poetry*, 23–75. New York: Norton.

Riley, Denise. 1999. Bodies, identities, feminisms. In *Feminist theory and the body: A reader*, edited by Janet Price and Margrit Shildrick, 220–226. Edinburgh: Edinburgh University Press.

Russo, Mary. 1994. *The female grotesque: Risk, excess, and modernity.* New York: Routledge.

Saxton, Marsha. 1998. Disability rights and selective abortion. In *Abortion wars: A half century of struggle (1950–2000)*, edited by Ricky Solinger, 374–393. Berkeley: University of California Press.

Scott, Joan Wallach. 1988. Gender as useful category of analysis. In her *Gender and the politics of history*, 29–50. New York: Columbia University Press.

Sedgwick, Eve Kosofsky. 1990. *Epistemology of the closet.* Berkeley: University of California Press

Silvers, Anita. 1995. Reconciling equality to difference: Caring (f)or justice for people with disabilities. *Hypatia* 10 30–55.

Spelman, Elizabeth, V. 1988. *Inessential woman: Problems of exclusion in feminist thought.* Boston, Mass.: Beacon Press.

Tuana, Nancy. 1994. *The less noble sex: Scientific, religious and philosophical conceptions of woman's nature.* Indianapolis: Indiana University Press.

Wald, Priscilla. 2000. Future perfect: Grammar, genes, and geography. *New Literary History* 31 (4): 681–708.

Williams, John M. 1999. And here's the pitch: Madison Avenue discovers the "invisible consumer." *WE Magazine*, July/August, 28–31.

Wolf, Naomi. 1991. *The beauty myth: How images of beauty are used against women.* New York: William Morrow and Co.

Young, Iris Marion. 1990a. Breasted experience. In her *Throwing like a girl and other essays in feminist philosophy and social theory*, 189–209. Bloomington: Indiana University Press.

———. 1990b. Throwing like a girl. In her *Throwing like a girl and other essays in feminist philosophy and social theory*, 141–159. Bloomington: Indiana University Press.

PART II

❦

Desire and Identity

Inseparable

GENDER AND DISABILITY IN
THE AMPUTEE-DEVOTEE COMMUNITY

☙

ALISON KAFER

In 1998, I attended a disability products fair in southern California. As I mingled with vendors and other participants, I thought about how wonderful it was to be in such a disability-friendly environment, and I found myself feeling at home. Not too long after arriving, I bumped into a man in his late sixties. He quickly introduced himself and asked me if I had lost my legs in a fire. (I had.) As he continued to question me about my disabilities, I asked him if he was an amputee too. "No," he said, "but I have a very good friend—about your age—who is." He gave me his card, and I continued touring the exhibits. Later, as I ate lunch, another man approached and asked if he could share my table. After we introduced ourselves, he told me that he knew me through a friend of his. Surprised and a bit confused, I asked him who his friend was.

"L—," he replied.

"But I don't know L—," I thought to myself. As the man talked about his business and what had brought him to California from Texas, I tried to remember someone named L—. Finally, I remembered that L— ran an amputee support group I had visited once several years ago. But why would he have told this man about me? And how could this man know who I was simply by looking at me?

And then it hit me: this man was a devotee. L— must be a devotee. All of these single men talking to me at this convention must be devotees: that's why they know so much about disability, why they all seem to have female friends with disabilities, why they're so friendly. I felt incredibly naïve.

Although my unexpected lunch date marked my first face-to-face encounter with a devotee, it was not my introduction to the phenomenon. I first stumbled onto devotees online; it was 1996, not long after my injuries, and I was searching

107

for information about amputees and disability. Devotees, I quickly learned, were men sexually attracted to women with disabilities, particularly amputees. Countless websites were dedicated to the phenomenon, offering everything from videos of amputee women to chatrooms where "amps" and "devs" could get to know each other. Some groups even sponsored weekend conferences at which amputees and devotees could socialize. I initially found the whole idea disturbing and tried to push it out of my mind. After my encounter with the man from Texas, however, and the realization that L— must have given his fellow devotees my name and physical description, I found it harder simply to ignore the issue of devotees. How and why were these men sharing my personal information? What was the nature of their relationships with amputees? What did other women with disabilities think about devotees? Like any hard-working academic, I decided to turn to the research.

Gender, Disability, and the Amputee-Devotee Community

The amputee-devotee community, consisting of women with amputations and the men sexually attracted to them, has been widely discussed within the disability community.[1] The nature of this conversation has frequently assumed the form of a debate: people either praise the amputee-devotee phenomenon, seeing it as a source of sexual expression for disabled women, or they oppose it, casting it as a site of objectification and exploitation.[2] The little academic research that has been done on the topic has been almost exclusively negative, with devotees portrayed as pathological predators suffering everything from castration anxiety to low self-esteem (e.g., Bruno, 1997). Lacking in the scholarly research, as well as in many popular discussions of the subject, is a systematic analysis of the gendered nature of this phenomenon. I want to expand the terms of this debate by examining the co-construction of disability and gender within the community. Rather than attempting to place an absolute value on this site, positive or negative, I want to examine its representation of gender, focusing in particular on the ways in which amputees' disabilities impact the construction of gender within the community.

I want to stress at the outset that I do not presume masculinity or femininity to be biologically determined states. Rather, I refer to masculinity and femininity as cultural constructs: femininity in Western culture typically connotes passivity, fragility, and dependence; masculinity, on the other hand, suggests aggressiveness, independence, and strength.[3] These stereotypes connect to cultural expectations about what "men" and "women" are, with men (and only men) expected to be masculine and women (and only women) expected to be feminine.

These expectations are rarely met, however, and they are rife with contradiction. There are massive ruptures in the construction of femininity and masculinity, ways in which a person can be both "feminine" and "masculine." The meanings associated with these terms are themselves inflected with histories of race and class, rendering certain bodies more or less feminine, and more or less masculine, than the ideal. Moreover, no single person can fulfill the gender roles expected of her or him; femininity and masculinity are constructed in such a way that they are unattainable ideals. I suggest that these gaps, these positions of transition and excess, are made explicit at the intersection of gender and disability, and can be seen quite clearly in the discourses of the amputee-devotee community.

Indeed, ideologies of traditional masculinity and femininity, compulsory heterosexuality, and (in)dependence are constantly being negotiated within this community. Amputee women are alternately praised as fragile, severely disabled women in need of male protection and, conversely, as independent, fiercely able figures triumphing over adversity. Devotees are equally contradictory about their own roles, wavering between seeing themselves as potent saviors of women and as stigmatized members of a sexual minority, desperate for the validation of disabled women. It is precisely these contradictions that I trace in this chapter. I argue that gender is fundamentally unstable within this community and that disability plays an integral role in that instability. Both the ideologies of conventional masculinity and femininity and the disruptions inherent in those conceptions are constructed through the interactions between disabled and nondisabled bodies. Disability and gender are inseparable; each is constantly negotiated through the other.

Drawing on correspondence from members of the community, as well as written analyses generated from within it, I examine the way "amputee" and "devotee" are gender-coded within these discourses. The chapter has two parts: First, I begin with an examination of the ways amputees and devotees are gendered traditionally, with men imagined as powerful subjects and women as passive objects. Then I move to an exploration of the ways amputees and devotees exceed these traditional definitions. In both sections, I point to the ways in which gender and disability are mutually informing.

Noble Gentlemen and Their Amp Ladies

The mutually constitutive nature of disability and gender is evident in the construction of devotees as prototypically masculine. It is through their encounters with women's disabilities that devotees are depicted as embodying the traditional role of man as the protector of women. For many devotees, the image of devotee as savior is integral to their sense of self. As one devotee explains, "The Good Lord put us here on this earth for a purpose—a good and noble purpose—to edify you special and unique people; . . . to share your burden; . . . to give you the love and admiration you so richly deserve."[4] His choice of words— noble, good, God-given—is not arbitrary; devotees here are chivalrous knights, masculine heroes. Their divinely inspired mission is to ease the disability-related burdens of female amputees.

Devotee David Cole (2000b) explains that devotees have an incredible

yearning to inform amputees of their protective feelings. Whenever he encounters a disabled person, he explains, "I . . . find myself wanting to somehow let
them know that I am on their side." Cole's expression of solidarity expands to
paternalism when he describes his reaction to a child with a congenital limb
anomaly. He details his desire to pick up this young girl, cradle her in his arms,
and tell her that he will always protect and keep her safe. Although such claims
to protection might be expected in regard to a small child, Cole uses this same
rhetoric in his descriptions of encounters with adult women. He writes of wanting to shield amputees from the hostile stares of the nondisabled, to reassure
them that they are appreciated, to comfort and cherish them. Men appear in these
accounts as women's protectors; it is through these women's disabilities that the
men are able to assert their position as masculine.

This positioning of male devotees as the protectors of women is not limited to the rhetoric of devotees. The structure of many amputee/devotee events,
such as ASCOTWorld's annual conferences, casts devotees as providers.[5] All
single amputees attend ASCOT conferences free of charge; male devotees, however, cover their own as well as the women's registration, food, and hotel costs.
The reasons for this policy are clear: many disabled women cannot afford to
pay their own way, and devotee men are quite willing to pay more to increase
the number of available women at the conferences. This policy sends other, more
subtle messages, however. It portrays men as financially responsible for women,
a responsibility that mirrors traditional male/female relations.

This image of man as chivalrous protector/provider is accompanied by the
image of man as sexual predator. The characterization of all devotees as predators is a gross generalization, but it is not entirely without merit. Some amputees have accused devotees of stalking or sexually harassing them; others have
complained of having their addresses, phone numbers, and photographs disseminated through the community without their knowledge or consent (Storrs 1996,
52–53; Gregson 2000). As a result, devotees have become infamous among segments of the disability community for stalking disabled women. Several amputee organizations, most notably the Amputee Coalition of America, have taken
action against devotees, issuing explicit privacy policies intended to prevent devotees from harassing amputees at their functions.[6]

Although cases of sexual assault by devotees are extremely rare, many
devotees admit to following disabled women. In some cases, the trailing is virtual: some amputees report being bombarded by email messages from devotees
whom they have never met. As a result, some women are reluctant to divulge
their disabilities online in order to avoid such unwanted attention. It is also a
common practice for devotees to pose as female amputees online in order to
meet other amputees (Nattress 1996, 18). Lurking on amputee listservs or posing as amputees in chatrooms gives devotees the opportunity to participate in
disabled women's conversations, unbeknownst to the women. Devotees recognize that posing as women allows them to develop close relationships with am-

putees, relationships that would be much harder to cultivate if their desires were made public (18–19).

Even more disturbing are stories about devotees following amputees whom they encounter in public. David Cole's webpage, for example, features several accounts of his trailing unknown and unknowing women (2000b). Similarly, *OverGround*, a British devotee magazine, showcases several essays in which devotees relate stories of following amputee women; a few are quite specific as to the place and time they located the amputee (e.g., John 2001).[7] According to devotees, however, following amputees does not constitute stalking; on the contrary, devotees insist, such behavior is harmless if one remains at a "respectful" distance from the amputee. As fellow devotee John Ollason (1996) explains, such behavior is typical of "male adolescents everywhere, racked with sexual desire in a society that gives them little opportunity to express their sexuality." Ollason accomplishes two things with this comment: first, he explicitly delineates this behavior as typically male, thereby asserting the masculinity of the devotees; second, he describes it as normal in an attempt to naturalize and justify such acts.

I turn now to the construction of femininity within this community, a construction that establishes femininity and disability as almost synonymous due to each concept's stereotypical association with images of passivity, powerlessness, and victimization. According to prevailing stereotypes, both "feminine" and "disabled" are adjectives suggesting one's need for aid, assistance, and reassurance; each is marked by the same lack of independence and self-assertion.

Disabled women often appear within the amputee-devotee community as "traditional" women. Indeed, many members of this community, male and female, refer to females exclusively as "ladies," reserving the term "woman" for lesbians.[8] This naming is not arbitrary; unlike "woman," "lady" evokes a time in which white females of a certain class were quiet, passive objects restricted to the home. "Lady" also implies a certain reverence, a placing of women on pedestals. Here, through this act of naming, women's fragile lady-like femininity serves to reinforce men's chivalrous masculinity.

Female amputees' association with the household is made explicit in videos for sale on the Internet that feature amputees doing housework. Indeed, some videos feature women engaged in banal activities like washing dishes or cleaning house while wearing peg-legs or other prosthetic devices. Although the videos often center around women donning and doffing their prosthetics or performing skin care on their stumps, the frequency of the housework scene demands scholarly attention. The popularity of these images suggests the deep desire of many devotees to watch disabled women perform gender-coded tasks, tasks which provide the devotees with visual proof of the women's simultaneous femininity and disability.

This focus on amputee women as the embodiment of traditional femininity is evident in the community's assumption that well-adjusted, normal women can only find happiness in heterosexual relationships; single women and lesbians are suspect. This belief takes a specific form in the amputee-devotee community, as women who refuse the attention of devotees are depicted as troubled individuals full of self-loathing. Ollason (1996) describes amputees who dislike or distrust devotees as people who "feel that being an amputee makes [them] ugly." Similarly, another devotee explains that his encounters with amputees rarely lead to relationships (or when they do, the relationships quickly end) because of women's insecurities about their disabilities. Women who are offended by devotees, he explains, are actually offended by their own disabilities. Once they learn to accept themselves, they will accept devotees. His narrative implies that all disabled women not involved with devotees must be unhappy and devoid of self-esteem.

Lesbians are also pathologized, cast as failures at heterosexuality.[9] Many in the community assert that devotees are incredibly valuable to women's well-being because too many amputee women become lesbians because of rejection from nondevotee men. This kind of rhetoric builds on the idea that women can only find happiness in the arms of a man by implying that amputees can never accept their disabilities until they succumb to the love of a devotee. Once again, the devotee emerges as the savior of disabled women.

Women's sexuality is feminized within the community because of its construction as passive, silent, and receptive. Nowhere is this more obvious than in the "collecting behavior" of devotees. Many devotees pride themselves on their massive collections of amputee memorabilia, including drawings, videos, photographs, and magazines (Duncan 1999; J. 2001d). The Internet is filled with websites containing thousands of images available for men's perusal.[10] This overabundance of images explicitly constructs amputee women as the object of the male gaze. Indeed, although many devotees proclaim that photographs are a poor substitute for a real relationship with an amputee, several admit a nagging feeling that they really prefer the photos; a relationship is too frightening, too much work (Storrs 1996, 52; Cole 2000b).

This positioning of women as passive sex objects is exacerbated by the plethora of "following" stories on the Internet. As I noted earlier, many devotees post accounts of their encounters with amputees, describing instances in which they trail amputees through stores or down streets. Often accompanying these stories are brief asides in which the devotee defends his behavior: he never gets too close to the women he follows, the women are unharmed by his acts, he isn't stalking them. In these accounts, in which "I followed her for hours" appears in tandem with "following amputees without their knowledge is harmless," amputee women are portrayed as silent targets of male sexual predation. Although few devotees would admit to seeing women in this way, their rhetoric describes women in precisely this manner. The incredible amount of time devotees spend justifying their tendencies to follow amputee women suggests that women are continually at risk of being stalked. As an amputee, it is difficult to listen to or read these explanations without growing paranoid because women appear in this discourse exclusively as the object of male sexual pursuit. Some men even go so far as to suggest that the stalking is women's fault; as one devotee explained to me, if amputees were more receptive to devotees, then there would no longer be any need for the devotees to engage in such clandestine behavior.

None of these associations are stable or monolithic, however, as constructions of gender are no more stable within the amputee-devotee community than they are outside of it. Characterizations of devotees as all-powerful protectors or of amputees as victims of sexual predation are often juxtaposed with narratives of amputees as powerful and devotees as victimized. In the following section, I turn to these kinds of stories.

Sexy Supercrips and Their Stigmatized Suitors

The representation of amputee women as silent sex objects is not without contradictions. Amputees themselves produce many of the images that are for sale over the Internet. Organizations like ASCOTWorld and CDProductions exist in part to assist women in making their own videos and photo-sets. Both of these groups are owned and operated by disabled women.[11] Moreover, all of the profit for the videos and photos is given to the models themselves.[12] It is through opportunities to identify themselves as actively sexual, such as those ASCOT-World and CDProductions offer, that amputees can be seen as exceeding the notion of traditional feminine passivity in the face of sex (Waxman-Fiduccia 1999). Indeed, these women can be seen as sexual aggressors, independently naming their sexual power.

Similarly, while disabled women may appear in relation to devotees as hyperfeminine fragile objects, they simultaneously appear—often in the very same discourses and contexts—as icons of strength and endurance. David Cole (2000b), who often describes amputee women as in need of male support, also extols these women for triumphing over amazing adversity. "Devotees," he writes, "feel a profound respect for an amputee's abilities and her independence." This sentiment is echoed in other devotees' insistence that they desire amputees not out of an interest in helpless women but out of a fascination for completely independent and powerful women. In a variation of the supercrip myth, amputees appear in these comments not as traditionally feminine "ladies," but as superhuman heroines.

In both depictions, however, women's disabilities are key to their representation. In the first case of women as victims, their disabilities hinder their independence and subjectivity, rendering them hyperfeminine objects reliant on male saviors. In the second case of women as pillars of strength, their ability to overcome their disabilities (presumably by accomplishing such mundane tasks as riding the subway independently and holding down a job) renders them less feminine because more independent. In both instances, women's gender and their disabilities are mutually informing, inextricable.

This assertion of amputees' independence has a corresponding effect on the gender construction of the devotees. While they frequently portray themselves as saviors of amputees, they occasionally slip into casting the amputees as saviors and themselves as the sufferers of gross injustice. "Tony," for example, explains that he lived most of his life shrouded in shame because of his secret desires. Friends and coworkers harassed him about his desire for amputees until he felt completely victimized and silenced by their reactions. It was not until he met an amputee and explained his attraction to her that he felt any sense of self-worth and dignity. Many amputees echo this construction of devotees as victims, criticizing the stigmatization of the men's desires and asserting their ability to affirm the devotees' self-esteem. Although this defense of devotees could be construed as the embodiment of the feminine commandment to "stand by your man," I suggest that this behavior actually exceeds such feminine loyalty. Because of the very real social stigma placed on these men's choices, and to their resulting desperation for female approval and validation, women assume here the masculine role of protector, while men assume the role of the feminine protected.

This gender reversal is made even more explicit in some devotees' concern that amputees will exploit them. Cole and other devotees worry callous amputees will exploit the men's desire, seducing devotees in exchange for money or expensive gifts. Rather than placing the devotee in the role of aggressive sexual predator, the amputee is presented as such (Cole 2000a). As a result, the devotee becomes feminized, the victim of sexual exploitation, while the amputee appears almost masculine, the sexual aggressor.

This contradictory, fluid sequence of interpretations and gender codings suggests the reasons why disability cannot simply be added to existing theories of gender. Although the construction of gender is unstable both within the disability community and outside it, the forms those contradictions take might be quite different. Feminist theorists, disabled and nondisabled alike, must begin to attend to the specific, local sites of the gendering process, must begin to acknowledge the ways in which gender is lived through disability and disability through gender.

Acknowledgments

I would like to thank all of the amputees and devotees who shared their thoughts and experiences with me, especially Jama Bennett and Kath Duncan. Thanks also to those who encouraged this research and helped me to negotiate its complexities: Dana Newlove, Sara Patterson, Ranu Samantrai, Ellen Samuels, Rosemarie Garland-Thomson, Zandra Wagoner, and Margaret Waller.

Notes

1. Although an overwhelming majority of devotees are men in search of women, there are also gay and lesbian devotees as well as female devotees attracted to male am-

putees. Because of space constraints, I discuss only heterosexual amputees and devotees here, and I focus on the male devotee-female amputee interaction.

2. This debate has most recently been performed at the conference "Sexuality and Disability in Culture: Societal and Experiential Perspectives on Multiple Identities" at San Francisco State University, March 17–18, 2000. See also the July and September 2000 editions of *Amputee-Online*, available at *www.amputee-online.com/amputation*.

3. In discussing the constructedness of gender, I do not mean thereby to suggest the naturalness or unconstructedness of sex. I am persuaded by Judith Butler's assertion that sex is no more "real," no less culturally mediated and constituted, than gender. See her *Bodies that matter: On the discursive limits of "sex"* (New York: Routledge, 1993).

4. Unless otherwise noted, all comments attributed to devotees have been culled from personal emails or conversations with the author. Because of the social stigma facing men with this attraction, many devotees are not open with their friends and family about their desires. They post to Internet sites often using pseudonyms or only their initials. As a result, I do not know the legal names of many of the men who contacted me. Out of respect for the privacy of those who did use their real names in their correspondence with me, all names in this chapter have been changed.

5. ASCOTWorld, or the Amputee Support Coalition of the World, is one of several organizations serving the amputee-devotee community. At least once a year ASCOTWorld hosts a conference for amputees and their admirers.

6. The Personal Rights and Privacy Policy of the Amputee Coalition of America (ACA) reads, in part:

> Individuals participating in ACA-sponsored events shall have the right to: enjoyment of ACA activities without disruption or interruption; treatment with respect in every encounter; freedom from harassment of any sort and freedom from any inappropriate behavior; personal privacy, which includes specific advance permission before being photographed by other than an ACA-sanctioned photographer; expect that any person will cease their activity upon the member or participant's first stated objection.

This policy was last revised in September 2000. See Ian Gregson, "The devotee issue: Part two—The opposing view," *Amputee-Online* [electronic journal], available at *http://amputee-online.com/amputation/sept00/sept00wissues.html*.

7. LeRoy Nattress compiled a list of the most common activities devotees do to meet amputees: (*a*) seeing a woman on crutches or limping, following her to verify her status as an amputee, and then learning as much as possible about her; (*b*) sitting in a public space where others have seen an amputee in the hopes of seeing, photographing, and possibly meeting her; (*c*) collecting photographs and articles about female amputees; (*d*) drawing pictures of amputee women or modifying existing pictures to make the featured woman into an amputee; (*e*) keeping a detailed list of female amputees that one has seen or read about; (*f*) developing programs or starting organizations that serve amputees, like shoe-exchange groups, self-help organizations, etc.; (*g*) calling female amputees that one has read about to learn how they cope with their disabilities, what their lives are like, etc., without ever talking about oneself; (*h*) carrying on extensive correspondence with a female amputee, often pretending to be a female amputee oneself; (*i*) asking an amputee one already knows

for the names and numbers of other female amputees; (j) writing fiction about amputee women or women who become amputees; (*k*) researching the amputee-devotee community or disability issues in order to meet disabled women; (*l*) possessing and providing information on wheelchairs, prosthetics, and other assistive devices to women with disabilities. Few devotees, Nattress stresses, partake in all twelve. See LeRoy William Nattress, Amelotasis: Men attracted to women who are amputees: A descriptive study, Ph.D. diss., Walden University, 1996, 18–19.

8. This difference between "woman" and "lady" was made clear to me during a discussion with a devotee. After listening to him talk about "ladies" for hours, I was surprised to hear him begin a story about "two women." My surprise faded, however, when I learned that the women were lesbians. This encounter marks the only time I have ever heard a devotee use the word "woman" to refer to a female.

9. Of course, this positioning of lesbians as failed heterosexuals is not unique to the amputee-devotee community but is a reflection of the heterosexism that pervades the larger culture.

10. Simply typing "amputee" and "devotee" into any search engine will bring up dozens of possible links. Some of the more well-known amputee image sites include: www.cdprod.com and www.ascotworld.com/ftpsite.html, which are both run by disabled women; and www.ampix.com and www.criptease.com, which, like the first two sites, require devotees to pay for the images. There are sites, many of them European, which offer images free of charge. The site www.d-links.com/indexa.htm offers links to many of them.

11. ASCOTWorld, I should note, offers services not only to devotees but to amputees as well. Jama Bennett, the organization's founder, posts information about shoe-exchanges, wound care, prosthetics, and skin care on her website. Unlike CDProductions, which operates almost exclusively as a sales site for videos and photos, ASCOTWorld functions more as a virtual community.

12. Unfortunately, at least one amputee has yet to see any financial benefit from the sales of her video. She has struggled with CDProductions for over a year, and her complaints have largely gone unanswered. "Lisa," Personal communication, November 13, 2000.

Bibliography

Asch, Adrienne, and Michelle Fine. 1988. Introduction: Beyond pedestals. In *Women with disabilities: Essays in psychology, culture, and politics*, edited by Michelle Fine and Adrienne Asch. Philadelphia: Temple University Press.

Bruno, Richard L. 1997. Devotees, pretenders, and wannabes: Two cases of factitious disability disorder. *Sexuality and disability* 15: 243–260.

Butler, Judith. 1990. *Gender trouble: Feminism and the subversion of identity*. New York: Routledge.

———. 1993. *Bodies that matter: On the discursive limits of "sex."* New York: Routledge.

Child, Margaret. 1996 [cited November 11, 1999]. What are disability paraphilias, and who are devotees? *OverGround* [electronic journal]. Available at http://www.overground.be/features/theory/whata.html.

Clare, Eli. 1999. *Exile and pride: Disability, queerness, and liberation*. Cambridge, Mass.: South End Press.

Cole, David. 2000a [cited February 20, 2001]. A few bad apples. *The Devotee Chronicles* [electronic journal]. Available at http://www.nthward.com/chronicles/frames.htm.

————. 2000b [cited February 20, 2001]. I, devotee. *The Devotee Chronicles* [electronic journal]. Available at http://www.nthward.com/chronicles/frames.htm.

Dixon, Dwight. 1983. An erotic attraction to amputees. *Sexuality and Disability* 6: 3–19.

Duncan, Kath. 1999. *My one-legged dream lover*. Sydney: Jennifer Cornish Media.

Elliott, Carl. 2000. A new way to be bad. *The Atlantic Monthly*. 286 (6): 72–84.

Elman, R. Amy. 1997. Disability pornography: The fetishization of women's vulnerabilities. *Violence Against Women* 3: 257–270.

Everaerd, Walter. 1983. A case of apotemnophilia: A handicap as sexual preference. *American Journal of Psychotherapy* 37: 285–293.

Frank, Gelya. 1988. On embodiment: A case study of congenital limb deficiency in American Culture. In *Women with disabilities: Essays in psychology, culture, and politics*, edited by Michelle Fine and Adrienne Asch. Philadelphia: Temple University Press.

Garland-Thomson, Rosemarie. 1997. *Extraordinary bodies: Figuring physical disability in American culture and literature*. New York: Columbia.

Gregson, Ian. 2000 [cited February 1, 2001]. The devotee issue: Part two—The opposing view. *Amputee-Online* [electronic journal]. Available at http://amputee-online.com/amputation/sept00/sept00wissues.html.

J. 2001a [cited May 5, 2001]. Against either-or-ism: The way to find the special friend. *OverGround* [electronic journal]. Available at http://www.overground.be/features/theory/aeior.html.

————. 2001b [cited May 5, 2001]. Devotees: Are they necessarily sexual harassers? *OverGround* [electronic journal]. Available at http://www.overground.be/features/theory/devot.html.

————. 2001c [cited May 5, 2001]. Interview with Jama Bennett. *OverGround* [electronic journal]. Available at http://www.overground.be/features/people/inter.html.

————. 2001d [cited May 5, 2001]. Interview with a collector. *OverGround* [electronic journal]. Available at http://www.overground.be/features/people/colle.html.

————. 2001e [cited May 5, 2001]. Twins: An exploration of the morality of the feelings of devotees. *OverGround* [electronic journal]. Available at http://www.overground.be/features/theory/twins.html.

————. 2001f [cited May 5, 2001]. W. and K.: A complementary couple. *OverGround* [electronic journal]. Available at http://www.overground.be/features/people/wandk.html.

————. 2001g [cited May 5, 2001]. What's wrong with pix' n' flix? *OverGround* [electronic journal]. Available at http://www.overground.be/features/theory/whats.html.

————. 2001h [cited May 5, 2001]. With friends like these . . . *Over Ground* [electronic journal]. Available at http://www.overground.be/features/theory/withf.html.

John. 2001 [cited May 5, 2001]. Sightings. *OverGround* [electronic journal]. Available at http://www.overground.be/features/people/sight.html.

Kafer, Alison. 2000. Amputated Desire, Resistant Desire: Female Amputees in the Devotee Community. *DisabilityWorld* [electronic journal]. Available at http://www.disabilityworld.org/June-July2000/Women/SDS.htm

Money, John. 1990. Paraphilia in females: Fixation on amputation and lameness: Two accounts. *Journal of Psychology and Human Sexuality* 3:165–172.

Money, John, Russell Jobaris, and Gregg Furth. 1977. Apotemnophilia: Two Cases of Self-Demand Amputation as a Paraphilia. *Journal of Sex Research* 13: 115–125.

Money, J., and K. W. Simcoe. 1984–1986. Acrotomophilia, sex, and disability: New concepts and case report. *Sexuality and Disability* 7: 43–50.

Nattress, LeRoy William. 1996. Amelotasis: Men attracted to women who are amputees: A descriptive study. Unpublished Ph.D. diss., Walden University.

Ollason, John. 1996 [cited November 11, 1999]. Why devotees sometimes behave badly. *OverGround* [electronic journal]. Available at http://www.overground.be/features/theory/whyde.html.

Shakespeare, Tom, Kath Gillespie-Sells, and Dominic Davies. 1996. *The sexual politics of disability: Untold desires*. New York: Cassell.

Storrs, Bob. 1996. Caveat dater: Devotees of disability. *New Mobility: Disability Culture and Lifestyle* 6–7 (28): 50–53.

———. 1997. Amputees, Inc. *New Mobility: Disability Culture and Lifestyle*. 8 (45): 26–31.

Waxman-Fiduccia, Barbara. 1999. Erotic? Perverse? Sexist?: Sexual imagery of physically disabled women. *Sexuality and Disability*. 17 (3): 277–282.

Fighting Polio Like a Man

INTERSECTIONS OF MASCULINITY, DISABILITY, AND AGING

༄

DANIEL J. WILSON

In the 1950s, polio was a young person's disease. Young men who contracted the disease often considered their struggle against the effects of the disease as a military battle or athletic contest. Their bodies and their futures as disabled men were the battlegrounds and athletic fields on which the contest was fought. Fighting polio like a man meant rejecting dependence and passivity in favor of actively resisting the limitations imposed both by a crippled body and by an unaccommodating society. Although the masculine myths of warrior and athlete helped many young male polio survivors recover maximum physical function and to make their way in an often hostile world, viewing a life-long disability as a battle or athletic contest had its own costs. The myths and images that sustained their youthful struggle with disability became less helpful as they grew older. As they aged and as their bodies tired and broke down, these polio survivors had to create new images of masculinity to sustain their struggle with disability. In writing about their polio and disability, men such as Leonard Kriegel, Lorenzo Milam, Hugh Gregory Gallagher, Wilfred Sheed, and Arnold Beisser have attempted to articulate masculine identities that both acknowledge the long battle they have fought and that permit a graceful withdrawal from the field.

As a disease, polio posed particular challenges to the masculinity of its male victims.[1] Polio struck suddenly, often reducing strong, athletic boys and men to total paralysis and complete dependence in a matter of days or even hours. In paralytic polio the virus damaged or destroyed the anterior horn cells of the spinal cord. These cells were part of the motor neuron system, and when their functioning was decreased or destroyed, the muscles controlled by the affected nerves were either temporarily or permanently paralyzed, depending on the extent of the damage (Paul 1971, 1–9; Halstead 1998, 1–19). Polio typically began like

119

a case of the flu; it was only if and when the virus left the intestinal tract and migrated to the spinal cord that paralysis occurred. Paralysis occurred in only a small percentage of polio cases; at mid-century, the number of paralytic cases ranged from less than one per 100 infections to 3.1 paralytic cases per 100 infections. The crippling associated with polio, although widely feared, was a relatively rare complication of a fairly common disease (Nathanson and Martin 1979, 681). However, when paralysis did occur, it struck squarely at a young man's conception of masculinity.

The polio epidemics of the 1940s and 1950s occurred at a time when many commentators believed that American manhood was in crisis. K. A. Courdileone, for example, has recently argued that this postwar crisis of masculinity was linked to the anxieties of the cold war. Cold war-era cultural critics worried that American men had lost their strength, vitality, and autonomy in becoming victims of "a smothering, overpowering, suspiciously collectivist mass society" (2000, 522). Political observers, such as Arthur Schlesinger, Jr., worried that these unmanned, feminized men lacked the strength and will to confront and defeat resurgent communism (Schlesinger 1962, 237–246; Courdileone 2000, 517–521). In addition, Schlesinger and others alerted Americans to the threat that the loss of self in mass society posed to gender identity. As Courdileone observed, "lurking beneath the crisis in masculinity was often the specter of an expansionist homosexuality" (529). Many psychologists at mid-century held that "homosexuality was in large part an acquired trait that resulted from men's 'adaptive failure' to cope with modern life" (530). Boys too much under the influence of their mothers and passive and dependent boys, especially sissies, were thought to be in particular danger of becoming homosexuals (Kimmel 1996, 243; Courdileone 2000, 530–31).

Prevailing mid-twentieth century conceptions of masculinity would have posed significant challenges to boys and young men stricken with paralytic polio even without the cold war and homophobic anxieties of the time. The mid-century masculine ideal was perhaps best summarized by the sociologist Erving Goffman in his classic *Stigma* (1963):

> In an important sense there is only one complete unblushing male in America: a young, married, white, urban, northern, heterosexual Protestant father of college education, fully employed, of good complexion, weight, and height, and a recent record in sports. Every American male tends to look out upon the world from this perspective. . . . Any male who fails to qualify in any of these ways is likely to view himself—during moments at least—as unworthy, incomplete, and inferior. (128)

Although few men would have met all of Goffman's criteria for masculinity, survivors of paralytic polio found it particularly difficult. As Robert Murphy notes in his study of the effects of paralytic illness: "Paralytic disability constitutes emasculation of a more direct and total nature. For the male, the weakening and atrophy of the body threaten all the cultural values of masculinity: strength, activeness, speed, virility, stamina, and fortitude" (1987, 94–95). Paralytic polio temporarily, at least, unmanned young men and boys. Their muscles were flaccid and atrophying, they often experienced temporary impotence, and they were bedridden and completely dependent on female nurses and attending staff. They were once again "dependent, childlike, and helpless—an image fundamentally challenging all that is embodied in the ideal male, virility, autonomy and independence" (Asch and Fine 1988, 3; Tepper 1999, 47).

A recent study of men with physical disabilities by Thomas J. Gerschick and Adam S. Miller uncovered three patterns in men's efforts to "display appropriate gender identity." Gerschick and Miller argued that the ways the men in their study constructed a "sense of masculinity" fell into one of "three dominant frameworks." They labeled these frameworks, "reformulation," "reliance," and "rejection." Men who reformulated hegemonic masculinity "redefined" the characteristics of manhood. Those who were reliant developed "sensitive or hypersensitive adoptions of particular predominant attributes." The third group rejected society's standards and either developed their own values or denied the importance of masculinity in their lives (1995, 185, 187). For the polio survivors whose memoirs are analyzed in this chapter, the dominant mode of response was a mixture of reformulation and reliance.

Ironically, the very cultural values that initially emasculated the paralyzed polio survivor also provided the means by which a young male could construct a sense of masculinity consistent with society's values and expectations. One of the best ways to confront and reduce the disabilities of paralytic polio was to fight it like a man. Recovery from paralytic polio was long, hard, and often painful. Tight spasmodic muscles had to be loosened with hot packs or hydrotherapy, therapists restored range of motion by painfully stretching muscles, and weeks, perhaps months, of physical therapy restored function in muscles whose nerves were spared or only damaged by the virus. Recovery from polio could easily be construed as a battle or a contest against the virus, against the doctors and therapists, even against one's own damaged body and sense of self. The cultural values of masculinity—strength, aggressiveness, toughness, activity, stamina, and fortitude—were allies in the struggle to recover muscle function and to achieve something approaching a normal life. As Leonard Kriegel recalled, everyone he knew believed "that you were better off struggling with the effects of disease as a man than as a woman. Polio . . . was a disease battled by being tough, aggressive, and decisive. And by assuming that all limitations could be overcome, beaten, conquered. In short, triumph over polio's effects lay in 'being a man.' One was expected to 'beat' polio by outmuscling the disease" (1991, 56). As Kriegel suggests, physical and psychological recovery was achieved, in part at least, through the remasculinization of the self. This new sense of manhood was constructed, or reconstructed, not on school athletic fields or on fields of battle but in the rehabilitation facilities and in the long, lonely hours of exercise.[2]

Although fighting polio like a man was functional in the sense that the prevailing masculinity valorized pushing the body against the physical limitations imposed by the destructive virus, these same values often forced these young men to contain or repress what Robert Murphy has described as "an existential anger, a pervasive bitterness at one's fate, a hoarse and futile cry of rage against fortune." As Murphy so perceptively observed, this often destructive anger is "expressed in hostility toward the dominant society, then toward people of one's own kind, and finally it is turned inward into an attack on the self." Murphy rightly suspected that this "anger is much greater among those suddenly disabled and the young, for their impairment happens too quickly to permit assimilation, and it clouds an entire lifetime" (1987, 106). For several of these polio survivors, this rage and anger was an ever-present undercurrent that the masculine values could not always successfully contain. Leonard Kriegel put it well when, some forty-five years after polio struck, he wrote, "I am still angry about the loss of my legs. I suspect I shall be angry when I draw my dying breath" (1991, xv).

Polio struck Leonard Kriegel in the summer of 1944 when he was eleven. He would spend more than two years in the hospital and at the New York State Reconstruction Home before he returned to the Bronx walking on braces and crutches. Polio was a demanding teacher; it taught him that if he was to survive, he "would have to become a man—and quickly" (1991, 55). His immigrant father reinforced the lesson, urging his son from the side of the hospital bed to "Be brave! . . . Be a man!" (193). Kriegel recalls that in the context of post-World War II America, fighting polio as a man was what the culture expected. As he later noted, "a man was expected to face adversity with courage, endurance, determination, and stoicism. With these, and with a touch of defiance, he might right the balance with his fate, however unjust and arbitrary that fate might appear" (55–56). Almost from the beginning, Kriegel understood his "war with the virus" as a struggle not only to recover physically but also to prove his manhood (4). His hope, and he believed the hope of the boys around him, was to acquit himself well in the rigors of rehabilitation. He hoped "to take whatever fate would mete out—and to take it as a man" (7). For Kriegel taking it as a man, being "manly," meant enduring hot baths to relieve painful and stiff muscles, learning to walk with braces and crutches and to fall safely, building a strong upper body to compensate for his paralyzed legs and finding ways to productively channel his anger and rage at the loss of his legs[3] (7). Reliance on the masculine standards of postwar America gave Kriegel a framework within which he could fashion the rehabilitation of his body. What had changed for Kriegel was not the masculine values he embraced but the locale in which they operated. Kriegel embodied masculine values not on the athletic field or on the field of battle but in the rehabilitation hospital and on the streets of Brooklyn as he struggled to rebuild his body and to confront the barriers of an unaccommodating society.

At fourteen when he had polio in 1953, Charles Mee was slightly older than Leonard Kriegel. He recalled that polio reduced him "from a healthy athletic boy weighing 160 pounds to a frightened child of 90 pounds" (1999, 17). The postwar male ethos was very much in evidence during Mee's rehabilitation. Mee remembers being told the stories of heroic youngsters who had overcome polio. The moral was very clear: "The way to win was to fight; the fight was up to us; and it was a test of character. The penalty for failure was to be a helpless invalid for life. On the other hand, success would be greeted not simply as a good thing, but as a wonderful and deeply satisfying thing" (85–86). Mee, however, did not entirely buy into this cultural belief that "any problem can be solved with will, determination, and ingenuity" (92). But the expectations of his parents, his physicians, his coaches, and his priest meant he had little choice but to play along. "This culture," he wrote, "made me feel, as a boy, that I needed to keep my chin up, reassure my parents about how well I was doing, never be sad, look to the future, be optimistic, perform a can-do persona even if I felt no connection to it. It made me live a lie, confuse myself about who I was and what I felt and how life was for me" (93). Even though Mee recognized the inauthenticity of the heroic narratives he was offered, he was not ready to dismiss their influence entirely. He recognized that "the stories of fighting and heroism were puffed-up entertainment for other people," but they still offered him some hope. As he recalled, "I knew, too, that I could help myself along if I bought in to them a little bit" (140). In recovery from polio, determination, willpower, and hard work often brought results. Some muscles could be restored to function, and ways could be found to compensate for those that remained paralyzed. As Charles Mee slowly discovered, fighting polio like a man, even if you weren't a true believer, often brought a marked improvement in one's ability to function.

Hugh Gallagher was in his first year of college when he contracted polio. He vividly remembers the "advancing paralysis, the searing fever, the body as battleground," but the more significant struggle was what he called the "inward tragedy taking place." "This," he wrote, "involved the collapse of a young man's life, the end of expectation, the passing down of a life sentence without hope of pardon or parole" (1998, 13–14). For Gallagher, "polio was a battleground, no less dangerous than any war." Despite the activity of doctors and nurses, Gallagher recalled that "the battleground was within me; the struggle was waged, the life-or-death decisions were made, within me" (28). When polio struck, Hugh Gallagher had been trying hard to break "the tight constrictions that bound [him] to [his] parents and their cultural values and mores" (14). Polio, however, reduced him to utter dependence upon his parents. In his later writings on his battle with polio, Gallagher recalled how difficult it had been for him to secure his independence, to become a man. "He wanted," he remembered, "to be an individual human being, a man in his own right. He did not want to be somebody's dependent. . . . He put it in his own thinking that he would be as much like other self-reliant grown-up men and women as possible" (154). Gallagher's efforts to become a man exacted a high psychic price, denial of his disability and his feelings of anger and rage at what had happened to him (4–5, 177–78). Twenty years after the onset of polio, and after twenty years of pretending that he had accepted his disability, Gallagher was overwhelmed by depression.

Wilfred Sheed had polio in 1945 when he was fourteen and in boarding school. He recalls an atmosphere in which he and the other polio patients were expected to avoid self-pity and to get on with the business of recovery. Sheed remembers that he and his fellow patients quickly stopped railing against their fate. "There was," he wrote, "no conscious decision about this or any special virtue in it: *none* of us felt sorry for himself, that I ever heard of. Polio victims didn't cry because (a) we were too busy trying to get better and (b) what was in it for us?" (1995, 26). Perhaps because his polio occurred at the end of World War II, Sheed writes of his illness and recovery in military terms. At Warm Springs, Georgia, where he spent five weeks, Sheed discovered the positive psychic benefits of rehabilitation: "[W]e were *doing* something, we were *going* places. Every day another muscle, and on to Berlin in the morning." He left Warm Springs sooner than he had initially intended because, as he put it, it was "a sleepy kind of place," and he wasn't convinced that they "shared [his] Churchillian enthusiasm for the blood, sweat, and tears of this thing" (27). Military metaphors shaped his experience of the disease and rehabilitation. Drawing on a commonplace from World War II, Sheed believed that as in foxholes, "there were no atheists in the polio ward either, because at that moment, whatever life remains in you rallies spontaneously like a volunteer army in a city under siege, and suddenly every last cell and corpuscle is at the barricades, and Faith is very much a part of the ensemble: I'll think of *some*thing; *some*one will think of something" (32). Rehabilitation was like a military campaign: "During that time you can keep racking up small victories, not matching the early spectacular ones in [his] case—the mighty battles of the back and stomach, both of which regions had been feared lost, and the prolonged fighting over the use of [his] right leg, a trophy that came out of the war almost as spindly as ever, but blessedly functional" (33). Like the soldiers who didn't talk about their experiences when they came home from Europe and the Pacific, Sheed tried to put the experience behind him and to get on with his life. As he put it, "the task is simply to make the world, and ourselves, forget for as long and as often as possible that there has ever been anything wrong with us: to be, in other words, 'great pitchers,' and not just 'great-one-armed pitchers'" (45).

Like Gallagher and Sheed, Lorenzo Milam envisioned his polio-wracked body as "the battlefield." Nineteen when he came down with polio in 1952, Milam saw himself as "Troy": "I have been sacked and looted and burned by the barbarians. The Huns came and devastated every street, every temple, every square" (1984, 66). Milam did not fully buy into the ideology of rehabilitation at Warm Springs, but, as he recalled, "I stand on that day (and every day thereafter) not because I am strong and brave and true and have to defy the nay-sayers with my natural tenacity; but rather I stand because it is what is expected of me" (72). The challenge for Milam when he left Warm Springs for home was to "normalize" himself in spite of his disability and his renewed dependence on his parents. As he recalled, he had once before "started out to be a man" and "moved out of [his] childhood home." But then he "sickened and paled and withered" and he was forced "back, a child again" (88). Polio had not only taken his muscles, it had also taken his manhood.

Arnold Beisser was twenty-four when he had polio in 1950. He had just completed medical school, was a nationally ranked tennis player, and on his way to report for active duty as a Navy reserve officer. The most severely paralyzed of these men, Beisser was paralyzed from the neck down and would spend a year and half in an iron lung and three years in the hospital. In addition to his very severe physical limitations, Beisser found the challenge to his masculinity hard to bear. He had, as he later recalled, "been thrust backwards in the developmental scale." His "dependence was now as profound as that of a newborn." He once again had "to deal with all of the overwhelming, degrading conditions of dependency that belong with infancy and childhood," while still considering himself a "mature adult" (1989, 21). Because he had been an active and successful athlete, he initially "tried to turn [his] disability into a competitive sport." Athletes and cripples [his word] "both require periods of serious training and retraining, and with both, performances are measured and records kept of how far one can go and how long it takes" (80). When he became disabled, Beisser was also imbued with what he called "the pioneer spirit": "the belief that if someone wanted something badly enough he could have it, and if you were willing to work hard enough for something, you could always get it." As he acknowledged, those values had "advantages" for they "promoted optimism and well-being," and were, in some cases at least, a "self-fulfilling prophecy" (117–118). For many years, he preferred "to see [his] disability as an adversary, an opponent or an enemy to be overcome and battled with." When he considered his disability "as an enemy, it [was] a male adversary." He tried "to face him squarely, to look him in the eye, and to hold [his] ground" (133). In spite of Beisser's continuing severe disability, surrendering the cultural values that had sustained him in his pre-polio life and through many years of rehabilitation "seemed a matter of cowardice, and [he] did not want any of that" (119). It took years for Beisser to find an alternative set of beliefs more appropriate to his lifelong disability.

Polio clearly posed a complex challenge to the sense of masculinity of boys and young men. The cultural values of mid-twentieth century America offered them only one masculine response: treat the disease as an enemy or adversary, fight it with all the strength you possess, resist becoming dependent, repress your emotions, and take it like a man. Each of these men accepted these cultural values to some extent, in part, at least, because they believed them and because they had no viable alternative. In addition, the treatment regime for polio survivors in the forties and fifties drew upon these cultural mores to motivate patients in the arduous process of recovery. Writing in the mid-fifties, the sociologist Fred Davis noted that "the treatment procedures" tapped into the "implicit faith of parents and children" in the "efficacy of 'will power' in overcoming adverse circumstances." Treatment for paralytic polio was the "quintessence of the Protestant ideology of achievement in America—namely, slow, patient and regularly applied effort in pursuit of a long-range goal" (1972, 115–16). Jessica Scheer and Mark Luborsky have more recently argued that embracing these values provided polio survivors with "one passage to normalization." However, they also recognize that while "the behaviors inspired by these messages were adaptive for regaining muscle strength and for participating in the mainstream, . . . they negated the psychological realities of physical loss, vulnerability, and long-term living with a disability" (1991, 1178–1179). While some polio survivors such as Leonard Kriegel wholeheartedly embraced the masculine ethos, others such as Charles Mee and Hugh Gallagher found themselves living a lie. Outwardly conforming to the ethos because they saw no alternative, they postponed confronting the psychological impact of permanent disability and of denying their feelings of anger, shame, and betrayal. The challenge for all of these men came as they matured and aged. The masculine ethos that had spurred their recovery could not always be sustained over a lifetime of living with a disability.

This enforced conformity to the mores of post-World War II masculinity became for some of these polio survivors a kind of performance for family, physicians, and therapists, and perhaps, even for themselves. Judith Butler has recently drawn our attention to the ways that gender is *"performative."* Individuals desire a coherent gender identity and that identity is produced "on the *surface of the body"* through "acts, gestures and desire" (1990, 136). She has also argued that gender performance becomes "a strategy of survival within compulsory systems," such as the hegemonic masculinity of post-World War II America. For polio survivors in the forties and fifties, gender was definitely "a performance with clearly punitive consequences" (139). When polio paralysis made it impossible for these men to perform masculinity in traditional ways—through athletics or war, for example—they performed masculinity in the one way left to them, how they fought their disease and disability. Because of the characteristics of their disability, displacing the values of hegemonic masculinity on to their project of physical rehabilitation fostered physical recovery. But as these narratives make clear, it was a performance that was only incompletely internalized. Despite Charles Mee's realization that the values of his family, religion, and society made him "live a lie," he pushed his body through the rigors of polio rehabilitation because he felt he had no choice and, in truth, because acting like a man brought some physical improvement (1999, 140). At a crucial point in his rehabilitation, Hugh Gallagher acknowledged to himself for the first time that he would "never again be beautiful, innocent, secure in health, strong in body, confident in mind. Everything had changed and [he] would be forever crippled" (1998, 55). That afternoon, the "young man" he had been, "rich in life and youth, died." He "retreated" into himself and "became again the cheerful patient, the dutiful son," but it was all performance, a performance that could not always be sustained (57).

The later consequences of denying their disability, of repressing the powerful emotions involving loss, dependence, and sense of masculinity included self-destructive behavior and serious episodes of depression. Although all of these men found ways to compensate for the loss of muscle function, finished their education, and had successful careers as writers, physicians, college professors, and government bureaucrats, the initial failure to deal with the psychological assault that accompanied polio's physical devastation left them vulnerable to later psychological problems. Charles Mee, Hugh Gallagher, and Wilfred Sheed each experienced a serious psychological breakdown after years of living an apparently well-adjusted life with a disability. And while Leonard Kriegel, Arnold Beisser, and Lorezo Milam seem to have escaped serious depression, they, too, found that they had to alter their relationship with their disability and their sense of manhood as they aged.

Writing more than forty years after polio took away his boyhood, Charles Mee recognized that polio damaged the psyche as well as the body. The "need to prove" himself, to live up to the prevailing masculine ethos, drove him to pursue "quick, striking success" as a young magazine editor. Preoccupied with his "own urges and insecurities and compensatory strategies," and "prey of [his] own unexamined fears and confusions and rages" he spent years "savaging [his] body with alcohol and drugs." He can now acknowledge that while "physical damage is easy to repair; the psyche takes longer." In his case, it took "years of heavy drinking, some drugs, a fall into a very deep depression, the love of more than one woman, three failed marriages, [and] a passionate life of writing history books" before he could achieve some kind of perspective on being disabled (1999, 213).

Like Charles Mee, Hugh Gallagher had for years repressed the strong emotions engendered by his disability. He had apparently overcome his disability in a successful career as writer and as an aide in the White House and the U.S. Senate. However, as he came to realize, "disability is far more complex, more profound than mere physical impairment." In his experience, "the emotional aspects of the loss have a greater and more persistent impact." His emotions became "a psychic wound that never heals" (1998, 2). His frequent statements to friends and acquaintances that he never gave his disability a thought were nothing more than pretense and denial. His disability was "*not* OK, it has *never* been OK. In fact, [he] keened over [his] disability all the time, everyday, all day" (4). In the summer of 1974, his "body and soul rebelled." He left work and never returned. He "had collapsed both mentally and physically" and found himself "in the grip of a deep situational depression" so severe he "spent the rest of the decade getting out of it" (110).

Unlike Mee and Gallagher, Wilfred Sheed does not directly attribute his depression and his addiction to drugs and alcohol in his mid-fifties to unresolved emotional responses to his polio. He describes himself having "to wade through the purely man-made swamp of addiction-depression," and he remains uncertain why he fell prey to his addiction to drugs and alcohol and to depression. While his physicians attributed his "condition, curse, spell," to "Denial," Sheed himself is less certain. He thinks his problems might have been the result of faulty "brain chemistry," although the final diagnosis from the doctors is that he had "an incurable personality disorder" (1995, 58–59). Although he does not explicitly make the connection, it is likely that Sheed's experience was at least partly related to his response to polio. He acknowledges that as a young man he had "taken the arts of concealment to . . . dizzy new heights." He admits, however, that he was "probably always a lot more handicapped than [he] let on, either to [himself] or to others. [His] knacks were all geared to the same end, a massive cover-up, a downright Watergate of the nerves and muscles, in order to pass inspection" (50).

The experiences of Mee, Gallagher, and Sheed suggest some of the psychic and emotional toll that the prevailing masculine ethos of post-World War II exacted from these polio survivors. The virus-induced paralysis had left these young men dependent and passive. It appeared impossible that they could ever live up to the dominant masculine values of strength, activity, virility, stamina, and fortitude. In part out of a fear that passivity and dependence bred homosexuality and in part because they could conceive no alternative to the hegemonic masculinity, parents, coaches, psychologists, and rehabilitation specialists offered these vulnerable young men only one option—be a man (Wilson 1998, 15). If one could no longer be an athlete or soldier, one could be a man in the way one fought back from polio's devastation. Anger, fear, anxiety were to be repressed, not spoken of, and certainly not addressed by professionals. Few hospitals for physical rehabilitation offered their patients psychological counseling to cope with their sudden disability, and I have found no evidence that polio patients received professional assistance to deal with the psychological and emotional burdens of their illness.[4] As Robert Murphy so astutely observed, this anger and rage, if left unchecked, "clouds an entire lifetime" (1987, 106).

Most polio survivors have not experienced major depressive episodes after decades of living with their disability, but many, if not most, have come to experience what is described as post-polio syndrome or the late effects of polio. After several decades of functioning at the level at which they left rehabilitation, polio survivors are experiencing new muscle weakness, increased fatigue, increased muscle pain, decreased endurance, and the loss of hard won function. Many are forced to return to wearing braces, using canes and crutches, and relying on wheelchairs and scooters. The causes of post-polio syndrome are uncertain, although there is some evidence that the symptoms are caused by "a progressive degeneration or impairment of motor units," and by "excessive wear and tear on different parts of the musculoskeletal system" (Halstead 1998, 7).

Whatever the cause, for many men, post-polio syndrome poses new challenges to their masculinity. The hard won victories of rehabilitation are slipping away, and the metaphors of battle and competition that sustained their youthful struggles against the disease have lost their power to inspire and motivate. After years of taking it like a man, of denying or dismissing their disability, of "faking it," these polio survivors are forced once again to redefine or reformulate their sense of masculinity.

After thirty-eight years of picking himself up after falling, Leonard Kriegel discovers, to his surprise, that he can no longer get to his feet by himself. He still had powerful arms, but there had been "a subtle, mysterious change" in his "sense of rhythm and balance." His body, he concluded, "had decided—*and decided on its own, autonomously*—that the moment had come for [him] to face the question of endings." It was he later concluded "a distinctively American moment." It left him "pondering limitations and endings and summations" (1991, 17). A few years later, Kriegel found himself returning to using a wheelchair full time. As a young man he had fought hard to leave the chair and to become a crutchwalker. Rejecting the chair had been part of his "true passion, the need to surmount whatever was difficult, to prove [his] worth by overcoming all obstacles in [his] way," and to succeed through "his own manly virtue" (38). He now, however, recognizes that "as one grows older, it becomes increasingly difficult to ignore the fact that one's inner being has grown tired—tired of defiance, tired of resistance, tired of the daily grind." One's drive, one's sense of purpose "just wears down, until one reaches the point where all that can be said is, 'To hell with it!'" He discovers that returning to the wheelchair was not "the spiritual death" he had feared (42–43, 45). After forty years of crutchwalking, forty years of struggle, defiance, and resistance, it was time to say "no more," and to recognize that he had put up a good fight but that the time for that particular fight had passed.

Like Kriegel, Charles Mee and Wilfred Sheed both sought to refashion their concept of masculinity as they aged and as their bodies lost the ability to endure pain and push ahead at any price. When Mee discovers "a whole new set of physical limitations" brought on by post-polio and aging, he still feels "the old anger welling up" and he "hates it." Still now, unlike his youthful days, Mee thinks he "can hate it and just get on with [his] life." He now understands that "sorrow and loss and regret and life and pleasure do not need to crowd one another out." Part of his new attitude is the recognition that what he is experiencing is part of "the aging that eventually overtakes us all." After years of struggle against the physical and psychological consequences of polio, Mee now feels that he can "contemplate" the changes in his body "with almost perfect equanimity—which is to say, with a fairly normal sense of dread and rage and bitterness and frenzy and despair at the prospect of losing strength and dying— and go on to luxuriate in the present" (1999, 221–222). He is "no longer interested in recovery or restitution," and concludes that "you don't recover from the events of life, you take them with you, you knit them in, you grow with them, and around them; they become who you are; they're life itself" (223). Wilfred Sheed is less explicit than Mee on the changes in attitude brought on by aging with polio, perhaps because severe addiction/depression and cancer complicated his experience. Nonetheless he recognizes that when post-polio syndrome struck in his "mid-fifties, it weakened the whole physical apparatus just enough to call [his] bluff on all fronts at once." He was surprised to "realize quite how much [he] had been faking it for all these years," and he could no longer pretend, even to himself, that he was not disabled (1995, 50). For both Mee and Sheed the new physical limitations that came with post-polio forced a reassessment of how they responded to their disability. They could no longer pretend not to be disabled, but more importantly, they no longer wanted to. The young man's need to prove himself capable of taking it, of overcoming all obstacles, of pushing through pain to perform as normally as possible, was no longer appealing. Now the challenge was finding ways to accept with dignity the changes the body demanded.

Arnold Beisser, perhaps because he is a psychiatrist, gave the most attention to finding alternatives to the masculine ethos of his youth as a way of dealing with his disability. He acknowledges that he had to grieve for what polio had forced him to give up. He had "to stop clinging to an obsolete image of [himself] as an athlete, as an able-bodied person, as a particular kind of lover, as a traveler" (1989, 125). But giving up these images of himself did not automatically provide him with a useful alternative. It was a long process of learning to "accept that new personal needs and desires are legitimate, even when they are out of the ordinary." Beisser had to learn "acceptance with dignity," which he described as "surrender without a sense of capitulation." The key was living "as if" one had "freely chosen the new life" (131). Acceptance, he acknowledges, does not come all at once; his relationship with his disability is lifelong and evolving. At times, he still sees his "disability as an adversary, an opponent or an enemy to be overcome and battled with." At these times, it is a "male adversary." There are other times, however, when he has to "to acknowledge" he "is helpless before" his disability and "there is no alternative to surrender." When Beisser recognizes the power of his disability over him, it no longer "dominates" him. Instead, they join together. Interestingly, when he surrenders, his "disability becomes female, and [they] are united in that special way that men and women can unite" (133). In his evolving relationship with his disability, Beisser has clearly moved beyond the manly competition that dominated his initial response. His language, however, especially when he speaks of surrendering, still bears vestiges of the masculine metaphors of his youth. Nonetheless, his relationship with his disability has become more complicated as he comes to recognize the limitations of the competitive masculine model. No matter how hard he competed, some things, like the extent of his paralysis, were never going to get better. But, if he put aside the masculine values with which he began and built a new life out of the possibilities left to him, he could find life, work, and love meaningful in ways he had never anticipated. When he embraced his disability instead of fighting it, when he approached it the way a man approached a lover, his world expanded. The masculine ethos of post-war America could, given the particular characteristics of polio, help heal the body, but a less adversarial conception of manhood was necessary to heal the person. Arnold Beisser was no less a man for these changes, for he had constructed a sense of masculinity more complex and subtle than he had known before.

When polio was at its height in mid-twentieth-century America, there was only one manly way to respond to the disease and its attendant disability. One had to fight it like a man—push ahead, endure pain without complaint, and repress any feelings of fear, anger, and loss. These values were reinforced by American culture in the person of parents, priests and ministers, coaches, family and friends. This masculine ethos was also consciously reinforced and employed by the rehabilitation regime of the era. Physicians and therapists used these masculine values and the shame of falling short to motivate their patients to cooperate in the long, hard, and painful process of recovery from polio. Most young men accepted on some level the repeated injunctions to have courage and to fight like a man. This was especially the case in the rehabilitation facilities where peer pressure was added to the urgings of the staff. Polio was in many ways the ideal disease for the masculine ethos because, in fact, taking it like a man, enduring pain, pushing beyond limits often worked. Progress was evident, some muscle function, at least, was restored, and one could stay outside the iron lung longer than before or take more steps unassisted.

Unfortunately, polio patients and rehabilitation specialists were often so busy healing the body that they neglected the emotions and the psyche. Few rehabilitation hospitals addressed the psychological needs of their seriously disabled patients, and nothing in the culture encouraged polio patients or their families to seek aid in dealing with the inevitable feelings of loss, fear, anger, and frustration. Although these emotions could be and often were repressed, they remained in place only to surface later when the façade of the well-adjusted, happy cripple could no longer be maintained. It was not uncommon for episodes of clinical depression, sometimes accompanied by alcohol or drug addiction, to emerge decades after rehabilitation had been completed.

Even men who escaped the more serious episodes of depression have more recently been forced to rethink their adherence to the manly codes of their youth. Post-polio syndrome, with its increased pain, fatigue, and loss of muscle function, has forced polio survivors to confront new limitations. Now, however, they face them with diminished strength and energy. The body is tired and so is the will. The daily battles that invigorated their youth no longer appeal. They seek to withdraw from the contest with their bodies and with society's expectations.

But even as they once again reformulate their relationship to their crippled bodies and social expectations, even as they recount their struggles to be a man—not just a crippled man—these polio survivors in their memoirs construct and perform their masculinity. These narratives perform masculinity by demonstrating how these men, in their own eyes and, they hope, in the eyes of their readers, became men by the way they fought polio. They are the aging warriors recounting the battles of their youth. Leonard Kriegel, for example, writes that his "essays also speak of my pride in my performance. All things considered, I have done well." His essays provide evidence that he "had made the only bargain with fate a cripple and writer could make. I had survived. And I would preserve that survival in the language of record" (1991, xv). Charles Mee discovers that as post-polio imposes new limits on his body, he can face the decline with the greater "equanimity" gained from the experience of a lifetime: "I've had a lot of practice at this sort of thing by now." Now the changes he is experiencing don't so much "set [him] apart from the rest of the world as . . . knit [him] in with others, with the aging that eventually overtakes us all. This is the common lot" (1999, 222). Even Hugh Gallagher manages to find a measure of solace in the experience of being disabled. He writes that "through our disability, we are granted—if we can stand it—the despair *and* the wisdom that springs therefrom, usually reserved for the old and dying. We must live with this knowledge." He comes to accept the fact that, as he puts it, "my broken-down body is not me. This is, of course, another sort of denial but it is closer to reality. I see it as life affirming" (1998, 3–5). These polio survivors want us to know that even though the field of battle was their own bodies and the cultural expectations of mid-twentieth century America, they acquitted themselves well. They were not just crippled men, but real men.

Notes

1. There is some evidence in the scientific literature that polio struck males more frequently than females. The consensus seems to be that the ratio was 1.3 males to 1 female, or about 4 males for every 3 females (Ruhräh and Mayer 1917, 63; Draper 1935, 57; Lewin 1941, 35).
2. I have discussed the construction of masculinity in the wake of polio more fully in "Crippled Manhood" (Wilson 1998).
3. Kriegel's memoir, *The Long Walk Home* (1964), recounts his efforts to prove his manhood through his life-long war with the polio virus. Many of the essays collected in *Falling into Life* (1991) and *Flying Solo* (1998) are reflections about and meditations on his manhood and his disability.
4. In the more than 150 polio narratives I have compiled, almost no one mentions psychological counseling early in their recovery or during their physical rehabilitation.

Works Cited

Asch, Adrienne, and Michelle Fine. 1988. Introduction: Beyond pedestals. In *Women with disabilities: Essays in psychology, culture, and politics*, edited by Adrienne Asch and Michelle Fine. Philadelphia: Temple University Press.

Beisser, Arnold R. 1989. *Flying without wings: Personal reflections on being disabled.* New York: Doubleday.

Butler, Judith. 1990. *Gender trouble: Feminism and the subversion of identity*. New York: Routledge.

Courdileone, K. A. 2000. Politics in an age of anxiety: Cold war political culture and the crisis in American masculinity, 1949–1960. *Journal of American History* 87: 515–45.

Davis, Fred. 1972. Definitions of time and recovery in paralytic polio convalescence. In *An introduction to deviance: Readings in the process of making deviants*, edited by William J. Filstead. Chicago: Markham Publishing Company. First published in *The American Journal of Sociology* 61 (1956): 582–587.

Draper, George. 1935. *Infantile paralysis*. New York: D. Appleton-Century Company.

Gallagher, Hugh Gregory. 1998. *Black bird fly away: Disabled in an able-bodied world.* Arlington, Va.: Vandamere Press.

Gerschick, Thomas J., and Adam S. Miller. 1995. Coming to terms: Masculinity and physical disability. In *Men's health and illness: Gender, power, and the body,* edited by Donald Sabo and David Frederick Gordon. Thousand Oaks, Calif.: Sage Publications.

Goffman, Erving. 1963. *Stigma: Notes on the management of spoiled identity.* Englewood Cliffs, N.J.: Prentice-Hall.

Halstead, Lauro S. 1998. Acute polio and post-polio syndrome. In *Managing post-polio: A guide to living well with post-polio syndrome,* edited by Lauro S. Halstead and Naomi Naierman. Washington, D.C.: NRH Press.

Kimmel, Michael. 1996. *Manhood in America: A Cultural History.* New York: The Free Press.

Kriegel, Leonard. 1964. *The Long Walk Home.* New York: Appleton-Century.

———. 1991. *Falling Into Life: Essays.* San Francisco: North Point Press.

———. 1998. *Flying Solo: Reimagining Manhood, Courage, and Loss.* Boston: Beacon Press.

Lewin, Philip. 1941. *Infantile Paralysis: Anterior Poliomyelitis.* Philadelphia: W.B. Saunders Company.

Mee, Charles L. 1999. *A nearly normal life: A memoir.* Boston: Little, Brown and Company.

Milam, Lorenzo Wilson. 1984. *The cripple liberation front marching band blues.* San Diego: Mho & Mho Works.

Murphy, Robert F. 1987. *The body silent.* New York: Henry Holt and Company.

Nathanson, Neal, and John R. Martin. 1979. The epidemiology of poliomyelitis: Enigmas surrounding its appearance, epidemicity, and disappearance. *American Journal of Epidemiology* 110: 672–92.

Paul, John R. 1971. *A history of poliomyelitis.* New Haven, Conn.: Yale University Press.

Ruhräh, John, and Erwin E. Mayer. 1917. *Poliomeyelitis in all its aspects.* Philadelphia: Lea & Febiger.

Scheer, Jessica, and Mark L. Luborsky. 1991. The cultural context of polio biographies. *Orthopedics* 14: 1173–1181.

Schlesinger, Arthur M., Jr. 1962. The crisis in American masculinity. In *The politics of hope.* Boston: Houghton Mifflin.

Sheed, Wilfred. 1995. *In love with daylight: A memoir of recovery.* New York: Simon and Schuster.

Tepper, Michael S. 1999. Letting go of restrictive notions of manhood: Male sexuality, disability and chronic illness. *Sexuality and Disability* 17: 38–52.

Wilson, Daniel J. 1998. Crippled manhood: Infantile paralysis and the construction of masculinity. *Medical Humanities Review* 12: 9–28.

"Disability" and "Divorce"

A Blind Parisian Cloth Merchant
Contemplates His Options in 1756

ₒⱼₚ

CATHERINE J. KUDLICK

In 1756, a Parisian cloth merchant named Jean-Denis Jameu filed a formal complaint against his wife "for having removed several pieces of furniture and precious effects from our household." The report issued by his lawyer, but presented as if written in his own words, noted that "this is a known and proven fact, so her condemnation should be inevitable" (Jameu, 209; hereafter only given as page numbers). Jameu was responding to his wife's petition for a *séparation des corps et de biens* (separation of person and possessions), the closest option to divorce in prerevolutionary France. Anne-Cécile Verset had accused her husband of twenty-seven years because of his "debauchery, drunkenness, and violence" (209). Blind since the age of five, Jameu had been forced at the time of his defense to take a small apartment in the enclave of the Quinze-Vingts Hospital, then the only residence for blind people in Paris seeking aid. Now that his wife was suing for separation, a wish he clearly did not share, the successful merchant wanted what he believed to be rightfully his. "Since until now nobody has made a scene [*jusqu'ici les mauvais procédés n'avoient point éclaté*], I have put up with it without complaint," he explained. "But since she has now dared to attack me, since she's distributing a public statement against me, I must defend myself" (210). Jameu and his lawyer thus issued a counterattack, in the form of a twenty-eight page printed pamphlet that was published and sold illicitly on the streets of Paris later in the century.[1]

This essay uses Jameu's response to his wife's petition for separation as a point of departure for considering blindness, gender roles, and class standing in mid-eighteenth-century France. While I have unfortunately been unable to locate Anne-Cécile Verset's own petition or even the judge's verdict, Jameu's detailed account of his life history written in response provides an unusual window into the world of a blind man in the merchant classes of the old regime. Even—and especially—as a manipulative plea for sympathy to obtain a decision in his favor, Jameu's statement gives a clear sense of social expectations surrounding blindness and marriage in the Parisian petite bourgeoisie. Interestingly, he uses his blindness to elicit sympathy in ways we might not expect.

Before taking up the details of Jameu's case, however, some cursory background information is necessary. Ecclesiastic law, reinforced by secular courts, forbade divorce until a 1792 law passed at the height of revolutionary excitement made it legal.[2] However, petitions filed at local judicial courts served as a means by which an unhappy spouse could appeal. Because men had more socially acceptable options if they wanted to end a marriage (such as placing an undesirable wife in a convent), the petitions for separation almost all came from women. These petitions had a formulaic character (which, reading through the lens of Jameu's responses, Verset appears to have followed to the letter), beginning with a narrative of the situation and moving on to outlining the nature of specific complaints in more detail. To be considered, petitions needed to demonstrate that a marriage had degenerated in one of several ways later laid out in the Enlightenment's compendium of all knowledge, the *Encyclopédie*, in its crusade for more liberal divorce laws: considerable violence and ill-treatment, a false accusation of dishonorable acts, a husband's having been convicted for having attempted to murder his wife, insanity (but only in cases where there was reason to fear for the wife's life), and concrete evidence of his having developed a deadly hatred (*haine capitale*) toward her. Filing such a petition proved to be quite costly, and as a result, they were somewhat rare. Thus, Verset must have had sufficient cause and wealth to do so, while for his part Jameu had equally compelling means and motives for responding (Phillips 1980; Traer 1980; Hanley 1997; Hardwick 1998).

That Jameu was blind surely played a part in how he and his unhappy wife dealt with the possible end to their long marriage. In the first half of the eighteenth century, few economic options existed for blind people. Those of noble birth could attain some education with the help of readers and tutors; some used this system to remarkable advantage, giving them respected careers in fields such as literature, mathematics, philosophy, and music. By contrast, we know very little about the lives of the vast majority of everyone else, even the merchant class to which Jameu belonged. In the century before Braille made it possible to read and write, blind people had even fewer options than their sighted counterparts for describing their lives. Moreover, until the pioneering work of Valentin Haüy in the 1780s, no systematic education or job training existed for the majority of blind people in France. Because most lacked Jameu's good fortune to be working productively in a trade, they lived from begging, a royal privilege uniquely granted to blind people since the inception of the Quinze-Vingts in the thirteenth century. As a result, it is easy to understand that Jameu's blindness placed him in a more precarious economic situation than that of a sighted man facing the dissolution of his marriage (Wilson 1821–1838/1995, Henri 1984, Weygand 1998).

At about the time that Anne-Cécile Verset began to contemplate dispensing with her husband's furniture, the philosophe Diderot was writing his soon-to-be revolutionary *Letter on the Blind for the Benefit of Those Who See* (1749). Considered by many to be the definitive text in establishing a modern attitude toward blind people, Diderot's *Letter* would invite Enlightenment thinkers to consider blindness as something that could make a significant contribution to understanding the world of ideas and perceptions. But beyond the questions he raised for sensualist philosophy, his text speaks to stereotypes and social values at the same time that he at least attempted to portray blind people as human beings. Thus, though he exoticized them, Diderot broke with the tradition of seeing the blind as pathetic wards of public charity. The central figure of his *Letter* (allegedly a real person) offered the image of blind man as an individual who in many ways personified a typical upper-crust bourgeois of the eighteenth century, both in his respectability and in his transgressions. Inadvertently, he also revealed a great deal about prevailing values that applied to mainstream bourgeois French society and how these values played themselves out in the married lives of blind people. Though Diderot's blind man belonged to a segment of the French bourgeoisie a few notches above Jameu, thanks to remarks the philosophe made in passing, we can get a sense of how someone such as Jameu was expected to fare in the marriage marketplace and what expectations he was to have of his wife.

Diderot's *Letter*, written to a learned woman, attempted to bring respectability to blindness by attributing to the Blind Man of Puiseaux qualities of learning, productivity, and order so valued by those most likely to read the text. Born blind, Diderot explained, "he is possessed of good solid sense, is known to great numbers of persons, understands a little chemistry, and has attended the botanical lectures at the Jardin du Roi with some profit to himself." The son of an acclaimed professor of philosophy in Paris, the blind man lived the comfortable life of a bourgeois who enjoyed an "honest fortune," but having had "a taste for pleasure in his youth," he squandered his money—and presumably his reputation—so that he opted to settle in the tiny village of Puiseaux (1749/1994, 140). Diderot admired how as "a friend of order" the blind man imparted to his wife and son the laudable habits of order and regularity; blindness, according to the philosophe, needed an orderly world, and humane sighted people could help keep it that way. Moreover, by using raised letters, the blind man could be a good father by reading to his son, a fact that revealed both the blind man's own education and his willingness to pass it on, thereby teaching the boy the value of letters. Even if he departed from the bourgeois ideal by beginning his day as the sun was setting and working through the night, Diderot's blind man more than compensated for this strange schedule. Not only could he work more productively because no one disturbed him, but he could also use the time to return everything that had been moved during the day to its proper place. Thus,

Diderot explained, "when she awoke, his wife would find everything neatly put away" (140). Though disabled and a bit of a recluse, the Blind Man of Puiseaux nonetheless adhered to credible bourgeois values by being an intellect, a good husband and father, and a man who did his share of the work.

Looking more closely at the marriage itself, the blind man both defied and maintained mid-eighteenth-century conventions. "He married to have eyes of his own," Diderot explained. "Before this he had an idea of taking a deaf man as his partner, to whom he could lend ears in exchange for eyes" (1749/ 1994, 146). Interestingly, a nondisabled man would never be considered an appropriate choice for an assistant, and a blind woman would be unthinkable.[3] Somehow, two men with seemingly complementary disabilities failed to threaten the social status quo in the way that a "mixed" pairing (able-bodied/disabled or disabled male/disabled female) might. Thus, the sighted wife proved key to the blind man's survival, even—as in Jameu's case—when he made a comfortable living.

As Adèle Husson, a blind writer steeped in the conservative values of Old Regime France would observe in the following century, "it is of utmost necessity that a blind man take a female companion, because since he can't get around on his own, she becomes his guide, his protector, his guardian angel" (Kudlick and Weygand 2001, 53). This placed a man such as Jameu in a socially awkward position, dependent as he was on a woman for his livelihood. Perhaps sensitive to this predicament, Diderot sought to restore a blind man's wounded manhood in other ways. According to Diderot, a blind man thus might use his impairment to trade up. "There is no risk of his mistaking his wife for another, unless he was to gain by the change," the philosophe coyly told readers (1749/ 1994, 146). In this way Diderot allowed that a blind man could enjoy the rights and privileges of manhood just like his sighted counterparts. Not only must his wife be his helpmate, but he could—and perhaps even should—reap the benefits of the double standard, whereby he could find pleasure with other women while his wife was expected to remain faithful. But for all his attempts to make the Blind Man of Puiseaux respectable, the philosopher-cum-proto-anthropologist suggested that blindness raised disquieting questions about manhood that someone such as Jameu would encounter as he responded to his wife's petition.

Jean-Denis Jameu began his memoir by recounting the history of his life. Dwelling but little on his childhood years, he noted only that he had been blind since the age of five and that his parents owned "a big cloth selling business" on the rue Poissonnière. At the age of fourteen "in order to shelter me from the surprises that the loss of sight would expose me," his parents sent him to live at the Quinze-Vingts Hospital (210–211). Begun in the mid-thirteenth century by Saint Louis, the Paris institution was intended to lodge three hundred (fifteen times twenty, i.e., *quinze-vingts*) needy blind people from throughout the kingdom. They lived in an isolated enclave administered by officials of the Catholic Church, sometimes learning a craft but more often remaining idle except to beg for alms on the streets of Paris (Bentounsi 1976). Since Jameu had grown up in a family of cloth merchants, he quickly mastered and even surpassed the rudimentary sewing skills offered by the institution's poorly qualified teachers. Thus, he proudly described how he became expert at telling the value of cloth and pricing it through touch. "I seemed to have eyes at the tips of my fingers," he explained with pride (211).

At twenty-eight, his family thought it high time to marry him off. Since blindness compromised his social standing and his parents feared that no one would see him as a suitable match, they fell upon the young Mlle Verset who had recently come to work at the shop and lodge with them. "She was a girl without parents, without possessions, without hopes," Jameu reported in his testimony, "but she had a talent for sales, and appeared to like working." As he tells it, she was desperate, seeing the marriage as her only means of survival. Things degenerated quickly after her true "spiteful and absolute" personality began to emerge (212). Jameu felt he had only two means for dealing with the situation, which he characterized as: "the tone and gestures that are in common use to return a woman to reason, and the second being to arm myself with patience" (212).

Jameu believed that by opting for patience he had helped accelerate the long and steady decline that increasingly characterized their marriage. For a time he thought that having children would help. But as often happened in this era before advances in hygiene and medicine, nearly all of them died young. On top of everything else, his wife showed a distinct dislike for their only surviving daughter, which only exacerbated the growing tensions within the household. Finally, after eight years of marriage, Mme Jameu made it known that she no longer wanted to sleep with him. As he put it in his puckish way, "she had her bed changed, taking instead one that was so narrow that it was not possible for me to share it with her" (213). He relegated himself to a far corner of the house with his harpsichord (which his wife detested) and a few other small items, including a mattress on the floor. To provide room for cloth workers whom she had hired on her own, Verset soon made Jameu unwelcome even in his own shop. Thus, he moved to the sales room where, according to his testimony, he lived for nine years sleeping on piles of cloth on the countertop without mattress or blanket (214).

Almost more troubling to Jameu than the physical discomfort he endured was the humiliation he had to face as rumors of this unusual sleeping arrangement raced through the neighborhood. "I didn't complain," he asserted. When neighbors scolded his wife, he claimed that she responded by saying that her husband wanted it that way, as a form of mortification. "Turning me into a saint so that she wouldn't have the reputation of being a wicked woman!" Jameu fumed, "now, if that isn't a tactless manipulation of the truth!"(214).

They came to real blows over the marriage of their only surviving daughter. Jameu claimed that he wanted her to marry the man she loved, while his wife sought a more profitable business match. For once, he said, he dug in his heels, refusing his wife's choice at any cost. He won a pyrrhic victory, at least in terms of his own life, for tensions had grown so high that he returned to live in his own apartment at the Quinze-Vingts as the marriage plans progressed. Because space was always limited and many desperate blind people sought to live within its protected walls, Jameu must have offered to pay his own way or he managed to make an extremely convincing case to the director. Just before the wedding day, he urged his wife to join him there in order to leave the house to the newlyweds as promised in the marriage contract. Not only did she refuse, but according to Jameu, she remained in the house making life so miserable for the young couple that they fled, only to return to find that she had removed most of the furniture. "Up to this point," Jameu concluded the story of his life, "there were insults and excesses, but they did not come from me. However my wife, who sensed how dreadful her conduct had been, took it upon herself to bring a formal complaint against me. . . . " (219).

Having outlined the story of his life, Jameu sought systematically to disprove Verset's charges against him. To her claim that he was "debauched and violent," he asked, "why did she suffer for twenty years without complaining? Did she need to wait until after robbing me to demand a separation?" (221). To her claim that he had wanted to separate years before and "have each of us enter a convent" because he hadn't been cut out for marriage, he retorted that he would have invoked his condition as a blind man (what he called "*mon état*") and never have gotten married in the first place. "If I got married," he asserted, "it was because this is what I really wanted" (223). To her claim that she suffered a miscarriage because of trauma she experienced upon seeing her husband fall while drunk, he reminded readers that a blind man does not have to be drunk in order to take a fall (223). And to her claim that he beat her on two occasions, once by supposedly kicking her in the stomach, and a second time by throwing a chair at her head so hard that after eight years she still had the marks to prove it, and alleging that he did so because she wouldn't accompany him to a fireworks display near the home of a prostitute he hoped to visit, he fumed, "Why didn't she say that I had hit her with a cane? My condition obliges me always to carry one, and this gesture would have been much more natural than throwing a chair at her head. Besides," he went on, "it is so easy to duck a punch and escape from a blind man, [so] her story simply isn't believable." Above all, he asked, "why would a blind man want to go see fireworks in the first place, especially if he had a lady friend in the neighborhood?" (227–228).

Far more troubling to Jameu was his wife's claim that she was doing him a good deed (*une grâce*) by marrying him. "I thank her" he said curtly, "but believe I have already more than paid her back" (223). He explained that

> as a blind man, I was a useful man about the house. As the loss of one
> sense profits the others, nature, who wishes to lose nothing, always finds
> a way to compensate us, and my wife knows this very well. What
> services didn't I provide, either in folding and unfolding merchandise,

or in blocking pieces of cloth or in sewing? All of Paris comes to admire my place [*mon adresse*] and since ordinarily this curiousness wasn't without motives [*cette curoisité n'étoit pas stérile*], this could only help our commerce. In a word, my wife may have had good eyes, but she had no possessions; I was blind, but I gave her an establishment. (224)

Or, as he put it in the bluntest possible terms: "Monsieur was of equal value to Madame" (224).

What can we learn from such a story about the attitudes toward blind people and gender expectations in old regime France? Clearly, Jameu found himself married to Verset for many of the same reasons that would influence a sighted man of his class standing: economic need and social convention. In the Parisian petite bourgeoisie of the Old Regime, marriage often resembled a business partnership more than the sentimental bond it would become later in the nineteenth century, and it was obvious from Jameu's defense that he viewed it as such. Thus, regardless of her husband's blindness, a wife such as Verset would be expected to help run a business, engaging in all aspects from bookkeeping to supervising employees. In many cases when a husband had been obliged to travel, it wasn't uncommon for a woman to manage a business on her own. But even as a wife played a valuable role in maintaining the household's economic livelihood, it remained clear that this was a partnership in which the husband dominated. Furthermore, in a traditional family, a wife was also expected to bear the children who would perpetuate the family name and carry on the business. Even if someone such as Verset ultimately broke with her only surviving daughter, the aggrieved wife did fulfill her social obligations by being a mother.

But Jameu's condition also made marriage different. Not eligible to join the clergy because of his blindness, he needed to be married to a sighted woman if he wanted to maintain his social standing and way of life. At the age of twenty-eight, his parents had married him off, much like they would a daughter to someone beneath them. They offered their shop almost like a dowry, expecting only a small one from his prospective wife; had Jameu not been blind, it's likely that the family would have wanted a woman with greater resources than Verset had to offer. Fearful that their blind son might remain dependent forever, the parents jumped at the first opportunity, a desperate boarder-employee already living under their own roof. If Jameu had been brought to the marriage like a woman, in many respects Verset conducted herself as a man once she got there. She hired and fired employees without consulting her husband, even though it would have been easy for her to seek his opinion, because he constantly worked in the shop. In fact, more often than not—at least according to Jameu—the "spiteful and absolute" woman dealt with him as an employee of inferior social standing. And if that wasn't enough, she treated him almost like a husband would treat a wife. She banished him to various parts of the house much like a man might have sent an unwanted woman off to a convent. She attempted to negotiate the marriage of their daughter without his consent. Forced by the circumstances of his blindness to endure these affronts to his manly role without complaint, Jameu finally cracked. Verset had petitioned for separation because, according to Jameu, he had started asserting his rights as a man. Put another way, the delicate topsy-turvy gender equilibrium of the Jameu marriage was destroyed when they each began to play the appropriate roles society had assigned to them as man and wife.

Not insignificantly, both Verset and Jameu each clung even more strongly to their assigned gender roles in their respective appeals. Verset followed the lead of generations of women before her to petition for separation and came up with the appropriate formula to make her plea; judging from Jameu's responses, she never invoked his blindness as an issue, only the manly acts of violence, drinking, and debauch sanctioned by custom and by law as part of the appeals process. For his part, Jameu spoke of entitlement, to his furniture, his pride, and his wife. "I'm told it's a matter of principle," he noted, "that the husband is head of his household [*le mari est maître de la communauté*], and as a consequence, the wife is not allowed to dispose of the furnishings that are a part of it without her husband's consent" (219–220). Her behavior, he testified, had crossed a line because she had lied in order to cover her crimes against him and also because she had undermined his manly authority.

Finally, the gravest insult, and the act that had prompted Jameu to write a twenty-eight page published defense, was that by bringing their story into the open, Verset herself had gone to the court of public opinion, thereby humiliating him and tarnishing his male honor. The decades before the French Revolution proved to be an especially ripe time for using court documents as a form of public entertainment, at the same time that cases such as Jameu's provided a forum of open discussion about everything from politics to gender roles. Growing literacy combined with a spectacularly litigious society to produce a new genre of published writing that simultaneously "seduced and instructed" a public that assumed an increasingly important role in French political culture (Maza 1993, 12). By the time it was published in 1769, Jameu's mémoire would be part of a genre that would outsell all others in the prerevolutionary decades. The spicy stories and the literary ambitions of the lawyers who wrote them played to a public hungry to read the lurid details of people who broke the law or the rules of social convention (Maza 1993). Responding to the fact that Verset had made their private conflict public, Jameu and his lawyer sought to produce a document that would use the same publicity to preserve his position as a man in the Old Regime.

In defending his manhood, Jameu also sought to maintain his social standing as a bourgeois Parisian merchant. The full title of his petition makes this clear, by referring to him as "Jean-Denis Jameu, Bourgeois de Paris." Surely the return to the Quinze-Vingts wounded his pride, forced as he was to leave his home and business only to find himself once again surrounded by the inferior masses of Parisian blind people. On several occasions in his testimony, for example,

Jameu stressed that he was not like the usual blind beggars that one saw in the streets; he even paused to give a brief narration of the different classes of blind inhabitants at the Quinze-Vingts, so that his readers would have a clear understanding that he belonged to the institution's elite residents. With some sympathy for those beneath him yet with obvious pride in his more elevated social standing, Jameu explained how the poorer blind people wore a uniform embroidered with the royal fleur-de-lys, which gave them a legitimate right to beg in the Paris streets. "People of my class," he noted, "wear neither the uniform nor the fleur de lys" (224–225). Moreover, he clearly took great pride in contributing so much to the success of his cloth enterprise, referring to it in elevated language such as "*mon adresse.*" He wanted it known that his wife would never have made it without him; not only did he inherit a successful business from his family, but, according to him, he was the one who gave it the order and respectability that attracted quality patrons. Because a husband's dominant position and significant contributions to running a family business would have been a given, a sighted man probably would not have drawn attention to his accomplishments in the same way or for the same reasons. Jameu seemed to understand as he knew his judges probably would: to speak of a blind merchant was not unlike speaking of a female merchant. To obtain a ruling in his favor, he had to strike a delicate balance between his independent manhood and his greater need for his wife's assistance so essential to maintaining his economic and social class standing.

Jameu also used his blindness to interesting advantage in order to defend his manhood. A century later when disability had become fully sentimentalized and rendered unquestionably feminine in a world with more strictly defined gender roles, a man in Jameu's predicament might have easily tugged at the heartstrings of his judges by invoking pitiful descriptions of his helpless state.[4] But in the decades before romanticism helped transform pity into a weapon, Jameu presented his blindness as the key element in a reasoned defense: a blind man carries a cane, a blind man aims badly, a blind man is useful because he takes advantage of other senses, therefore a blind man could not possibly have done what his unruly wife accused him of doing. In using his blindness logically rather than emotionally, Jameu discussed it matter-of-factly at the same time that—unconsciously, anyway—he wrote against the feminized position in which it placed him. Thus, viewed through Jameu, blindness could not be easily categorized even as it played a vital role in fixing a blind man in a complex gendered social order.

Jameu's story reveals how a disability—in this case blindness—can offer a new perspective on ideas about gender and the expectations the Parisian bourgeoisie attached to it. Interestingly, disability has a contradictory relationship with the status quo. On the one hand, Jameu taught us, blindness reinforced existing values, in effect providing a pretext for keeping things as they always were. Jameu and Verset each returned again and again to traditional gendered arguments to underscore the severity of the wrongs that had been done them. In this way, they each sought to make blindness more normal so that Verset's appeal and Jameu's response might follow the appropriate channels for winning the case or, at the very least, public opinion. On the other hand, Jameu's blindness undeniably forced the couple to have a relationship that—were it not for his disability—parts of which would have been condemned as socially inappropriate. Clearly, Jameu depended upon his wife more than most "normal" men would; he married Verset out of the same needs that would have motivated a woman seeking a partner, and he relied on her far more than a traditional husband would admit. Moreover, he seemed to accept his wife's affronts to his manhood virtually without complaint, at least compared with what one might expect from a male ideal that didn't freely succumb to women's wishes.

It would be hard to know to what extent this unusual dynamic explained the failure of their marriage, if living out of step with the rest of the Parisian petit bourgeoisie proved to be too much of a strain on a couple trying to be respectable and respected in the highly competitive cloth trade. It's possible that had they been better suited personally, the Jameus would have offered the numerous customers who came to admire their shop a different option for how a man and a woman could function in the world. But in the turbulent decades on the eve of the French Revolution that would raise so many difficult questions about gender and class, this may have been too much to ask. Perhaps it was the search for stability in anticipation of this great social and cultural upheaval that made Parisian men and women nervously chuckle over the odd story of a blind man snubbed by his wife's narrow bed.

Acknowledgments

The author wishes to thank Sara Maza, Suzanne Desan, and her friends at he Coronado Center for the Blind for comments on earlier drafts.

Notes

1. Because this account appeared in a collection entitled *Causes amusantes et connues* in 1769, it was probably published illicitly but had sufficient appeal to enjoy public distribution. For a discussion of the genre, see Sarah Maza (1993). For a discussion of the clandestine press more generally during the Old Regime, see Robert Darnton (1982).
2. The Napoleonic Code restricted divorce until it became illegal again under the Restoration and remained so until 1884.
3. A blind woman, by contrast, was never expected to marry, an idea discussed in greater detail for the nineteenth century in Kudlick and Weygand (2001).
4. Though France has its variants on nineteenth-century sentimentality (see, e.g., Margaret Cohen, *The Sentimental Education of the Novel*, Princeton, N.J.: Princeton University Press, 1999), the links between sentimentality and blindness have been more fruitfully explored for America, particularly with respect to women. See James Emmett Ryan, The Blind Authoress of New York: Helen DeKroyft and the Uses of Disability in Antebellum America, *American Quarterly* (June 1999) and Mary Klages,

Woeful Afflictions: Disability and Sentimentality in Victorian America (Philadelphia: University of Pennsylvania Press, 1999).

Works Cited

Bentounsi, Yasmine. 1976. Les Quinze-Vingts dans la Second Moitié du XVIIIe Siècle (1742–1799). Master's Thesis, Université de Paris X, Nanterre.

Cohen, Margaret. 1999. *The sentimental education of the novel*. Princeton, N.J.: Princeton University Press.

Darnton, Robert. 1982. *The literary underground of the old regime*. Cambridge, Mass.: Harvard University Press.

Diderot, Denis. 1749/1994. Lettre sur les aveugles à l'usage de ceux qui voient (Letter on the blind for the benefit of those who see). In *Philosophie*, vol. one of *Ouvres*. Paris: Editions Robert Laffont.

Hanley, Sarah. 1997. Social sites of political practice in France: Lawsuits, civil rights, and the separation of powers in domestic and state government, 1500–1800. *American Historical Review* 102 (1): 27–52.

Hardwick, Julie. 1998. Seeking separations: Gender, marriages, and household economies in Early-Modern France. *French Historical Studies* 21 (1) (winter): 157–180.

Henri, Pierre. 1984. *La Vie et l'oeuvre de Valentin Haüy*. Paris: Presses Universitaires de France.

Jameu, Jean-Denis. 1769. Mémoire pour Jean-Denis Jameu, Bourgeois de Paris: Contre Demoiselle Anne-Cecille Verset, sa femme. Reprinted in *Causes amusantes et connues* (1769). Compiled by Robert Estienne. Berlin: Anonymous.

Klages, Mary 1999. *Woeful afflictions: Disability and sentimentality in Victorian America*. Philadelphia: University of Pennsylvania Press.

Kudlick, Catherine J. 1999. The helpless and the hopeless in cross-cultural context: Narratives of little blind girls in nineteenth-century France and America. Paper presented at Berkshire Conference of Women Historians. Rochester, New York.

Kudlick, Catherine J., and Zina Weygand. 2001. *Reflections: The life and writings of a young blind woman in post-revolutionary France*. New York: New York University Press.

Maza, Sarah. 1993. *Private lives and public affairs: The causes célébres of prerevolutionary France*. Berkeley: University of California Press.

Phillips, Roderick. 1980. *Marriage and family breakdown in eighteenth-century France: Divorce in Rouen, 1792–1803*. Oxford: Clarendon, Oxford University Press.

———. 1988. *Putting asunder: A history of divorce in western society*. Cambridge, Eng.: Cambridge University Press.

Ryan, James Emmett. 1999. The blind authoress of New York: Helen DeKroyft and the uses of disability in antebellum America. *American Quarterly* (June).

Traer, James. 1980. *Marriage and the family in eighteenth-century France*. Ithaca, N.Y.: Cornell University Press.

Weygand, Zina. 1998. La Cécité et les aveugles dans la société française: représentations et institutions du moyen age aux premières années du XIXe siècle. Doctoral Thesis, Université de Paris I, Panthéon Sorbonne, U.F.R. d'Histoire.

———. 1999. La Lettre (1749) et ses Additions (1782): La parole aux aveugles. *Voir Barré: Périodique du Centre de recherche sur les aspects culturels de la vision* 18, 16–29.

Wilson, James. 1821–1838. *Biography of the blind*. Washington, D.C.: Library of Congress; reprint 1995.

Bodies in Trouble

IDENTITY, EMBODIMENT, AND DISABILITY

⚜

KRISTIN LINDGREN

As many feminist philosophers have observed, there is a long history in Western metaphysics of devaluing the body.[1] In the *Phaedo*, Plato articulates a view that has shaped this history of somatophobia:

> the body provides us with innumerable distractions in the pursuit of our necessary sustenance; and any diseases which attack us hinder our quest for reality. . . . It seems that so long as we are alive, we shall continue closest to knowledge if we avoid as much as we can all contact and association with the body . . . and instead of allowing ourselves to become infected with its nature, purify ourselves from it until God himself gives us deliverance. (1969, 111)

What interests me in this familiar passage is Plato's explicit naming of disease as an impediment to philosophy. While he welcomes death as the moment of the soul's release from embodiment, Plato seems to view disease as further debasing a body that is, by its very nature, a source of contamination. If the healthy body, with its unruly needs and appetites, inevitably distracts the philosopher from the pursuit of knowledge, then the diseased body, even more unpredictable and unruly, must surely halt the project of philosophy altogether.[2]

In an essay entitled "On Being Ill," first published in 1930, Virginia Woolf observes that literature, like philosophy, aspires to transcendence. She notes that "literature does its best to maintain that its concern is with the mind; that the body is a sheet of plain glass through which the soul looks straight and clear" (1948, 9–10). Woolf aims to overturn this view of the body as a transparent medium, asserting: "All day, all night the body intervenes; blunts or sharpens, colours or discolours. . . . The creature within can only gaze through the pane–

smudged or rosy; it cannot separate off from the body like the sheath of a knife or the pod of a pea for a single instant; it must go through the whole unending procession of changes, heat and cold, comfort and discomfort, hunger and satisfaction, health and illness" (10). It seems to me no accident that Woolf's meditation on embodiment, and her claim that the "creature within" can experience the world only in and through its body, occurs in an essay about illness. In health it may be possible to ignore the body, but in illness it demands acknowledgement and attention. Both Plato and Woolf recognize the difficulty of disavowing a diseased body, but they make very different valuations of physical experience. While in the *Phaedo* Plato finds the life of the body a distraction to philosophers and an unfit subject for philosophy, Woolf finds it "strange indeed that illness has not taken its place with love and battle and jealousy among the prime themes of literature." She calls for a literature that describes the "daily drama of the body" and, specifically, the experience of illness (9–10).

Nearly three-quarters of a century after Woolf lamented the paucity of writing about illness, there is a rich autobiographical literature chronicling the experiences of illness and disability.[3] In the first major study of the body of literature she terms "pathography," Anne Hunsaker Hawkins asserts: "As a genre, pathography is remarkable in that it seems to have emerged *ex nihilo*; book-length accounts of illness are uncommon before 1950 and rarely found before 1900" (1993, 3). Though there are several examples of this genre penned in the nineteenth century, and its longer history can be traced in works such as John Donne's *Devotions Upon Emergent Occasions*, published in 1624, it is undeniable that the genre has flourished in recent years. Its current proliferation and popularity can be attributed to several factors, including the rise of the literary memoir, the growing interest in previously marginalized voices, and the culturally sanctioned questioning of medical authority. Narratives of illness and disability are also, perhaps above all, products of a cultural moment in which talk of bodies and selves saturates both academic and popular discourse.[4]

These autobiographical narratives claim bodily experience as an important epistemological category. They support neither Plato's view of the unruly body as an impediment to knowledge nor a view of the body as a transparent medium through which the self enacts its projects. Rather, they suggest that embodied experience generates knowledge and crucially shapes these projects. Moreover, they characterize living with what Nancy Mairs (1996b) calls a "body in trouble" as itself a conscious project, one that demands a strategic rethinking of self-identity. First-person accounts of illness and disability demonstrate that knowledges produced by bodies in trouble can contribute in unique ways to theories of identity, subjectivity, and embodiment.

Our Bodies, Ourselves

In recent years, theorists in many disciplines have been thinking about bodies, and feminist theorists in particular have worked to reclaim the value of the body and its experiences. However, the body in trouble has too often remained unexplored terrain. Feminist theory, even as it aims to privilege bodily experience, sometimes reenacts Plato's devaluation of the diseased body. Because women have historically been seen as more embodied than men, first-wave feminist thinkers working to demonstrate that "anatomy is not destiny" often advocated the idea of transcending or exercising control over somatic experience.[5] Recent feminist approaches to the body can also perpetuate the devaluation of a body that does not conform to certain norms or ideals.[6] When a body is both female and diseased or impaired, it can be viewed, and experienced, as doubly corporeal, doubly devalued, and, as Nancy Mairs (1996a) suggests, doubly shameful. Men with disabilities do not escape devaluation; a disabled male body is often feminized, seen as both vulnerable and darkly powerful.[7] Without a sustained consideration of the experience and representation of illness and disability, theories of embodiment, including feminist theories, too often depend on an abstract idea of a normative body rather than on the widely varied forms and experiences of actual bodies. A focus on the body in trouble can contribute to the feminist project of revaluing bodily experience and to the development of more nuanced and inclusive theories of the body.

In thinking about embodiment, feminists have often challenged the mind/body dualism that is a prominent feature of Western philosophy. For example, Elizabeth Grosz calls for the development of a more fluid way of conceptualizing the relationship between body and mind, a relation hinted at by the terms "*embodied subjectivity*" or "*psychical corporeality*" (Grosz 1994, 22). Recontextualizing a metaphor she borrows from Lacan, Grosz suggests the Möbius strip as a model for the constantly shifting relationship she posits between body and mind, one that she characterizes as "the torsion of the one into the other, the passage, vector, or uncontrollable drift of the inside into the outside and the outside into the inside" (xii). Illness narratives offer a resonant site for testing this metaphor. People who live with illness or disability are often compelled to rethink the relation between body and mind or body and self; in so doing, they both support and challenge Cartesian dualism, revealing the potential fluidity of the mind/body relation but also the persistent power, and sometimes the practical usefulness, of ideas of disembodiment and transcendence.

In developing new models of embodiment, many feminist theorists have looked to the tradition of existential phenomenology, particularly the work of Maurice Merleau-Ponty.[8] A phenomenological approach, which locates consciousness and subjectivity in the body and emphasizes lived experience and perception, contributes crucial insights both to theories of embodied subjectivity and to our understanding of the experience of illness. Most phenomenological accounts of illness or disability, however, rely on hypothetical cases or on third-person accounts by physicians or psychoanalysts. Autobiographical narratives, in contrast, provide descriptions of phenomena and reflections on embodiment from the point of view of the person who has lived the experience. In arguing for the importance of first-person narratives, I do not intend to suggest that they offer unmediated access to the body's truths. Experience is mediated by language and by sociocultural and historical forces, and these accounts of bodily experience are also shaped by literary choices and conventions. Narrative representations of lived experience can, however, deepen and complicate our understanding of the phenomenology of illness, pain, and disability and can reshape our views on embodiment.[9]

Incorporating the perspective of people with illnesses and disabilities into our models of embodiment and subjectivity has important implications for how we conceive of self-identity. Anyone who lives with illness needs to develop both practical and theoretical strategies for living with a body that no longer provides a stable ground for self.[10] For many people, living with a radically unpredictable body, or a body that has lost functions or parts, calls into question the stability and continuity of identity. The rhetoric of "my old self" and "my new self" pervades autobiographical narratives of illness and disability. These narratives make clear that illness represents not only a crisis in the body but also a crisis in self-identity. Hawkins contends that first-person accounts, by confronting the reader with the "pragmatic reality and experiential unity of the autobiographical self," challenge postmodern skepticism about the status of the self (1993, 17). I argue, in contrast, that these accounts, rather than solidifying a humanist idea of the self as stable and unified, often support postmodern ideas of selfhood and ground these ideas in bodily experience.[11]

In the narratives I examine here, the new self constructed in the wake of illness is often described not as a distinct, bounded entity entirely separate from the old self but as a fluid configuration in which elements of old and new, self and other, inside and outside, exist concurrently. This configuration, which recalls Grosz's metaphor of a Möbius strip, challenges a model of identity predicated on excluding the other, a model that underlies some of the discriminatory beliefs and practices that affect those of us with disabilities. The paradigms of selfhood that emerge from these narratives contribute to the development of models of identity that incorporate difference and change.

In the next section of this chapter, I draw on both phenomenological and autobiographical accounts of illness to discuss the ways in which the lived experience of illness and disability reshapes the relation between body and self. I then turn to a discussion of immunity and identity to show that the dominant models of both are defined by what they exclude. This logic of exclusion, I suggest, coupled with the lived experience of one's body in illness as alien or unfamiliar, often leads us to conceptualize disease as an alien invader within the self. Turning again to autobiographical narratives, I explore the ways in which the authors of these accounts explicate, question, and reshape the powerful metaphor of alien invasion, and I suggest that their uses of this metaphor have important implications for reimagining both identity and illness. In examining the experience and representation of illness and disability, I draw on contemporary essays and memoirs by Robert Murphy, Susan Wendell, Nancy Mairs, Amy Ling, Judith Hooper, and Reynolds Price.

Disembodiment, Transcendence, and Reembodiment

In his phenomenological account of embodiment, *The Absent Body* (1990), Drew Leder argues that the healthy, normally functioning body disappears from awareness. This lived experience of bodily absence, he suggests, contributes to the conceptual power of Cartesian dualism (3). According to Leder, it is often at times of bodily dysfunction, such as pain or disease, that our bodies come to conscious awareness. He goes on to examine how these experiences of dysfunction transform one's relation to one's body: "In pain, the body or a certain part of the body emerges as an *alien presence*. The sensory insistence of pain draws the corporeal out of self-concealment, rendering it thematic. No event more radically and inescapably reminds us of our bodily presence. Yet at the same time pain effects a certain alienation . . . The painful body is often experienced as something foreign to the self" (76). Thematization of the body at times of dysfunction, a phenomenon he terms "dys-appearance," leads to an awareness of the body as "separate from and opposed to the 'I'" (88). Thus, in Leder's account, the experiences of both health and disease, each in a distinct way, seem to support the principle of mind/body dualism.

There are important differences, however, between a healthy body that is absent from consciousness and a diseased one that is negatively present to consciousness. In health, the split between body and mind is experienced as a positive or neutral absence; in illness, this split can be accompanied by a sense of the body as an other to the self, a problematic object that interferes with the self's projects. For Leder, as for Merleau-Ponty, the body can never be an object like other objects; a person is never without a body, and the self that observes or objectifies the body is always an embodied self (Merleau-Ponty 1962; Leder 1990). Nonetheless, he suggests, pain or disease (as well as other experiences of rapid bodily change, such as puberty, pregnancy, aging, or the acquisition of new skills) can engender a certain objectification of and alienation from one's body: "Whenever our body becomes an object of perception, even though it perceives itself, an element of distance is introduced. I no longer simply 'am' my body, the set of unthematized powers from which I exist. Now I 'have' a body, a perceived object in the world" (Leder 1990, 77). The distinction between "being" a body and "having" one is at the heart of debates about the nature of embodiment. As Leder recognizes, experiences of bodily dysfunction can illuminate these debates; he notes that "such disruptive experiences have . . . a certain phenomenological power and demand quality that makes them central in shaping our views on embodiment" (70).

In an account that supports many of Leder's claims, the anthropologist Robert Murphy describes in *The Body Silent* (1990) his experience of becoming progressively paralyzed by a benign tumor growing in his spinal column: "My impairment . . . is a precondition of my plans and projects, a first premise of all my thoughts. Just as my former sense of embodiment remained taken for granted, positive, and unconscious, my sense of disembodiment is problematic, negative, and conscious. My identity has lost its stable moorings and has become contingent on a physical flaw" (104–105). Murphy's description suggests that the experience of disabling illness not only brings the body to consciousness but also reveals the extent to which our sense of a stable identity is dependent on an unchanging, taken-for-granted body. Bodily dysfunction can create a fracture between self and body that demands a rethinking of the relation between them. Murphy asserts that people with paraplegia or quadriplegia, most of whom are not born with these conditions, "have to become reembodied to their impairments. And if their condition is grave enough, they may even have to become disembodied" (100).

As Murphy's condition progresses to quadriplegia, he traces his own gradual process of disembodiment. He comes to view his body as a "faulty life-support system, the only function of which is to sustain my head," and he employs a strategy of "radical dissociation from the body, a kind of etherealization of identity" (1990, 101). Describing how this plays out in practice, Murphy observes that he refers to his own limbs as "*the* leg or *the* arm" and that his caretakers follow his lead, saying, for example, "'I'll hold the arms and you grab the legs'" (100). He adds that "the paralytic becomes accustomed to being lifted, rolled, pushed, pulled, and twisted, and he survives this treatment by putting emotional distance between himself and his body" (101). As Murphy's narrative reveals, the body can become other to the self not only through belief systems that devalue it or cultural practices that discipline it, but also through an experiential rending of the unity of body and self or an adaptive response to physical disability.

The disidentification of body and self can help a person with disabilities not to feel reduced to her body. The philosopher Susan Wendell, who lives with CFIDS/ME,[12] gives another example of conscious dissociation:

> In general, being able to say (usually to myself): 'My body is painful (or nauseated, exhausted, etc.), but I'm happy,' can be very encouraging and lift my spirits, because it asserts that the way my body feels is not the totality of my experience, that my mind and feelings can wander beyond the painful messages of my body, and that my state of mind is not completely dependent on the state of my body. . . . In short, I am learning not to identify myself with my body, and this helps me to live a good life with a debilitating chronic illness." (1996, 174)

As Wendell points out, such a strategy is not the same as ignoring her body (173), nor is it the same as being alienated from bodily experience (177). Recognizing the importance of gender in shaping our views on embodiment, she suggests that feminist theorists often reject ideas of transcendence because they are seen as rooted in a long history of devaluing women's bodies and somatic experience in general. She contends that feminists overlook the importance of bodily suffering as a motive for wanting to transcend the body and calls for a new understanding of transcendence grounded in strategies of disembodiment, strategies that in her view do not limit freedom of consciousness but rather increase it.

Wendell's version of transcendence, rather than stemming from a desire to control the body or to purify the self from its appetites and demands, grows out of a respect for bodily experience, even that which causes suffering. This idea of transcendence is grounded in her observation that the experience of pain and disease "can teach consciousness a certain freedom from the sufferings and limitations of the body" (1996, 172). Like Murphy, Wendell emphasizes the alteration of identity that accompanies disability. Noting that illness has brought not only pain and limitations but also new interests, knowledges, and projects, she asserts: "my body has led me to a changed identity, a very different sense of myself, even as I have come to identify myself less with what is occurring in my body" (175).

Murphy's and Wendell's accounts illustrate that illness and disability can lead not only to a heightened awareness of the body, as Leder argues, but also to a conscious negotiation of the relation between body and self, a negotiation that leads them to practice, and to see the value of, strategies of disembodiment, disidentification, and transcendence. For poet and essayist Nancy Mairs, disability leads to a very different strategy; in the essays "Carnal Acts" and "Body in Trouble" she describes her struggle to "embrace [her]self in the flesh" (Mairs 1996a, 96), to *identify* with a body crippled by multiple sclerosis and with a female body from which cultural values operate to alienate her. Explaining that disability has forced her to rethink the relation between body and self, she supports Leder's account of the connection between health, bodily awareness, and dualist paradigms: "The physical processes of a perfectly healthy person may impinge so little on her sense of well-being that she may believe herself separate from and even in control of them. From here it's a short leap to the conviction that cerebral phenomena are of a different, generally higher, order than other bodily events"(1996b, 41–42).

At the same time, Mairs counters Leder's description of the split between body and self experienced by a person living with pain or disease. She claims, instead, that living with MS has challenged her culturally instilled assumptions about embodiment and forced her to locate her self firmly in her body: "This, for me, has been the most difficult aspect of adjusting to a chronic incurable degenerative disease: the fact that it has rammed my 'self' straight back into the body I had been trained to believe it could, through high-minded acts and aspirations, rise above. . . . I *have* a body, you are likely to say if you talk about embodiment at all; you don't say, I *am* a body" (1996a, 84). Mairs asserts that illness has led her to identify more completely with her body, to embrace the idea of being a body rather than having one. In her view, the body cannot be teased apart from or transcended by a sovereign self; it *is* the self. This is not to say that Mairs would reject Wendell's notion of transcendence of bodily suffering but rather that she rejects an idea of transcendence that assumes we are in control of our bodily experiences. The notion of *having* a body implies that the self exercises control over and even ownership of the body.[13] Illness and disability reveal that the body has a mind of its own.

In Mairs's account, the experience of disabling illness does not support the body/mind split of dualist metaphysics; indeed, she suggests that heightened awareness of the suffering body can work to repair this split. She writes: "The body in trouble, becoming both a warier and a humbler creature, is more apt to experience herself all of a piece: a biochemical dynamo cranking out consciousness much as it generates platelets, feces, or reproductive cells to ensure the manufacture of new dynamos" (1996b, 42). Mairs's assertion that bodily dysfunction leads her to experience herself "all of a piece" stands in contrast to the analyses of Leder and others who stress dysfunction as a moment of fracture and fragmentation. One reason for this difference is that Leder fails adequately to consider the experience of people with chronic or degenerative illness; for these people, bodily breakdown marks not a moment of altered awareness but a continuous process. The same person may experience her body quite differently at the onset of illness and months or years later, and she may employ varying adaptive strategies at different points in her illness.

Mairs's writings make clear that her still uneasy identification with her crippled body is a strategy she has developed over time. Her description of one aspect of this process of identification reveals the conscious will behind it and illustrates, in its initial resonance with and later divergence from Murphy's strategy of dissociation, that negotiation with disability takes widely differing forms:

> For years after I began to have symptoms of MS, I used language to avoid owning them: "The left hand doesn't work anymore," I said. "There's a blurred spot in the right eye.". . . Only gradually have I schooled myself to speak of "my" hand, "my" eyes, thereby taking responsibility for them, though loving them ordinarily remains beyond me. (1996b, 43)

Replacing the distancing rhetoric of "the left hand" with the more intimate language of "my hand," Mairs moves toward experiencing herself as someone who is "all of a piece." However, this experiential unity is not naive or unconscious; rather, it is a consciously developed response to living with disability. Mairs's writings suggest that it is still possible, in illness, to experience oneself as *being* a body, but it is no longer possible to do so in a taken-for-granted, unconscious way. Living with MS has impelled Mairs consciously to reassemble herself.

Mairs's insistence that living with MS has led her newly to envision and experience herself as a unified being also points to a larger problem with phenomenology's emphasis on disease as a time of fracture and alienation. As I have been arguing, people who live with illness or disability often reconceptualize the relationship between their selves and their changing bodies. In so doing, they establish a new body image or corporeal schema; in Murphy's terms, they "become reembodied to their impairments" (1990, 100). This new corporeal schema may or may not be experienced as negative or lacking. Mairs contests the notion that suffering bodies must be seen as "broken," "embattled," or "spoiled" rather than as "human variants" (1996b, 47–48). In a society that embraced a wider variation of bodies and bodily experience as normative, disease and impairment would less frequently be experienced as disruptive and deviant. Adopting the rhetoric of difference rather than brokenness can enable us to see more clearly the knowledges and self-constructions engendered by illness and disability without denying the suffering these conditions sometimes cause.[14]

Over time, chronic illness and disability demand that we develop ways of living our bodies and of thinking about embodiment that facilitate rather than impede our ability to carry out our projects. The distinction between having a body and being one is not only a theoretical issue but also a conundrum of daily life. The differing strategies Murphy, Wendell, and Mairs employ make clear that there is no single way of experiencing or conceptualizing disabled embodiment. Perhaps, as Terry Eagleton has written, "it is not quite true that I have a body, and not quite true that I am one either" (1993, 7). What these strategies share, however, is the rethinking of the relation between body and self in response to changes in the body. Whether it leads to Murphy's "radical dissociation" (1990, 101) or Mairs's "radical materiality" (1996b, 60), disability radically revises views on embodiment and identity. These narratives offer a complex, nuanced account of embodiment, one that recognizes both our embodiedness and our capacity for transcendence. They suggest that in illness, one's self, like one's body, can no longer be unconscious and taken for granted; constructing and reconstructing a self in relation to a body becomes a conscious and continuous project.

Identity and Immunity

This project of self-construction takes place in a sociocultural context and is shaped by interactions with others and by cultural discourses about body, self, and illness. In Western culture, representations of illness and disability are often marked by a form of apotropaic thinking that works to protect healthy and nondisabled people from the ever-present possibility—indeed, the overwhelming likelihood—that they too will someday live with a body in trouble. These representations manage the fear of disease and impairment by constructing distinct boundaries between healthy, able bodies and ill or disabled bodies. As Sander Gilman explains: "[T]he fear we have of our own collapse does not remain internalized. Rather, we project this fear onto the world in order to localize it and, indeed, to domesticate it. For once we locate it, the fear of our own dissolution is removed. Then it is not we who totter on the brink of collapse but rather the Other" (1988, 1). In the age of AIDS, images of containment and contamination have proliferated, and images of threatened borders pervade representations of disease and disability. These representations are always predicated on the notion of a stable body/identity that can be defended against invasion, contamination, or change.[15]

The dominant models of both identity and health rest on what they exclude. The way in which these models reflect each other and become intertwined is revealed by the language of modern immunology, which employs the terms "self" and "nonself" to distinguish between cells belonging to the body and those belonging to foreign matter—harmful bacteria, viruses, or anything else that threatens the health and integrity of the body. This terminology suggests that concepts of self-identity crucially shape the representation, and, I would argue, the experience of disease processes. Like the conceptual distinction self/other, the biomedical distinction between cells labeled "self" and "nonself" presupposes a clearly demarcated boundary between the two, one which, in the prevailing military metaphor of immunity, can be patrolled and defended. The anthropologist Emily Martin, in her study of cultural representations of the immune system, *Flexible Bodies* (1994), makes a link between this popular view of the body as a "defended nation-state" and the protection of individual identity: "In this picture, the boundary between the body ('self') and the external world ('nonself') is rigid and absolute. . . . The maintenance of the purity of self within the borders of the body is seen as tantamount to the maintenance of the self" (52–53). Martin notes that the dominant images of immunity draw either on metaphors of warfare or on representations of the body as a police state that checks identity papers and excludes or executes illegal aliens (54). In both metaphors, the protection and solidification of self-identity is central.

According to the self/nonself model of the immune system, its role is to prevent or overcome disease by attacking anything categorized as "nonself" that threatens the body's boundaries. Autoimmune disease, on the other hand, is the result of an immune system that can no longer distinguish between self and nonself and attacks the body's own tissues as if they constituted a threatening outsider. Within the framework of the self/nonself model, disease is conceptualized either as the failure of the immune system to protect self from nonself or as its misrecognition of self as nonself. In either case, disease is caused by the breakdown of the clear boundary between self and other, inside and outside.[16]

The paradigm of a body defending itself against foreign elements persists even within models of the body based on systems theory and information technologies. Martin traces the development of an alternate model of immunity that she characterizes as "complex, nonhierarchical systems embedded in environments composed of other complexly interacting systems" (1994, 65). Like Martin, Donna Haraway examines changing concepts of the body through immune system discourse; she asserts that the paradigm she describes as a "hierarchical, localized, organic body" has been replaced by a model of the body as "a semiotic system, a complex meaning-producing field" (1991, 211). On this model, bodily systems, including the immune system, communicate through processes similar to those of information technologies, and disease is viewed as "a subspecies of information malfunction or communications pathology . . . a process of misrecognition or transgression of the boundaries of a strategic assemblage called self" (212). Although Haraway's representation of self as a "strategic assemblage" differs markedly from the humanist model of a unitary self, the idea of a self with clear but transgressible boundaries survives in her information model of disease.

Neither Martin nor Haraway addresses how these representations of the immune system and of the body in general shape the lived experience of our bodies; neither examines at any length the perspective of those who live with disease.[17] Autobiographical accounts of disabling illness reveal how powerfully these models of immunity shape the experience and representation of disease and reinforce the idea that the self, as well as the body, is threatened by disease. At the same time, they demonstrate that the lived experience of illness or disability can lead us to question these representations of both identity and health and to generate new models and metaphors.

The Alien Within

The pervasiveness of biomedical and popular images of illness as a foreign agent, coupled with the lived experience of one's body as unfamiliar or alien, makes it very likely that we will imagine illness as an other within the self. This concept of illness is based on a notion of the self as prior to and distinct from the disease that invades it. Thus, a person who becomes ill or disabled, especially as an adult, can experience these conditions as threatening an established sense of self. The desire to defend a threatened identity can produce a strategy of dissociating the self from the disease, similar to the practice of disidentifying self and body discussed earlier in this chapter. While this strategy can sometimes be a useful one, it can also lead to strained and even comical locutions, such as Ronald Reagan's comment after successful surgery for cancer: "I didn't have cancer. I had something inside of me that had cancer in it and it was removed" (qtd. in Sontag 1989, 154). For many people living with chronic or degenerative illness, it becomes difficult to separate the "I" from the "it." When these terms can no longer be disentangled, it is necessary to rethink the structure of selfhood.

Autobiographical writings about illness and disability employ a variety of models and metaphors to reconceptualize the self; frequently, they represent subjectivity as split or doubled, as comprising both self and other. For example, Robert Murphy, paralyzed by a spinal tumor, writes: "I can only liken the situation [of disabling illness] to a curious kind of 'invasion of the body snatchers,' in which the alien intruder and the old occupant coexist in mutual hostility in the same body" (1990, 108). He invokes the metaphor of the "alien intruder" to represent not only the agent of disease but also the unfamiliar self and the altered sociocultural position created by illness or disability. He asserts that a person with disabilities has "been alienated from his old, carefully nurtured, and closely guarded sense of self by a new, foreign, and unwelcome identity" (109). Further, he claims that this altered identity estranges the person with disabilities from his social world: "In my middle age, I had become a changeling, the lot of all disabled people. They are afflicted with a malady of the body that is translated into a cancer within the self and a disease of social relationships. . . . They have become aliens, even exiles, in their own lands" (111). Murphy traces a process whereby disease, represented and experienced as an alien object within the body and self, transforms the ill person into an alien within the social body. This process, experientially familiar to many of us who live with illness, depends on a continuing opposition, or in Murphy's stronger terms, "mutual hostility" between invader and invaded.

The paradigm of illness as an alien other within the self becomes more troublesome and complex when the person living with illness is already viewed as, or experiences herself as, an excluded other. I would suggest that this model is inherently problematic for women, who have historically been positioned as the other, as well as for those seen as others by virtue of race, ethnicity, class, or sexual orientation. In her essay about breast cancer, entitled "The Alien Within" (1999), poet and scholar Amy Ling writes: "labeled a cancer, harboring cancer, fighting to eliminate cancer—these are all positions—sometimes sequential, sometimes simultaneous, and always paradoxical—that I have known" (114). Born in China, Ling and her family were labeled "illegal aliens" in this country when their visitors' visas expired. Although she became a naturalized citizen, Ling reports: "having once been labeled 'undesirable alien' and 'foreign intruder,' I have felt my American identity to be a somewhat tenuous thing" (115). Ling is denied tenure at one institution on the basis of blatantly biased arguments, and her job directing an Asian American Studies program is later threatened by a committee report advising the elimination of interdisciplinary programs, a report that she says "made us sound like a cancer growing at the expense of the legitimate body" (120).

Having been perceived, in multiple contexts, as a threatening intruder, Ling is uncomfortable with the concept of cancer as an alien invader and with treatments based on what she views as military principles and a "scorched–earth policy." More sympathetic to so-called alternative treatments based on the idea that cancer is not a foreign invader but an imbalance that can be righted, Ling reluctantly chooses the conventional Western treatment that Dr. Susan Love has famously termed "slash, poison, and burn" (1999, 124). Trying to eliminate the cancer to save her life, Ling is always aware of the paradoxes of her position and resolves that she "must live with contradictions" (132). If she is to envision herself fighting off an alien invader, she must take up a normative subject position she has never claimed and subscribe to a concept of clear and defensible boundaries that has often worked against her. For Ling, cancer is not only a somatic crisis but also a crisis of conflicting identities. She asks: "How can one survive being both the cancer and the body politic?" (132).[18]

Ling's question points to the need for new ways to conceptualize illness and the altered identity it engenders. Judith Hooper, also writing about breast cancer, imagines her cancer as a mutiny from within rather than an invasion from outside. In "Beauty Tips for the Dead" (1994), Hooper envisions a scenario in which one of her cells "got bored" and instigated a mutiny: "Screw the system! *Viva la revolucion*! Then, like a microscopic Che Guevara, it talked other cells into going along with this. 'We want to build a different kind of cell. *We* have a better idea for a cell'" (127). Reconfiguring the dominant metaphors of alien or military invasion, Hooper's image casts the cancer cells as already part of her body, though a part that has split off from the rest. Her tongue-in-cheek strategy is one of negotiation and compromise rather than hostile engagement: "I try to talk to them. 'Hey cells,' I say. 'Enough already. If there is something you want, let me know; maybe we can come to some sort of compromise'" (127–128). Hooper's images mark a distinctly different approach to conceptualizing disease; like Murphy, she uses a model of split subjectivity, but she emphasizes that the split subject comprises versions of the self rather than a threatened self and an alien invader.

The split subjectivity described by people with illnesses and disabilities can be an alienated one, most clearly represented by metaphors of warfare and alien invasion. However, this split subjectivity can also signal an identity that is predicated on fluid boundaries between self and other. One model of a fluid construction of self grounded in bodily change exists in feminist accounts of pregnancy. For example, Iris Marion Young, drawing on the tradition of existential phenomenology and foregrounding the viewpoint of the pregnant woman, claims that the experience of pregnancy can reconfigure the relationship between inside and outside, self and other, body and mind. Through the shifting of bodily boundaries and the recognition of her body as both "herself and not herself," the pregnant subject, in Young's account, is "de-centered, split, or doubled" (1990, 160). At the risk of seeming to endorse a pathologized view of reproductive processes or of failing to recognize crucial differences between pregnancy and illness, I want to suggest that Young's account of pregnant subjectivity can contribute to conceptualizing the subjectivity of a person who lives with illness or disability.[19] As in Young's description of a pregnant woman experiencing her body as both "herself and not herself," a description of illness or disability from the point of view of the person living with these conditions often includes the experience of one's body as both self and other, as a site of blurred boundaries and decentered subjectivity.

To be sure, when the metaphor of pregnancy is explicitly invoked in relation to disease, it is sometimes used to describe a dark inversion of a desired pregnancy. Susan Sontag notes a tradition of representing cancer as a "demonic pregnancy" (1989, 13). A recent essay by Dr. Jerome Groopman, in which he describes his treatment of a male cancer patient largely through metaphors of battle and commodities trading, notes his physical findings in these terms: "His abdomen was bulging as if he were in his last month of pregnancy, filled with malignant ascites, a mixed brew of protein-rich fluid, that had weeped from his liver, spleen, and lymph nodes and nourished schools of swimming cancer cells" (1997, 16). Groopman's patient takes up and undoes the metaphor of pregnancy and nourishment, saying: "'I had hoped it would be a replay of *The*

Exorcist. . . . Remember how the priest took the demon child out, bloody, ugly creature? I thought the surgeon would do the same'" (13). The jarring image of a demon child suggests not only that this cancer patient and his physician feminize his diseased body but also that he experiences his cancer as a malevolent subject rather than an alien object.[20]

When an illness is life threatening, there can be no easy coexistence of the person and the disease. Nonetheless, some accounts describe an effort to coexist with disease or to incorporate it into the self. In a memoir recounting his treatment for cancer of the spine, the novelist Reynolds Price registers a tension between two ways of imagining this perilous coexistence. He employs two central metaphors to describe the tumor in his spinal cord: "an alien and deadly eel" and a "virtual twin" (1994, 52, 36). The first image evokes a frightening, invasive other, the second a familiar doppelganger. Both representations are based on what he knows about the tumor: that it is long and narrow, shaped like an eel, and that it may have been growing slowly, without causing symptoms, since birth or even in utero. Throughout his narrative, Price juxtaposes these two images. While the image of the eel supports the notion of disease as an alien invader, the metaphor of tumor as twin reveals the often uncanny nature of disease, evoking an entity that is at once familiar and alien, me and not-me. Always aware of the threat it poses, Price nonetheless goes to some lengths to imaginatively incorporate this "twin." His language is striking in its attribution of agency and subjectivity to the twin who inhabits his body; he writes of "sharing the tumor's ongoing life" (56) and of his "sense of the cancer as a thing with its own rights" (36). He continues: "Now it sounds a little cracked to describe, but then I often felt that the tumor was as much a part of me as my liver or lungs and could call for its needs of space and food. I only hoped that it wouldn't need all of me" (36). Only when it unambiguously threatens his life does Price's characterization of his twin become less accepting: he then describes the tumor as "a guest who'd become a kind of lethal twin," and a "ravenous twin" (56–58).

Price's description of the tumor/twin who shares his body, while never explicitly referring to pregnancy, evokes the image of a pregnant woman trying to accommodate the needs and demands of another within her body. Whether a woman has actually experienced pregnancy or not, the awareness that her body likely has the capacity to harbor another living being makes this image a familiar one, one that may be a part of her body image. For a man to summon up the image of being inhabited by another body is a quite different metaphoric leap. It suggests not only that Price may experience illness as a feminine modality of bodily experience but also that this image uniquely conveys the phenomenon of altered boundaries and his uncanny sense of his body as both himself and not himself.

While surgery and radiation successfully halt the growth of Price's tumor, the treatment itself leaves him with paraplegia and searing chronic pain. As he had earlier tried to incorporate the tumor's existence, he now incorporates pain and disability into a transformed sense of himself. His advice to those newly confronted with disabling illness is to find a way "to be somebody else, the next viable you" (183); he characterizes his memoir as an account of a journey "toward the reinvention and reassembly of a life that bears some relations with a now-dead life but is radically altered, trimmed for a whole new wind and route" (189). The title of Price's book, *A Whole New Life*, suggests not only that he has reinvented himself but also that he is newly whole; however, his altered self and reassembled life are constructed from fragments of both old and new, fragments that often exist in tension and contradiction. Although he is free of cancer, Price continues to experience his transformed self as comprising both self and other.

Nancy Mairs, while affirming the experiential truth of disabled subjectivity as split or doubled, aims to repair this split. In "Carnal Acts," she describes her experience of the symptoms of multiple sclerosis:

> In effect, living with this mysterious mechanism feels like having your present self, and the past selves it embodies, haunted by a capricious and mean-spirited ghost, unseen except for its footprints, which trips you even when you're watching where you're going, knocks glassware out of your hand, squeezes the urine out of your bladder before you reach the bathroom, and weights your whole body with a weariness no amount of rest can relieve. An alien invader must be at work. But of course it's not. It's your own body. That is, it's you. (1996a, 83–84)

Mairs's description of the disease process as a "ghost" and an "alien invader" initially reinforces the paradigm of disease as an unwelcome other that has mysteriously invaded the self. Yet she immediately declares this model to be a false one, asserting not only that the imagined invader is simply "your own body" but also that "it's you." On this view, the boundaries dividing invader and invaded, inside and outside, self and body, are illusory. This dissolution of boundaries represents neither a nostalgic desire for a unitary subject nor a sense of collapse. Rather, it extends the idea that illness is uncannily both me and not-me. In this sense, Mairs's image of the self haunted by an invisible ghost can be seen as affirming the uncanny doubleness suggested by Price's metaphor of the twin. Instead of conceiving of her body as a battleground between self and alien invader or as one body enclosing another, Mairs incorporates the not-me into the me, claiming a capacious subjectivity that is always acknowledged to be multiple and shifting, to contain both a "present self" and "past selves."

These descriptions of disease and impairment, like the varied strategies for reconceptualizing the relationship of body to mind or self that I discussed earlier, suggest that there is no single way of conceptualizing disabled subjectivity and self-identity. However, the metaphors Murphy, Ling, Hooper, Price, and Mairs employ reveal that disability often produces a subjectivity that is experienced and represented as split or doubled, as comprising both self and other. Whether the relationship between these entities is characterized as one of hostility, coexistence, or incorporation, these accounts represent illness and disability as challenging the idea of a stable, unified subject and an unchanging identity.

They also question the dominant representation of disease. The metaphor of disease as an alien invader, like the prevailing biomedical paradigm of immunity, reinforces the concept of health as the protection of the boundaries of the body against invasion from outside. These authors, while acknowledging the power and the experiential truth of this metaphor, also recognize its paradoxes, and they reshape it, question it, or provide alternatives to it.

On a model of identity or health based on exclusion of the other, illness and disability can be banished to the margins and the stability and purity of identity can be maintained. However, if the body in trouble is a site at which the distinction between self and other founders, then a model of identity predicated on exclusion founders here too. The altered paradigms of identity and subjectivity that emerge from these first-person narratives are more closely aligned with feminist relational models of the self, and with postmodern versions of subjectivity, than with the humanist concept of a unitary, stable, and exclusionary self.

The lived experience of illness or disability, as it is represented in these autobiographical essays and narratives, demands that we rethink the dominant paradigms of embodiment, identity, and health. The experience of their bodies/selves as constantly in flux, and of the boundaries between self and other, mind and body, inside and outside, as shifting, leads the authors of these narratives to develop a variety of practical, metaphorical, and theoretical strategies for reimagining these concepts. Their accounts suggest that acknowledging the specificity and importance of disabled experience, and valuing the knowledge it engenders, is critical to the development of theories of identity, subjectivity, and the body. Feminist theories and phenomenological accounts of embodied subjectivity can be useful in articulating models of disabled experience; conversely, an examination of the body in trouble, particularly when it foregrounds the viewpoint of people who live with illness and disability, enlarges and complicates the projects of both phenomenology and feminism. Sustained attention to the lived experience and representation of illness and disability can ground theories of embodiment in the widely varied experience of actual bodies, contribute to rethinking the relationship between body and self, and foster the development of models of identity that incorporate difference. The rich autobiographical literature of illness and disability provides a fertile ground both for efforts to conceptualize disabled experience and for the production of richer, more specific, and more inclusive theories of bodies and selves.

Acknowlegments

I would like to thank Michelle Friedman, Anne Dalke, Juana Rodriguez, and Carol Bernstein for their helpful comments on an earlier version of this essay.

Notes

1. See especially Elizabeth V. Spelman, "Woman as Body, Ancient and Contemporary Views" *Feminist Studies* 8 (1982): 109–131; Susan Bordo, *Unbearable Weight: Femi-*

nism, Culture and the Body (Berkeley: University of California Press, 1993); and Elizabeth Grosz, *Volatile Bodies: Toward a Corporeal Feminism* (Bloomington: University of Indiana Press, 1994).

2. I am grateful to Richard J. Bernstein for pointing out that Plato puts forth a different view in the *Phaedrus* and the *Symposium*. While acknowledging that in some of his dialogues Plato celebrates the body, especially the body of the beloved, in the service of philosophy, I am most interested in the strain of somatophobia in his writings. This strain, most fully expressed in the *Phaedo*, continues in the work of Augustine, Descartes, and others.

3. I consider illness, whether chronic, acute, or terminal, to be a category of disability. While my focus in this chapter is on disabling physical illness, the broader category of disability includes, for example, congenital or acquired physical differences such as visual, hearing, or mobility impairments; mental illness, brain injury, and cognitive impairments; learning differences; and the gradual losses of function associated with aging. In my view, the experiences of chronic and acute illness need to be more fully integrated into the study of disability.

4. There are three excellent book-length studies of autobiographical and biographical accounts of illness and disability: Anne Hunsaker Hawkins's *Reconstructing Illness: Studies in Pathography* (West Lafayette, Ind.: Purdue University Press, 1993); Arthur W. Frank's *The Wounded Storyteller: Body, Illness, and Ethics* (Chicago: University of Chicago Press, 1995); and G. Thomas Couser's *Recovering Bodies: Illness, Disability, and Life Writing* (Madison: University of Wisconsin Press, 1997). Each author discusses a variety of reasons for the current popularity of this genre. In their introduction to *Disability and Culture* (Berkeley: University of California Press, 1995), Benedicte Ingstad and Susan Reynolds Whyte comment on the cultural specificity of these accounts: "Both the form of these narratives as autobiographical accounts of disability and the content with its emphasis on self and body through time appear to be characteristic of European and North American culture" (20).

5. Simone de Beauvoir's *The Second Sex*, translated by H. M. Parshley (New York: Knopf, 1953; reprint Vintage, 1989) offers an example of this approach.

6. See Susan Wendell's *The Rejected Body: Feminist Philosophical Reflections on Disability* (New York: Routledge, 1996), especially Chapters Four and Seven, for an extended discussion of feminism's resistance to thinking about the suffering body.

7. See, for example, Rosemarie Garland-Thomson's analysis of Melville's Ahab, in *Extraordinary Bodies: Figuring Physical Disability in American Culture and Literature* (New York, Columbia University Press, 1997), 44–46.

8. See especially Chapter Four of Elizabeth Grosz's *Volatile Bodies: Toward a Corporeal Feminism* (Bloomington: Indiana University Press, 1994); Helen Marshall's "Our Bodies, Ourselves: Why We Should Add Old Fashioned Empirical Phenomenology to the New Theories of the Body," In *Feminist Theory and the Body: A Reader*, edited by Janet Price and Margrit Shildrick (New York: Routledge, 1999); and Iris Marion Young's *Throwing Like a Girl and Other Essays in Feminist Philosophy and Social Theory* (Bloomington: Indiana University Press, 1990).

9. In drawing on first-person narratives, I am influenced by Susan Brison's work on trauma and identity, which uses autobiographical accounts of traumatic experiences, including her own. See Brison's "Outliving Oneself: Trauma, Memory, and Personal Identity," in *Feminists Rethink the Self*, edited by Diana Tietjens Meyers (Boulder, Colo.: Westview Press, 1997). Also see Wendell 1996. For a feminist reading of the

problem of experience as a category of knowledge, see Joan W. Scott, "The Evidence of Experience," *Critical Inquiry* 178 (3): 773–797.

10. Throughout this chapter, I have chosen to focus on diseases and impairments that are commonly viewed as primarily affecting the body rather than the mind. While this distinction (diseases of mind vs. diseases of body) works against the larger and necessary project of questioning such a division, medical nosology generally continues to categorize diseases in this way. I have not foregrounded narratives of neurological or psychiatric illness because in these cases, alteration of self-identity can sometimes be a symptom of the illness, and even a criterion for diagnosis. I want to demonstrate that identity is transformed even when illness is not considered prima facie to alter the mind or self.

11. My different emphasis suggests the richness and variety of the genre. While Hawkins considers a large number and wide variety of pathographies, my smaller selection favors narratives written by those who were writers or academics before they became ill or disabled and includes works that combine personal narrative and critical analysis. This selection necessarily shapes my argument.

12. Chronic fatigue and immune dysfunction syndrome, as it is known in the United States, or myalgic encephalomyelitis, as it is known in England, Canada, and Australia. CFIDS/ME is a complex and as yet poorly understood illness that affects many different body systems, including the neuroendocrine and immune systems.

13. Rosalyn Diprose, in Chapter Six of *The Bodies of Women: Ethics, Embodiment, and Sexual Difference* (New York: Routledge, 1994), argues against the idea that the self's relation to the body is one of ownership, an idea she traces to John Locke. She suggests that this view of the self, as well as the idea that the self is separate from the body and that it remains the same even through radical changes in the body, underlies biomedical and reproductive ethics. To challenge these ideas of the self, Diprose draws on phenomenological accounts, including Leder's. She contends that a change in the body may represent a change in the self per se and that this view has profound implications for bioethics, property rights, and contract law. For example, in discussing the ethics of contracts for surrogate pregnancy, she argues that "the woman who made the promise at the time of conception is not the same self who is asked to keep it"(117). Diprose's work has shaped my thinking about the body and self in illness and disability.

14. The sociocultural construction of disability is a foundational idea in disability studies. For discussions of this model, see, for example, Lennard J. Davis, *Enforcing Normalcy* (London: Verso, 1995); David Mitchell and Sharon Snyder, eds., *The Body and Physical Difference: Discourses of Disability* (Ann Arbor: University of Michigan Press, 1997); Simi Linton, *Claiming Disability: Knowledge and Identity* (New York: New York University Press, 1998); and Colin Barnes, Geof Mercer, and Tom Shakespeare, eds. *Exploring Disability: A Sociological Introduction* (Cambridge, England: Polity Press, 1999).

15. For discussions of AIDS in relation to social and national boundaries, see especially Catherine Waldby, *AIDS and the Body Politic: Biomedicine and Sexual Difference* (London: Routledge, 1996); Julia Epstein, *Altered Conditions: Disease, Medicine, and Storytelling* (New York: Routledge, 1995); and Thomas Yingling, *AIDS and the National Body*, edited by Robyn Wiegman (Durham, N.C.: Duke University Press, 1997).

16. This model of immunity includes a mechanism called "self-tolerance" and other forms

of "tolerance" that prevent the body from mounting an immune response to something that would normally be considered nonself. In a normal pregnancy, for example, fetal cells are accepted through the mechanism of tolerance. For biomedical accounts of immune theory, see Julius M. Cruse and Robert E. Lewis, eds., *Atlas of Immunology* (New York: CRC Press, 1999); and William E. Paul, ed., *Fundamental Immunology,* 4th ed. (Philadelphia: Lippincott-Raven Publishers, 1999).

17. In her fieldwork, Martin interviews scientists, physicians, alternative practitioners, and laypersons, some of them intravenous drug users at high risk of HIV infection, asking individuals in each of these groups to articulate their understanding of health, disease, and the immune system. Almost without exception, these subjects explain their concepts of immunity as it operates to ward off disease and only hypothetically imagine what it might be like to experience the failure of this system.

18. While Ling's essay raises the question of non-Western treatments, my purpose is not to address alternative therapeutic modalities or the alternate models of health and disease on which these are based. Eastern medicine, in particular, frequently conceives of disease as an imbalance within the body rather than an infiltration or attack from outside its borders. However, what interests me here is how people implicated in the discourses and practices of Western biomedicine (although these same people can, and often do, employ alternative methods of treatment) represent their experience of disabling illness and its challenge to identity.

19. When I became ill and had to accustom myself to new and unpleasant physical sensations, sensations that made me feel inescapably and negatively embodied, I often thought of my pregnancy two years earlier, which was another time of inescapable but mostly pleasurable embodiment. It seemed to me then that these two conditions were phenomenologically related. Drew Leder, Iris Marion Young, and Rosalyn Diprose draw connections between these conditions. However, there are important differences between pregnancy and illness. Pregnancy is a time-limited condition; a woman knows from the outset that it will end. While medical complications do sometimes occur, pregnancy is not in itself a disease state—though it has often been seen as such. Most important, many middle-class women in industrialized countries actively choose pregnancy, and some women take pleasure in the bodily changes it produces, but people do not actively choose illness.

20. In recent years, discourses of fetal subjectivity have led to the representation of the pregnant woman as housing not only an other but also a subject whose interests may not coincide with her own. See Susan Bordo's "Are Mother's Persons?: Reproductive Rights and the Politics of Subject-ivity," in *Unbearable Weight: Feminism, Culture and the Body* (Berkeley: University of California Press, 1993).

Works Cited

Barnes, Colin, Geof Mercer, and Tom Shakespeare, eds. 1999. *Exploring disability: A sociological introduction.* Cambridge, England: Polity Press.

Bordo, Susan. 1993. *Unbearable weight: Feminism, western culture, and the body.* Berkeley: University of California Press.

Brison, Susan J. 1997. Outliving oneself: Trauma, memory, and personal identity. In *Feminists rethink the self,* edited by Diana Tietjens Meyers. Boulder, Colo.: Westview Press.

Couser, Thomas G. 1997. *Recovering bodies: Illness, disability, and life writing.* Madison: The University of Wisconsin Press.

Cruse, Julius M., and Robert E. Lewis, eds. 1999. *Atlas of immunology*. New York: CRC Press.

Davis, Lennard J. 1995. *Enforcing normalcy: Disability, deafness, and the body*. London: Verso.

de Beauvoir, Simone. 1953/1989. *The Second Sex*. Translated by H. M. Parshley. New York: Knopf. Reprint, New York: Vintage.

Diprose, Rosalyn. 1994. *The bodies of women: Ethics, embodiment and sexual difference*. New York: Routledge.

Eagleton, Terry. 1993. Review of Peter Brooks's *Body work*. *London Review of Books* 15 (10): 7–8.

Epstein, Julia. 1995. *Altered conditions: Disease, medicine, and storytelling*. New York: Routledge.

Frank, Arthur W. 1995. *The wounded storyteller: Body, illness, and ethics*. Chicago: The University of Chicago Press.

Garland-Thomson, Rosemarie. 1997. *Extraordinary bodies: Figuring disability in American culture and literature*. New York: Columbia University Press.

Gilman, Sander L. 1988. *Disease and representation: Images of illness from madness to AIDS*. Ithaca, N.Y.: Cornell University Press.

Groopman, Jerome. 1997. *The measure of our days*. New York: Viking Penguin.

Grosz, Elizabeth. 1994. *Volatile bodies: Toward a corporeal feminism*. Bloomington: Indiana University Press.

Haraway, Donna J. 1991. *Simians, cyborgs, and women*. New York: Routledge.

Hawkins, Anne Hunsaker. 1993. *Reconstructing illness: Studies in pathography*. West Lafayette, Ind.: Purdue University Press.

Hooper, Judith. 1994. Beauty tips for the dead. In *Minding the body: Women writers on body and soul*, edited by Patricia Foster. New York: Doubleday.

Ingstad, Benedicte, and Susan Reynolds Whyte, eds. 1995. *Disability and culture*. Berkeley: University of California Press.

Leder, Drew. 1990. *The absent body*. Chicago: The University of Chicago Press.

Ling, Amy. 1999. The alien within. In *Living on the margins: Women writers on breast cancer*, edited by Hilda Raz. New York: Persea Books.

Linton, Simi. 1998. *Claiming disability: Knowledge and identity*. New York: New York University Press.

Mairs, Nancy. 1996a. *Carnal acts*. Boston: Beacon Press.

———. 1996b. *Waist-high in the world: A life among the nondisabled*. Boston: Beacon Press.

Marshall, Helen. 1999. Our bodies, ourselves: Why we should add old fashioned empirical phenomenology to the new theories of the body. In *Feminist theory and the body: A reader*, edited by Janet Price and Margrit Shildrick. New York: Routledge.

Martin, Emily. 1994. *Flexible bodies: The role of immunity in American culture from the days of polio to the age of AIDS*. Boston: Beacon Press.

Merleau-Ponty, Maurice. 1962. *Phenomenology of perception*. Translated by Colin Murphy. London: Routledge.

Mitchell, David T. and Sharon L. Snyder, eds. 1997. *The body and physical difference: Discourses of disability*. Ann Arbor: University of Michigan Press.

Murphy, Robert F. 1990. *The body silent*. New York: W.W. Norton.

Paul, William E., ed. 1999. *Fundamental immunology*. 4th ed. Philadelphia: Lippincott-Raven Publishers.

Plato. 1969. *The last days of Socrates*. Translated by Hugh Tredennick. Harmondsworth, England: Penguin Books.

Price, Reynolds. 1994. *A whole new life: An illness and a healing*. New York: Penguin Books.

Scott, Joan W. 1991. The evidence of experience. *Critical Inquiry* 178 (3): 773–797.

Sontag, Susan. 1989. *AIDS and Its Metaphors*. New York: Farrar, Straus, and Giroux.

———. 1990. *Illness as metaphor and AIDS and its metaphors*. New York: Doubleday (reprint as combined work).

Spelman, Elizabeth V. 1982. Woman as body: Ancient and contemporary views. *Feminist Studies* 8: 109–131.

Waldby, Catherine. 1996. *AIDS and the body politic: Biomedicine and sexual difference*. London: Routledge.

Wendell, Susan. 1996. *The rejected body: Feminist philosophical reflections on disability*. New York: Routledge.

Woolf, Virginia. 1948. On being ill. In *The moment and other essays*. New York: Harcourt Brace and Company.

Yingling, Thomas E. 1997. *AIDS and the national body*. Edited by Robyn Wiegman. Durham, N.C.: Duke University Press.

Young, Iris Marion. 1990. *Throwing like a girl and other essays in feminist philosophy and social theory*. Bloomington: Indiana University Press.

Disabled Masculinity

EXPANDING THE MASCULINE REPERTOIRE

ℐℛ

RUSSELL P. SHUTTLEWORTH

The existence of multiple masculinities and femininities, and indeed what some sexuality researchers refer to as third genders, complicates any analysis of gender (see, e.g., Herdt 1993; Connell 1995). Connell argues that multiple masculinities exist in relationships of contest and negotiation with one another. His model of research "studies various projects of masculinity, the conditions under which they arise and the conditions they produce" (1995, 39). Yet in any society, ideal standards of masculinity constitute a hegemonic form. These culturally specific masculine ideals or expectations exert their power in everyday social interaction and, depending on the context, can often restrict the expression of alternative masculinities. Certain typical masculine expectations such as initiative, competitiveness, self-control, assertiveness, and independence, incorporated as dispositions to varying degrees, manifest in bodily comportment and corporeal and interpersonal negotiations and practices and are critical aspects of U.S. society's hegemonic masculinity. These expectations pervade our social being-with-each-other and are generally perceived as essential in business, sports, and dating, among other contexts, and symbolize male potency in U.S. cultural imaginary. Noncompetitive, tentative and also disabled men are not generally located in our society's images of masculinity. In this chapter, I discuss how some disabled men with whom I recently conducted ethnographic fieldwork contend with these masculine expectations in their search for sexual intimacy. Rather than rendering simplistic models of rejection or reliance, I show how those men who are most successful in love assume a flexible gender identity and expand their masculine repertoire of orientative-ideals and embodied, interpersonal practices beyond those associated with hegemonic masculinity.

Masculinity and Disability

Research on gender and disability has focused primarily on women (e.g., Asch and Fine 1988; Gill 1996; Rousso 1996). A few disability studies scholars, nevertheless, have noted the dilemmas that disabled men confront in the face of masculine expectations such as initiative, competitiveness, self-control, assertiveness, and independence, among others, which are prevalent in the United States (Hahn 1989; Gerschick and Miller 1996; Tepper 1999) and also in the United Kingdom (Shakespeare 1999).[1]

These accounts, however, neglect several important issues. One issue is how in everyday interaction the comportment of the body and sundry corporeal habits and interpersonal practices are seen as expressing gender (see, contra, Ferris, 1998; Valentine, 1999). In Bourdieu's (1977, 1990) terminology, men and women incorporate a gendered habitus involving gender specific dispositions that manifest as masculine and feminine corporealities and gendered bodily and interpersonal practices. Yet, in research on masculinity and disability, there is minimal critical examination of the implications for physically disabled men of not being able to effectively assume some of these dispositions in body and in practice (Shuttleworth 2000a, 2000b).

Men with impairments that restrict their bodies in terms of nondisabled carnal contexts and codes of meaning (Hughes and Paterson 1999), including verbal or communicative contexts, may not be able to, in Butler's terms, effect a normative masculine performance (Butler 1990, 1997a, 1997b), that is, the macho swagger, asking someone out on a date, initiating a kiss, and so forth. For Butler

> gender is in no way a stable identity of locus of agency from which various acts proceed; rather it is an identity tenuously constituted in time— an identity instituted through a stylized repetition of acts. Further, gender is instituted through the stylization of the body and, hence, must be understood as the mundane way in which bodily gestures, movements and enactments of various kinds constitutes the illusion of an abiding gendered self. (1997b, 402)

If we take Butler seriously and her view that performativity is the "vehicle through which ontological effects are established" (1997a, 236), then a corporeal ability to bring gender into being in repetitive social performances would appear to constitute a critical dimension to being perceived as gendered by others and feeling gendered oneself.[2] The notion of embodying masculinity refers to the incorporation of masculine standards and dispositions and also the sense of masculinity conveyed by one's corporeality and social performances in-the-world.

The meaning that effectively brings into being some version of masculinity or femininity was most explicitly brought home to me on a conference trip several years ago. I was accompanying a male friend with cerebral palsy as his personal assistant to a conference devoted to users of augmentative communicative devices with speech output. There were about ninety or so disabled people there, most of whom were using these speech devices, and quite a few significant others and personal assistants. Although my friend was comfortable using his head pointer and board, he was also curious about the new speech devices coming on the market. Among disabled people with speech impairments, the communicative body is understandably a central concern.[3] On a women's issues panel, one woman panel member asked the question via her speech device why men had more choices in their selection of a masculine voice and added that the few voices available for women did not sound different enough from the men's voices. There was much concurrence from the women in the audience. Clearly, the personal and sociocultural significance that speaking in a feminine voice held for these women was profound. Yet, I am certain that the men's reaction would have been similar if they had felt that their voices did not sound masculine enough. For this woman unable to embody a feminine voice, the availability of computerized speech not only opened up the possibility of conveying information in a normatively communicative way but also of conveying her identification with what she perceives as femininity through performative utterances. What this woman was objecting to was that her computerized verbal performance would not be recognized as feminine but would be subsumed under a masculine sense.

The second lacuna in research on disability and masculinity is that unless it is an account of lived experience, this work tends to remain at an abstract level of analysis.[4] What I mean by this is that despite discussion about the incompatibility of disability and masculine ideals, no sustained attempt shows how disabled men try to negotiate this dilemma during their interpersonal communication and embodied practice. This critique can especially be made of what is perhaps the most ambitious attempt to theorize disabled masculinity, the work of Gerschick and Miller (1996). Their tripartite model presents disabled men as relying on, reformulating, or rejecting hegemonic ideals of masculinity. Though acknowledging that all the disabled men they interviewed probably used a combination of the above modes of what they refer to as coping strategies (which situates their analysis clearly within a psychological model that shares the stage with adaptation), they never really connect masculinity to the lived experience of interpersonal relations. For example, they supplied their informants "with a list of characteristics associated with prevailing masculinity . . . and asked them to rate their importance to their conception of self." They continue, "Both positive and negative responses to this portion of our questionnaire guided our insight into how each man viewed his masculinity" (54). Subsequently, they took at face value their informants' accounts based on only one full-length interview and a brief thirty-minute follow-up. As seasoned ethnographers will tell you, however, informants' stories often change over the course of repeated interviewing, and at least some participant-observation is advised to provide context for informants' accounts.[5]

The performance of gender occurs in sociocultural contexts (including imagined social interaction) in which people are invested in various ways in the outcomes of their encounters with others; during everyday interaction, interpersonal stakes involving identities, self-esteem, and quality of life are often very high. Gerschick and Miller (1996), however, approach their work both methodologically and theoretically at a distance from these embodied practices, interpersonal negotiations, and the existential immediacy of the construction of gender identity and the evaluation of stakes in the lived moment. In all likelihood, Gerschick and Miller's informants, initially guided by an abstract gauge of their identification with "characteristics associated with prevailing masculinity" (54), geared their interview answers to an ideal sense of their relationship to typical masculinity.

Embodying Masculinity in the Pursuit of Sexual Intimacy

Recently, I conducted a series of modified life history interviews with fourteen men with cerebral palsy, all who live independently in the San Francisco Bay Area, 148 interviews in all, especially focusing on their history of interpersonal encounters and the ways in which they attempted to establish intimacy and sexual relationships with others. I noted the details of their accounts of these attempts, their successes and failures, what they thought were impediments, and what they thought helped. I kept an ethnographic journal while living with and working as a personal assistant for one of the men, a longtime friend, and also included notes from time spent socializing with several other men in the study. I also interviewed seventeen relevant others such as wives, girlfriends, former girlfriends, parents, siblings, personal assistants (PA's), and physical therapists for their perspectives on these men's sexual situation. The fourteen men who make up the primary sample were between the ages of eighteen and fifty-one when I began interviewing them. They all have some degree of mobility impairment: eleven men use wheelchairs, one man uses crutches, and two men limp when they walk. Eleven have speech impairments, and four of these use augmentative communicative devices such as an alphabet board or computer with speech output. Nine men are white, two are Latino, and three are black. Eleven men are heterosexual, one man is gay, one man identifies as primarily heterosexual but has experienced several brief sexual encounters with men, and one man identifies as bisexual and is in a group marriage with a man and a woman but always appeared more sexually interested in women during our interviews. In this chapter, I am concerned with the construction of masculinity in terms of these men's heterosexual experiences.

Embodying Masculinity

How to adequately embody and negotiate masculinity emerged as one of the most salient issues for these disabled men. For them, confronting the dilemma of how to be masculine when one is disabled is felt most acutely during their interpersonal attempts to establish sexual intimacy with others. That is, the dilemma of disabled masculinity comes to the foreground during their interactions with those to whom they are sexually attracted. In the heteronormative model, during interpersonal relations that prelude sexual intimacy, male initiative takes the form of asking a woman for a date, making the first physical moves, and so forth. This initiative is expressed via verbal negotiations and physically with confident, controlled bodily actions that progressively try to move a relationship with a woman toward sexual intimacy (e.g., putting an arm around a date, attempting a kiss, etc.) and is most often complemented by a masculine bodily bearing cast from the hegemonic mold (Shuttleworth 2000a).

Depending on the degree of impairment for the men I interviewed, they felt excluded from moving the body in typical masculine ways that expressed this initiative. For instance, Josh[6] muses, "It is funny because if a girl came up to me, would I know what to do? Like I do not kiss very well. Or because my arms are down here [by his sides], I cannot very well try to hold her hand. So what the hell do I do?" During another conversation, he said: "I think women like to be touched and hugged; I cannot very well do that. It drives me nuts."

In fact, not being able to meet expectations of masculine embodiment may make disabled men less appealing as romantic and sexual partners for some nondisabled women. For example, a former girlfriend of one of the men in the study caved in to the social pressures, primarily coming from her girlfriend, who kept asking her how she could be with a man who couldn't put his arm around her. Several of the more significantly impaired men in the study also said that they had been told at one time or another that no one would want them because they could not embrace or hold a partner (Shuttleworth 2000a, 2000b). Listen to Dirk:

> *Dirk*: I remember at one point when I was getting interested in [a girl], the staff member who was the attendant noticed that and said to me, you know, Debbie isn't going to be interested in you because she's going to want somebody to put her arms around, who can put out their arms around her.
>
> *Russell*: Is this a woman who said that?
>
> *Dirk*: Yes, and cuddle her, we were both in wheelchairs, we could get out of them easy enough and do whatever we could do. And I remember you know, feeling very bad, but I also remember it making sense.
>
> *Russell*: Why did it make sense?
>
> *Dirk*: Because of this sort of exchange shit, because I couldn't give her that, she probably wouldn't want me. And I guess it was true.

In the following quotation, Ed reveals how masculine embodiment is also symbolically linked to the image of the functional or potent phallus in the larger cultural imaginary:

> *Ed*: . . . her and I dated for almost a year and she had a few girlfriends and she told me that they said, why are you with him? They thought I wasn't

functional. Of course when we first started to get to know each other, she asked me, can I, can I? And I said, I can and all of the sudden these girlfriends said all this, they didn't ask, can he? They just assumed, I can't. And her family was like, why? Why don't you find a real man?

Russell: She said that's what they said to her?

Ed: Yeah, no one's ever said that directly to me. That and I kind of feel that like when I go out to the bars and some of these women feel that way. They just kind of don't want to, they want some action and I ain't going to give it to them.

Russell: You see them as not taking you into account as a person perhaps, as a man who could do that?

Ed: Right, it's kind of the whole thing, sexually and just the how, I would assume most women kind of want to be taken care of, that kind of thing, I guess. And I think that women see me in a chair and say, I can't do that.

Similarly, interviews with other men often revealed an intimate connection between their sense of manhood and their sexuality. This is not only due to their own incorporation of masculine expectations but also to other's responses to them (Shuttleworth 1996, 2000a, 2000b, 2001). For instance, Josh said to me one day:

Josh: It is like I don't have any maleness.

Russell: Do you really have a lack of maleness?

Josh: Women see me as asexual.

Russell: When do you feel a lack of maleness? At what times?

Josh: I see how girls look at me and treat me. When girls talk to me they do not seem interested in that way. . . . The feeling they give off. I feel blocked. I know I do not stand a chance. They just want to be my friend.

For the disabled men with whom I talked, the dilemma of how to embody and negotiate masculinity also involves important stakes: the possibility of having a sexual experience, of perhaps destroying a friendship, of not wanting to spend another Saturday night alone, and so forth (Shuttleworth 2000a). Negotiating how to be a man occurs within the context of these human social and sexual desires. Sociocultural and interpersonal challenges to these men's masculinity and sexuality within this context met with a variety of responses from research participants: from the cultivation of an extreme, hyper-aggressive masculinity to an expansion of their masculine repertoire of orientative-ideals and embodied, interpersonal practices (Shuttleworth, 2000a, 2000b). It is the latter men who I want to focus on here.

Expanding the Masculine Repertoire

There was another story that emerged from my talks with some of the men, as well as from my interviews with several women—girlfriends, former girlfriends, and wives of study participants (a total of five). In fact, these women told me that they appreciated their partner's masculinity as embodied in his unique bodily movements and practices. For instance, one man gave back rubs with his highly dexterous feet because he did not have use of his arms and hands. He had used the line, "Would you like a backrub?" for years on his dates and was sometimes successful in furthering relationships with it, most significantly with his wife of five years. Employing his body in this nontypical but for him more natural way, he was able to convey a masculine sense of initiative to his dates.

In fact, not being able to use their bodies in conventional ways may have given some men impetus to go beyond hegemonic masculinity and to focus on alternatives, both in terms of their corporeality and also the orientatative-ideals that guided their behavior and practices. A former girlfriend of one of the significantly impaired men who has also been romantically involved with several other disabled men said that "it is what men have to communicate not how they communicate, their positive attitude and the look in their eyes that attracts me to a man." She claims that whether he is disabled is irrelevant and that in fact men with disabilities make much more sensitive lovers than nondisabled men. The latter statement was echoed by several men in the study who said that because their bodies could not move in typical ways, it spurred them on to become innovative in their sexual techniques and to also focus more on their partner's pleasure than they thought nondisabled men did (Shuttleworth 2000a).[7]

Several men also told me that they would always wait for the other to make the first moves toward sexual intimacy, inhabiting what might be described as a passive interest. For instance, Ed, who uses a wheelchair, has often visited nightclubs in the past in the hopes of meeting potential partners. Quite a handsome man, he always lets women make the moves on him, albeit he makes it known that he is interested. This has resulted in some sexual encounters as well as a couple of relationships:

> *Ed*: . . . when Pablo and I went to this club in Fremont, and I met this woman and just talked. I started to think, okay, she's interested. She asked me to dance and we danced and then she went off with her friend for awhile. I guess it was because I was playing that I wasn't interested. . . . I guess she thought that I wasn't interested so she went off with her friend and I thought they left. On occasion, I looked around to see if she was still there and I didn't see her, and then she showed up again. And I said, I thought you left. She said, well, my friend found a guy, and I said, okay. And then she asked me to slow dance, I think she asked if I can slow dance . . . as soon as I said yeah, she dragged me on the floor. So she kind of stood real close and put my arm on her hip and I held her hand and she kind of swayed so my chair did the movement. . . . So after the club closed, we agreed that we would go to a restaurant where we can eat and talk where we can hear each other. And we went there and had a good talk . . . when we left the restaurant

she came in the van with me. I was thinking, okay, should I give her my number and I said, what the hell and I did.

Russell: She gave you her number?

Ed: I think she did after I gave her mine. But that following morning she called me, and we made a date. . . . We went out and had dinner. I asked her if she was tired and wanted to go home, because it was like ten o'clock or something. And she said, no I'm fine. So do you want to go somewhere and talk, I think that's what I said. Anyway, she ended up telling me where this park was that we parked way down the parking lot and started talking, maybe like an hour. And then she just kissed me and then it was all over. We were there for probably two hours rolling around in the van.

Russell: So you made love?

Ed: Yeah, basically. I knew once she told me that she wasn't tired that she had the tone and look like she wanted sex. So, you know, I said okay in my head. If the woman wants to have sex, she has to make the first move.

Ed waits for the woman to make the move in most of the steps in this seduction process—and notice how he does not ask for her number, he asks if she wants his number. Ed has had luck with this alternative in the past, and he was quite strategic in using it. Sometimes he might whiz by several women in his wheelchair a few times, trying to catch one of their eyes and then sit on the periphery of the dance floor or by the bar waiting.

Most of the men in this study also contrasted with the typical view of masculine sexuality as more about sexual objectification and less about emotional intimacy. These men came to the conclusion that emotional intimacy was imperative to their sexuality. Fred, for example, made this the basis for an entire philosophy of living. Even as a teenager and young adult, Fred knew he desired intimacy more than simply sex for its own sake.

Fred: I never wanted just sex.

Russell: What do you want with sex?

Fred: Intimacy.

Russell: How do you define intimacy, what is it?

Fred: Living with people in an intimate way.

Russell: Close?

Fred: Yes.

Russell: What about emotions, do they come into it at all?

Fred: That was why I did not try hookers.

Fred makes emotional intimacy central to a meaningful sexuality in his life and he has been very successful in establishing intimate sexual relationships with others using this foundation.

A significant finding that came out of this research is that those men who measured themselves against typical masculine ideals and who obsessed on their inability to adequately embody them were more apt to remain emotionally immobilized during their interpersonal encounters. In other words, they could not take risks. They were also more liable to socially withdraw when they fell short. These men tended to primarily blame their inability to measure up to masculine ideals as the reason for their failure in love. Those men, however, who perceived hegemonic masculine expectations as less a total index of their desirability and who could sometimes draw on alternative ideals and embodied, interpersonal practices (such as massaging dates with their feet, prioritizing emotional intimacy, interdependency, becoming friends first, allowing the other to sometimes make the first move when necessary without feeling less of a man) could better weather rejection and remain open to the possibility of romantic connection and sexual intimacy. Some of these alternatives are of course associated with femininity in our culture, but they take their place alongside more typical masculine images and dispositions in some disabled men's psyches and corporeal and interpersonal practices (Shuttleworth 2000a, 2000b).

In her study of seven mobility impaired people's sexual meanings, Anne Guldin (1999, 2000) found that the disabled men in her study assumed feminine communication styles, while women seemed to become more masculine in their approach, especially regarding flirting behavior. She suggests that perhaps disabled men attract women who are tired of hypermasculine men; that is, nondisabled women might see dating a disabled man as a symbolic balancing of culturally unbalanced male/female power relations. Thus, disabled men may attract women who are interested in an equal relationship. On the other hand, a disabled woman may tend to attract men who want an even greater power imbalance in male/female relations and who mistakenly perceive disabled women as needy or helpless. Therefore, disabled women may be more likely to attract overly aggressive men who do not respect their boundaries.

Guldin's hypothesis was not supported in the present research. Though some of the men certainly did utilize approaches and interpersonal strategies in trying to negotiate relationships that could be characterized as feminine, those who were successful in love appeared to pragmatically expand their masculine repertoire to incorporate these alternative approaches when the context called for them. Thus, in those contexts in which they could not be typically masculine, they incorporated alternative ideals and practices. Yet, in those contexts where they could exercise traditional masculine approaches, they often did so. In fact, an ability to move fluidly between different self-identities, as typically masculine or as incorporating a divergent sense of masculinity, was significantly related to sexual self-esteem and success in establishing sexual relationships. Successful men at love generally hooked up with partners who appreciated their expanded masculine repertoire rather than an inflexible ideal. Also in contrast to Guldin's findings, several of the men in this research could certainly occasionally come across as hypermasculine, for example, aggressively pursuing women when they clearly were not interested. Interviews with the five women who were currently or had been lovers of the men in this study revealed a variety of types, not simply those who were tired of hypermasculine men. What appeared to be common among these women was that they were less evaluative and were able to appreciate alternative forms of masculine embodiment and practice (Shuttleworth 2000a).

Though I find much in Guldin's work to commend, indeed it is indicative of a new critical-interpretive approach to disability and sexuality (see Shuttleworth 2000a), I think she runs a significant risk by prematurely considering the reasons why nondisabled people establish relationships with disabled people. The situation she describes may well characterize those in her study, albeit her analysis and interpretation are only based on several interviews with each informant. Yet, she implies that this situation may prevail more generally; that is, the attraction of nondisabled people to disabled people can only be predicated on ulterior motivations and the exercise of power relations that are sexist. In other words, disabled people can never hope to establish relationships that aren't tainted in some way by overtly sexist relations: women who are attracted to disabled men are escaping hypermasculinity and men who are attracted to disabled women are attracted for exploitative reasons. I have no doubt that these dynamics can sometimes come into play. Yet, too hastily theorizing why nondisabled people choose to be with disabled people deprives disabled people of the possibility that a nondisabled person will love them not for escape or exploitation but for who they are as whole persons. It was clear to me that the loving relationships that I witnessed between several of the participants in the present research and their wives/girlfriends were based on significantly more than the playing out of gender power relations, albeit these were not entirely absent.

Conclusion

Disabled men in this study often felt rejected because of their inability to meet hegemonic masculine expectations and to adequately embody masculinity. Yet, obsessing on their distance from what they perceived as a desirability index was a dead-end street in terms of negotiating relationships. Instead, the development of a flexible gender identity by several of these men, whereby they expanded their masculine repertoire of orientative-ideals in their embodied, interpersonal practices and were comfortable in sometimes using their bodies in alternative ways garnered them some success in establishing sexual intimacy with others. The example of these men lends support for the view that gender identity is not fixed but is situationally constructed. Moreover, using the body in alternative ways and emphasizing alternative ideals that diverge from those associated with strict hegemonic masculinity were not sexual liabilities but rather sexual assets for these disabled men. Indeed, there are persons, both disabled and nondisabled, who do not necessarily desire lovers who rigidly mirror hegemonic masculinity. I will conclude by presenting a final example illustrating the situational and pragmatic construction of gender identity. Men who were successful in love were more apt to feel comfortable in letting the nondisabled other do some of the more physically demanding work in their romance (grasping a hand, initiating a hug or kiss, etc.) and/or with the logistics of positioning for sexual intercourse. These men, however, could also be typically masculine by managing their romantic and sexual endeavors, either verbally or via use of their alternative mode of communication.[8]

Acknowledgments

The research in this chapter was assisted by a fellowship from the Sexuality Research Fellowship Program of the Social Science Research Council with funds provided by the Ford Foundation.

Notes

1. There are, of course, local masculine differences within both the United States and the United Kingdom, especially in terms of ethnicity and class, as well as between the two nations generally. Nevertheless, similarities can also be seen. For example, both nations to some degree foster the development of autonomy and competitiveness in men.
2. For Butler, performativity does not refer to a theatrical or even interactional sense of the self's performance, rather gender reality (or the reality of any other identity) is created through repetitive social performances. While I support Butler's notion of the construction of identities, including gender identity, as performative, I do not go so far as conceding human agency fully to this constructive process. One does not have to believe in the sovereignty of the subject to see that one's basic feeling states (e.g., feeling open or closed, extending one's self, or withdrawing into one's self), albeit shaped by different sociocultural milieus, are fundamental, intentional stances of a human organism responding to its environment as an emotional agent (see Buytendijk 1950; Freund 1990; Shuttleworth, 2000a, 2001).
3. When referring to embodiment in this chapter, I also incorporate the communicative dimension of human experience; that is, explicit communication either verbally or by other means is also an embodied act.
4. See Ferris (1998) for an excellent reflexive account of his lived experience of masculinity in relation to his impaired body via the vehicle of a nude photo shoot.
5. Whereas Gerschick and Miller interviewed each research participant face-to-face only once and followed this up with a brief telephone conversation, I met with participants repeatedly until I felt I had exhausted their understanding of their search for sexual intimacy. During the series of interviews, I continuously asked participants how particular experiences felt at the time and how they were affected by them. What I was attempting to apprehend was how subjects negotiated and embodied their masculine identities in the face of a plethora of sociocultural and interpersonal barriers to establishing sexual relationships with others and how they existentially integrated their experience. How they constructed their masculinity was thus revealed in their responses to particular sociocultural and interpersonal challenges that had concrete stakes (e.g., the possibility of a sexual experience, of perhaps destroying a friendship, of spending another Saturday night alone, etc.). Moreover, as the study unfolded, while I was living and working with Josh, I became convinced that participant-

observation is crucial to understanding informants' worlds and their day to day experiences. This is of course an anthropological principle, but I think it bears repeating for an interdisciplinary audience. Without an intimate, living-with association to Josh's everyday context, and to a lesser extent other disabled men with whom I worked and also socialized, some of the major insights of this research would not have been fathomed.

6. All names are pseudonyms.

7. This is in fact a common finding in disability and sexuality research. Guldin (1999) sees it as an inversion of the ability/disability binary. While on one level I would agree with this analysis, I think to see it simply as inversion diminishes the achievement of an actual expansion of creative sexual practice that can occur at an individual level.

8. While I am sympathetic with feminist and queer theorists' attempts to radically subvert the current gender binary of masculinity/femininity, I am also sensitive to the question of how disabled people can pragmatically access sexually intimate relationships, of course, taking into account their multiple identities. For the primarily heterosexual men in this study, it appears that an expansion of their masculine repertoire was a worthwhile avenue to pursue. That is, not simply a reliance, reformulation or rejection of hegemonic masculinity but a more contextually sensitive, pragmatic application of typical masculine orientations and the incorporation of alternative ideals and dispositions in one's interpersonal, embodied practices.

Works Cited

Asch A., and M. Fine, eds. 1988. Introduction: Beyond pedestals. In *Women with disabilities: Essays in psychology, culture, and politics*. Philadelphia: Temple University Press.

Bourdieu, P. 1977. *Outline to a theory of practice*. Cambridge: Cambridge University Press.

_____.1990. *The logic of practice*. Stanford, Calif.: Stanford University Press.

Butler, J. 1990. *Gender trouble: Feminism and the subversion of identity*. New York: Routledge.

_____. 1997a. Gender as performance: An interview with Judith Butler for radical philosophy. In *Identity and Difference*, edited by Kathryn Woodward. London: Sage Publications.

_____. 1997b. Performative acts and gender constitution: An essay in phenomenology and feminist theory. In *Writing On the Body: Female Embodiment and Feminist Theory*, edited by Katie Conboy, Nadia Medina, and Sarah Stanbury. New York: Columbia University Press.

Buytendijk, F.J.J. 1950. The phenomenological approach to the problem of feelings and emotions. In *Feelings and emotions: The Moosehead Symposium in cooperation with the University of Chicago*, edited by M. L. Reymert. New York: McGraw Hill.

Connell, R. W. 1995. *Masculinities*. Berkeley: University of California Press.

Ferris, J. 1998. Uncovery to recovery: Reclaiming one man's body on a nude photo shoot. *Michigan Quarterly Review* (summer): 503–518.

Freund, P.E.S. 1990. The expressive body: A common ground for the sociology of emotions and health and illness. *Sociology of Health and Illness* 12: 452–477.

Gerschick, T., and A. Miller. 1996. Gender identities at the crossroads of masculinity and physical disability. In *Toward a New Psychology of Gender*, edited by M. M. Gergen and S. N. Davis. New York: Routledge.

Gill, C. 1996. Dating and relationship issues. In *Women with physical disabilities: Achieving and maintaining health and well being*, edited by D. M. Krotoski, M. A. Nosek, and M. A. Turk. Baltimore: Paul H. Brookes Publishing Co.

Guldin, A. 1999. Claiming Sexuality: Mobility-Impaired People and Sexualities in American Culture. Master's paper, Department of Anthropology, University of Iowa.

———. 2000. Self-claiming sexuality: Mobility impaired people and American culture. *Sexuality and Disability* 18: 233–238.

Hahn, H. 1989. Masculinity and disability. *Disability Studies Quarterly* 9 (3): 1–3.

Herdt G. 1993. *Third sex, third gender: Beyond sexual dimorphism in culture and history*. New York: Zone Books.

Hughes, B., and Paterson, K. 1999. Disability studies and phenomenology: The carnal politics of everyday life. *Disability and Society* 14: 597–610.

Rousso, H. 1996. Sexuality and a positive sense of self. In *Women with physical disabilities: Achieving and maintaining health and well being*, edited by D. M. Krotoski, M. A. Nosek, and M. A. Turk. Baltimore: Paul H. Brookes Publishing Co.

Shakespeare, T. 1999. The sexual politics of disabled masculinity. *Sexuality and Disability* 17: 53–64.

Shuttleworth, R. P. 1996. An anthropological perspective on sexual and physical disability. Paper presented at the 95th American Anthropological Association Meeting, San Francisco.

———. 2000a. The pursuit of sexual intimacy for men with cerebral palsy. Dissertation in medical anthropology, University of California, San Francisco and Berkeley.

———. 2000b. The search for sexual intimacy for men with cerebral palsy. *Sexuality and Disability* 18: 263–282.

———. 2001. Symbolic contexts, embodied sensitivities and the lived experience of sexually relevant, interpersonal encounters for a man with severe cerebral palsy. In *Semiotics and dis/ability: Interrogating categories of difference*, edited by L. Rogers and B. Swadener. New York: SUNY Press.

Tepper, M. 1999. Letting go of restrictive notions of manhood: Male sexuality, disability and chronic illness. *Sexuality and Disability* 17: 37–52.

Valentine, G. 1999. What it means to be a man: The body, masculinities, disability. In *Mind and body spaces: Geographies of illness, impairment and disability*, edited by R. Butler and H. Parr. New York: Routledge.

PART III

Arts and Embodiment

Helen Keller's Love Life

✑✑

GEORGINA KLEEGE

Come on, Helen. You knew I'd have to get around to him eventually. One of the hazards of leading a life as public as yours is that even the events you'd rather forget are a part of the public record. The records of the Boston registry office, to be exact, an application for a marriage license signed by one Peter Fagan and one Helen Adams Keller.

That's a fact, Helen. Here are other facts.

Sometime in 1916, Peter Fagan was hired to be your secretary. You'd been acquainted for a while. He was a friend of a friend of John Macy's, someone from the same literary political circle. He was to assist you with your correspondence and other writing and to perform whatever clerical tasks you needed. He also accompanied you to lectures and other functions to act as interpreter when Teacher was too tired.

Teacher's health had become a problem, now aggravated by the stress of the breakup of her marriage. On top of that, she had developed a respiratory condition presumed to be tuberculosis. It was decided that she would go for the cure at Lake Placid, taking Polly with her. You were to go spend the time with your sister, Mildred, in Montgomery. Then your mother, who had come north to help close up the house, received a phone call, then read a newspaper story, reporting that you and Fagan had applied for the marriage license. There was a discussion. Soon afterward, Fagan was gone. The Wrentham household divided as planned. After only a few weeks at Lake Placid, Teacher and Polly left for Puerto Rico, where they stayed until the following spring. You remained in Montgomery. It is rumored that Fagan resettled in Florida, but you never heard from him again.

Or almost never. Your sister reported that while you were staying with her in Montgomery, Fagan showed up. One morning she saw you talking to a stranger on the front porch. It was a young man, and he was spelling into your hand. She summoned her husband, Warren, who in time-honored Southern male fashion, got his gun. There was some heated talk, and finally the man went away. A few nights later, Mildred heard a noise and roused Warren. He went and investigated, then came back with a bemused smile. He said you were out on the porch again, dressed for travelling, with a packed suitcase beside you. In the morning you were still there.

The only other recorded event that might have some relevance was that there was a fire in the house while you were staying there, a fire that started in your room. The family had to evacuate, the fire department was called, etc. You claimed the fire was an accident—faulty wiring or something. But given the state of mind you must have been in, I'm wondering if something else happened. Were you burning something, Helen—his love letters or other keepsakes? But this is only a detail.

So those are the facts. The obvious interpretation of these facts is that you, naive and sheltered as you were, found yourself swept off your feet by this young man, while Teacher and your mother could see him for what he really was. They saw him as an interloper and opportunist, ready to take you away from them and exploit your earning power to his own advantage.

Of course, there's a possibility that while they claimed to be protecting your interests, they were actually protecting their own. You were the bread-winner. You supported the Wrentham household, were still sending money home to your mother, and who knows? maybe even a few bucks on the sly every now and then to John Macy. They may have been worried that your marriage would alter those arrangements, might leave them in the lurch.

Or did they view Fagan in a more neutral light? Maybe they believed he was in earnest, that he really loved you, and wanted you as a wife rather than as a cash cow. So their worries were about you. They didn't know how well you would manage in domestic life. And (here's the ugly part) they were worried about what would happen if you had children. As I mentioned weeks ago when we started this topic, even today, Helen, the world is not thrilled by the prospect of disabled people reproducing. In your day, even people who had an enlightened view, people who should have known better, might have balked at the idea. Your old friend Alexander Graham Bell was a leader in the eugenics movement. Even you published a few lines here and there advising the "afflicted" not to have children. Really, Helen! Where was your head? The "afflicted" who live on after you are still dealing with that. For instance, people take for granted that I don't have children because I don't want to reproduce my defective genes. Who would want to risk bringing a blind child into the world? On two separate occasions in my life, women have told me that they would abort a fetus if they knew it would grow up to be blind. As I told you when we started this discussion, people will say the damnedest things to us. There's no topic too intimate, no statement too insensitive. But I wasn't going to argue with these women about their manners or their reproductive choices. If they felt that way about blindness, what kind of mothers would they be for those blind children?

But back to you. Whether or not Teacher and your mother assumed that you would have produced a disabled infant (your condition was caused by illness, not genes), I surmise they assumed you could not be trusted to care for a child yourself. How would you know when it was crying? What if it rolled under the sofa and got stuck; how would you ever find it?

Not that they would have said that to you. I sense the discussion never got that far. What exactly did they say? "Sorry, Helen. We can't let this happen. You can't have this man and he can't have you because . . . " Because what— that's what I want to know. I don't doubt that their motives were muddled, if not impure. But I'd like to know how they presented them to you. Whether or not you believed them is another matter.

So leave yourself out of it if you want. Give me their side of the argument and leave your words blank. I'll settle for that.

July 23

I imagine your mother found the situation especially distressing. She may have assumed that your blindness and deafness made you unmarriageable, so she was utterly unprepared to consider this man, or any man, as a suitable husband for her daughter. This is a confrontation she might have expected to have with your sister but never with you. I imagine her sitting alone in the front parlor of your house, trying to think what to say to you. What words will she find to express what's wrong with this union? How will she even begin? None of her inner turmoil appears on the surface, however. The surface is serene. She is the very image of the well-bred Southern lady. She is an Adams, who claims kinship with the first family of that name—something she never lets anyone forget. She sits in the small wingback armchair by the empty hearth. Her spine is straight, but not rigid. A very keen observer (like you, Helen, if you could see) might notice that her glances—first at the window, then at the mantle clock— are rather too quick and furtive. But an ordinary observer would only see a middle-aged woman at rest. Then there is a sound at the front door and she rises, then sits again almost in the same second. The movement is so rapid it could be taken for a weird, full-body spasm, an all-over twitch. But the sound is only the rather clumsy housemaid polishing the door knocker.

Your mother connects the shock she feels with the sound of the reporter's voice on the telephone, the rapid-fire questions, the crude roughness of his tone. Despite all the time she's spent with you up North, she's never quite gotten used to Yankee speech. This has less to do with the harsh, flat, unlilting sounds of the words than with the brutal quickness, the rough, overloud immoderation of it. And this was no ordinary Yankee on the telephone, but a newspaper man, bent, she realizes after the fact, on getting her to admit something without meaning to. Her husband, the Captain, was a newspaper man too, of course, but of a different sort altogether. He always instructed his reporters on rules of etiquette, especially when addressing a lady. But this one had shown no such deference. In fact, she thinks now, his rudeness may have even been a deliberate ploy meant to shock her into making an unwitting quotable quote.

She could have said much. She never quite approved of bringing Mr. Fagan into your household. Sitting there now, she draws some strength from this. She went so far as to voice her objections at the time. His political views were even more radical than Mr. Macy's, not to mention the fact that it was Mr. Macy who recommended him in the first place. Out of respect for Miss Sullivan (she never got used to calling her Mrs. Macy) she did not harp on this explicitly before. But now she steels herself with the intention to say it again if the need arises, not so much an "I told you so" as a "Don't blame me." Even leaving aside his politics and other connections, it always seemed to her not quite proper to bring a young man into the household in that capacity, and to put him in that kind of constant contact with you, Helen. Not that she dislikes him. In fact she finds him rather charming, certainly very polite, even courtly in a way she supposes some find old-fashioned. And the past few months, his presence in the house and on tour has created a different atmosphere, a more spontaneous and cheerfully chaotic hustle-bustle. Still, it never ceased to make her pull up short to walk into a room and see him there beside you, his fingers moving inside your cupped palm. And once (your mother won't admit this to Miss Sullivan, of course) one late afternoon sitting in the garden, she watched the two of you moving through the flower beds, your hands touching as you chatted idly, then your hand reaching to touch his lips and throat, to feel him speak the name of some flower. It made her dreamily conscious, and almost (this the part she doesn't even admit to herself) pleased that an unknowing passerby would see the young couple and read these gestures as the innocent explorations of new love.

But what shocks her most, Helen, is you. Once she finally hung up on that reporter, she went to find you, but could not bring herself to say anything. You were where you usually are, at your typewriter, answering letters. As occasionally happens, you were so engrossed in your work you didn't notice her presence at first. She stared down at your face, scanning every familiar feature, and was shocked to discover she could see there no sign of your—what else could she call it, Helen? —your deception. You looked as you always looked. It made her wonder, and there was longing in this of course, the hope that the newspaper man on the phone had gotten it all wrong. Because it's almost intolerable to her that you could be keeping this secret from her, that you could be capable of keeping any secret at all. Since you are so dependent on others for access to the outside world, it seems impossible that you could preserve anything on the inside that they did not know. And this came to your mother in the words, "She's lying to me. My Helen is lying to me!"—an ugly revelation most mothers have and get over when their child is three. And thinking the thought again, mouthing the words again, a throb rises in your mother's throat, which might have escaped as a sob except that at that moment the door is flung open and Miss Sullivan comes in.

She strides across the room in the deliberate, almost mannish way of hers that your mother always finds disconcerting. She straightens herself, swallows the sob, composes her feelings, as Miss Sullivan continues across the room. And she recalls briefly the first alarm of seeing this woman, almost thirty years ago, climbing down from the train and striding across the platform, her spine so straight it almost made a person curious about the skeletal structure underneath. Your mother was prepared to like the Yankee girl. Her heart swelled to see the small, erect figure wearing the unseasonably heavy wool dress. She imagined herself taking this poor but courageous girl under her wing as a companion, a confidante, a surrogate sister.

But when they shook hands there at the station, the courageous girl looked past your mother, looked through her, in a way that was not merely shy or socially awkward but downright rude. Her bearing showed she was eager to bypass these formalities and get down to business. Her indifference showed clearly that she saw your mother as all but irrelevant to the enterprise she was undertaking. Mrs. Keller was merely "the mother." The best she could do was to stay out of the way.

She has that same bearing still, your mother can't help noticing. And the observation stokes her fears. In the same instant she remembers something else about that first day, the look in her husband's eyes as he took in the newcomer's appearance. "Why did they have to send a beautiful one?" she'd thought at the time, and thinks again now, deflating further.

Teacher is no longer beautiful, of course. The years have really taken it out of her, or rather, piled it on her. She has taken on flesh, as women will in middle age. But on Teacher it seems more an unnatural swelling, an all-over puffiness. And while you flourish under the rigors of your life—the endless correspondence and other writing, the constant stream of new people, the meetings, and lectures, and receptions—they have drained her dry. Her eyes give her trouble all the time now. The skin around them is puckered in a permanent squint. All the extra weight impairs her movements. Sometimes her ankles are so swollen she can barely hobble across the room. In bad weather all her joints ache. And now there's this new respiratory complaint. Still, when riled as now, there is something startling about her, something that catches the breath. Because what people are aware of when they see her is not her face or body, but the energy animating them. Watching her now, your mother sees the layers of swollen flesh peel away, along with the wrinkles and graying hair, and the small, erect, vibrant body of thirty years ago steps free.

Then your mother notices the newspaper the other woman is carrying. She drops it into the armchair opposite your mother's, as if she is not only done with it but has found nothing of interest there. Your mother rises slowly to reach for it, but stops, afraid of what it will contain. So the two women face each other again, as for the first time. Miss Sullivan lifts off her hat, pats her hair, jabs the pin back into the band, and without a word of greeting, says again as she did that first day at Ivy Green, "And where is Helen?"

Your mother does not answer. She takes the paper and pulls it open. "It's all there," Miss Sullivan tells her wearily. She leans against the mantle briefly, then begins pacing the floor.

Your mother sinks back into her armchair again. She finds the short article but cannot focus her eyes on the newsprint. It is a relief to have the pages held up around her face so she isn't obliged to watch Miss Sullivan pacing back to the door, then back to the hearth, and back again. She hears it, though, and marvels again that a woman supposedly in such poor health, can throw down each step with such strength that the very walls rattle.

Your mother is trying not to cower. She's trying to summon her rehearsed speeches, but is not doing very well with it. "As you may remember, I always had my doubts about the wisdom, the propriety, of engaging . . . employing a young man to . . . "

But Miss Sullivan is not listening, only pacing. She stops in the middle of the room now. She blinks at your mother as if surprised to see her there and says, "I didn't think to check the other papers. I suppose they'll all have the story now."

Even in her trepidation, it occurs to your mother that there really was no need for Miss Sullivan to walk all the way down to the station just to buy the paper. She could have sent one of the servants. They are a rag-tag bunch, your mother thinks, undisciplined and strange. But surely one of them could have been trusted with a task as simple as that. But it is precisely the sort of thing Miss Sullivan is prone to do. She martyrs herself to fuel her own indignation. In another minute the exertion will make her start coughing.

"The first thing we'll have to do is call the paper and have them print a retraction," she says, on the move again, mumbling. Then she stops, turns, glowers down at your mother. "Exactly what did you say to that reporter?"

"Well I hardly had time to catch my breath. I . . . " Your mother feels an agitated sob rising in her voice now, a shrill, hysterical quaver. "I disengaged the line at once, as soon as I realized . . . I neither confirmed nor denied anything. He telephoned back but I told Polly to say I was home to no one."

"Good," Miss Sullivan says, and your mother can't help but feel a flush of pride at being praised. Then this is replaced by a sting of resentment that this woman feels it her right to praise her, your mother. She is not the pupil here, after all. But Miss Sullivan is musing now, holding her chin in her hand. "That's right. So he has no actual corroboration. Only a signature on a marriage license, which could be a forgery. Could be anyone. Surely Helen Keller is not such an unusual name. And the clerks at such places are not terribly observant. They must see a hundred couples a day. And the fact that she was silent the whole time would not necessarily . . . "

She stops again, her words trailing off into silence. Your mother looks at her, then looks where she is looking. And together they see you, Helen, gliding down the stairs. And though they knew you would be coming down any minute, it's as if they're shocked to see you there. They are simultaneously struck breathless by you, your appearance, how lovely you are. Not pretty. Even your mother would be quick to acknowledge that. But you have a quality. You've always had it. A quality that draws the gaze. And the quality is heightened by the dress you have on, which is newer and fancier than your usual day-at-home outfits. And your hair seems slightly more elaborate than usual, or maybe it's just the way the humidity has curled a few stray tendrils to make a hazy frame around your face.

They haven't been paying attention. You've been looking this way for weeks, if not longer. It's understandable they didn't notice while you were on tour, since on tour you are expected to make a good appearance. But even since you've been home, you've been more conscious of how you look. You've been uncharacteristically fussy about it, asking four and five times a day, "Do I look all right? Is my hair all right? Do these gloves go with this hat?" What they realize, suddenly, is that you've started dressing for a man. You've started making an effort to make yourself visually appealing, a vision of loveliness, a feast for the eyes, for him.

As they watch you glide across the room, each of them recalls a hundred minor instances of altered behavior that should have tripped an alarm. You have been eating less and smiling more. You've been embracing them more often than usual. Your letters to friends have been more effusively affectionate. You've even taken to hugging the dogs with such fervor that they yelp in fear.

You cross the room to stand near them. Your mother watches the other woman watching you. Without warning, something in Teacher's look sparks a maternal instinct in her, the same instinct that compels a mother to steer an eager toddler away from an open flame. But she knows it's already too late to intervene.

You stop near Teacher. Your nostrils flare slightly, and you say lazily, "Have you been out already?"

"Yes," she spells to you and says aloud for your mother, "I've been to get the paper. There's some rather distressing news."

The words "distressing news" are almost a code between you. She's always used them to prepare you for tragedy. She used them to announce the death of your first dog, Lioness, when you were ten, and the death of your father when you were sixteen. But your mind is elsewhere. "What news? News from Europe? The war . . . ?"

"No. News from home," she says. "Domestic news. Guess who's getting married."

Your first thought is John Macy. You know that there's been no formal divorce yet, but it would be like John to get mixed up with some woman and allow the rumor to be circulated before legal matters were finalized. You can imagine him speechifying about Byzantine divorce laws and bourgeois morality in a way that would make you laugh, if only it were about other people. John, remarried, you think, but who? But it's been so long since his name has been spoken in this house, you hesitate and say only, "Who's getting married?"

Teacher says, "You are, Helen."

Your hand jerks away from hers and dangles by your side for a full two seconds. Then you sweep it up to rest on your chest, and contort your face into a clownish mask of mute astonishment. Your mouth gapes, your eyebrows hoist your lids so high, your eyeballs protrude dangerously from their sockets. Good try, Helen, but the gesture needs work. Because you have never seen it done correctly, you don't know that those two seconds of hesitation give it all away. Your performance is so unconvincing that even your mother can't help but say, "I can't believe she's trying to deceive us this way."

Of course, you're oblivious to all this. You break your pose with a kind of gasp and ask Teacher, "Who do they think I'm marrying?"

"Whom," Teacher corrects automatically, then replies, "Peter Fagan of course."

"Peter!" you say. Your brain is on a treadmill. It pumps and strains but gets nowhere. You've talked about this, you and Peter, discussed how best to deliver the news to them. You've rehearsed various speeches. But the possibility that they might find out on their own never occurred to either of you.

Some of this mental activity may show on the outside, but I'm not sure. They are both studying your face, your mother because she still can't believe you're trying to pull this off and Teacher because she wants to watch you sweat. Finally she takes your hand. You feel the new tension there as she says firmly, "Tell us what happened, Helen."

But you surprise everyone, even yourself. You shake your free hand in the air as if you're wearing bells on every finger, and say, "It's silly. It's just a silly mistake." Then you break free of her and start waltzing around the room, fingering small objects here and there, smoothing a doily under a table lamp, fluffing the bouquet of flowers. You do a remarkable rendition of coy denial while the two of them look on, amazed.

Teacher says, "I wouldn't have thought it possible."

Your mother says, "My baby!"

The anguish in her tone makes Teacher turn on her. "We can't afford to get emotional now," she snaps.

Your mother adjusts herself in her chair, dabs her eyes with her crumpled handkerchief. "What ever shall we do?" she asks softly.

"We'll simply have to confront the man."

Meanwhile, you've come to a standstill in your flounce around the room. You're standing a little behind your mother's chair. You know they are talking about you. You feel the telltale air currents, or you smell the breath that propels their words. You rest one elbow on the mantelpiece, trying to strike a casual pose, still stalling for time. With your free hand you spell in the air, a careless, nonchalant question: "What are you talking about?" Then you allow your hand to fall and hang within easy reach of your mother.

But they don't answer. Your mother is not looking at you, and Teacher is deliberately ignoring you, perhaps because she feels she cannot trust herself to contain her anger. And why should they answer; you know what they're talking about.

You emit a strange breathy gasp that you hope sounds like light laughter, which makes them both look at you. Then you take up your mother's hand and say, "Mr. Fagan and me? It's just silly. He would never . . . he could never . . . he's engaged to someone else."

"What?" your mother says after repeating your words out loud.

"Yes. He confided it to me. He's engaged to someone else but must keep it a secret because the young lady's family does not approve."

You have no idea where these words are coming from. You suspect they come from one of those romance stories Polly is fond of reading to you to pass the time on trains. You never really pay attention to those stories but you think you've got the basic plot right. There's always a disapproving family on one side or the other, always the need for secrecy. You're hoping your mother, who occasionally dips into those magazines herself, will buy it.

"Engaged to another girl?" Teacher says. She exhales a snort through her nose. She arches her eyebrows and tells your mother, "Ask her, 'Who is this other girl?'"

"I cannot say. I promised . . . "

Teacher lets out a groan, steps forward and takes your hand. She positions it on her face to read her lips and enunciates slowly, "But the reporter saw your name on the license. Your name, Helen." Then she flings your hand away and says to your mother, "You see what he's done to her!"

Your mother's face is completely flushed now. She presses both hands to her cheeks and says, "Oh, I wish the Captain were still alive."

Teacher actually rolls her eyes at this, then repeats, "We'll simply have to confront him. He's probably waiting for it. He'll deny it too at first. For the effect."

Her tone makes your mother even more uneasy. "What do you mean?"

"I mean," Teacher says, "there's a script such men follow. First denial, then confession, then . . . " She shrugs her eyebrows with dismissive disgust.

"Then what?" your mother gasps, almost afraid to ask.

You are still standing there between them. You know you flubbed your lie and are now at a complete loss. You can feel Teacher's rage billowing out of her, and find yourself edging toward your mother for safety. Teacher stares straight at you, her eyes blazing, or glaring, or bulging (whatever it is eyes do), her jaw set, her lips pinched together. Then she looks at your mother again. "Extortion, of course. He'll expect some sort of payment," she says. "A lump sum, I'm hoping, and not a lifetime annuity."

"What?" your mother gasps. "Mr. Fagan? Surely not . . . "

You reach for your mother's hand and ask, "What is she saying?"

Your mother starts to respond, her fingers tentative, but suddenly you don't have your usual patience for her lack of fluency, and you fling yourself forward, aiming where you know Teacher to be. You lift her hand from her side, and repeat the question, the knuckles and tips of your fingers tapping hard against her parched palm. But she does not answer. She pushes your hand away, speaking to your mother. "Of course. What else? What else do you suppose he expects?"

"What are you saying?" your mother says. Despite her reservations about him she has to believe he's not capable of that.

"What are you saying," you spell in the air.

They ignore you so you reach for Teacher's hand again, but again she pushes you away. As she did when she wanted to punish you when you were a child, she turns her back, strides away, and throws herself onto the settee. You follow her, guided by the momentum of her movements. You plop down beside her, but she folds her arms away from you, clasps her hands in her armpits. Undaunted, you spell into her face. "All right, it's true. We are engaged. I love him and he loves me. I have a right to happiness, a right to marry the man I love. You can't stop me!"

But Teacher dodges your speaking hands, rocking her upper body from side to side so she can still speak around you to your mother. "What else would he want, a man like that? Why else did he come here? He came to take advantage of us, to exploit us." She throws back her head and lets out a single syllable of bitter laughter. "Surely you don't believe that reporter found this out on his own? If Fagan truly intended to marry her, he would have taken her away somewhere." She unclasps one of her hands to wag a finger in the air. "Mark my words. That reporter was tipped off. It was a warning, Fagan's way of letting us know he expects us to pay for his silence. Just think of the stories he could tell them if we don't . . . "

Abruptly, a new sound escapes Teacher's throat. When your mother looks she sees Teacher's hand over her mouth in an uncharacteristic posture of astonishment. She rises and moves swiftly back to your mother's chair. She says, "Is it . . . is she . . . ?" Words elude her. She sputters, seems on the verge of a coughing fit, and steadies herself, laying a hand on the back of your mother's chair. She leans toward her, as if to whisper. Then she straightens, and speaks the words distinctly, "Are we going to have to consult a physician?"

At first your mother doesn't get it. This has been the farthest thing from her mind. Then she too emits a gasp, and they both stare at you, sitting there, your hands in your lap now. And they both notice again that quality they saw when you came down the stairs. Despite your agitation they still see it. You are, in fact, glowing. There's a flush on your cheeks, but beyond that there's a luminosity around your head, your whole body. Their minds race ahead. Teacher's counting months, weighing options. Is it better to get a shotgun and force the man to do the honorable thing, or . . . ? While your mother, tears flowing down her cheeks now, is recalling your infancy, before the fever, the sweet freshness of your body. An ache starts in her arms, her breasts.

A baby? Good grief, Helen, a baby! Is this what you're not telling me? I don't know how I could have missed it. But now that I've gone through it, thought it through moment by moment, what else could it be?

Give me a minute to get my mind around this, Helen. And prepare yourself. You have some explaining to do.

Note

Writing Helen Keller is a series of letters written by me to Helen Keller, about events in Keller's life, events in my life, and other issues of concern to people with disabilities today. It is a work of imagination not a biography or scholarly study. I have written what seems to me to be possible or plausible, not what I can prove to be true. This excerpt treats an event that took place in 1916, when Keller was thirty-six and was briefly engaged to a man named Peter Fagan who had been hired to work as her secretary. Because this text represents a letter addressed to Helen Keller the pronoun "you" refers to her and not to the reader. "Teacher" was Keller's nickname for Anne Sullivan and is used here interchangeably with "Miss Sullivan." Other characters mentioned here include: John Macy, the Socialist, literary critic and Sullivan's estranged husband, and Polly Thomson, a young woman recently hired to be Sullivan's assistant.

Feeling Her Way

AUDRE LORDE AND THE POWER OF TOUCH

♪♪

SARAH E. CHINN

The Problem of Skin

How can we talk about how lesbians have sex with each other? This is no trivial question—if sexual connection with other women is at the core of lesbian identity,[1] then in some way accurately representing our sexuality is as close to a culture-making activity as we can get. That's not to say that there aren't pages and pages of descriptions of lesbian sex, from the "wave upon wave" vanilla of Naiad paperbacks to the hardcore daddy fantasies of S/M.[2] But very little of it is compelling, not because it is not sufficiently explicit but because it rarely succeeds in getting under a reader's skin.

Perhaps it's the skin itself that's the problem, or perhaps how to describe what sexuality does to it. In a related vein, Elaine Scarry has argued that there is no language for pain, no way of representing it. In language that strongly resembles the way we might think about sexuality, she argues that in the description of physical pain, "the events happening within the interior of [another] person's body may seem to have the remote character of some deep subterranean fact, belonging to an invisible geography that, however portentous, has no reality because it has not yet manifested itself on the visible surface of the earth" (1985, 3). Sexual desire, the sensation of sexual contact seem part of that subterranean world, outside our abilities to express ourselves. After all, how do we describe the electricity of lovemaking, of the loss of self in concert with (indeed dependent upon) an intense sensory awareness of self? As Elizabeth Grosz points out, "the most intense moments of pleasure and the force of their materiality cannot be reduced to terms that capture their force and intensity"(1995, 226).

Needless to say, this problem is hardly unique to lesbian sexuality—it is characteristic of sexual experience between people of any gender, or alone. In this chapter, I hope to tackle this conundrum by working with Audre Lorde's representations of lesbian sexuality, both in her "biomythography" *Zami* and in some of her theoretical work. Though I don't think Lorde gives us all the answers (or even that answers are necessarily what we need to explore how sexuality shapes us and our approach to the world), I do believe that *Zami* comprises a series of experiments in representing lesbian sexuality and human interconnection from which we as readers, lesbian and not, can learn. Consequently, my focus on lesbian sexuality here does not preclude analogy to other kinds of sexual practice; indeed, my larger argument is that Audre Lorde's representations of lesbianism can provide a key to thinking about sexuality and bodily experience more generally.

The sense that most people rely on primarily for information about the world around them—vision—is virtually useless when it comes to figuring out and describing the experience of sexual pleasure. Despite innumerable attempts to the contrary (and the well-stocked shelves of adult films in video stores attest to this), visual representations of sexual pleasure inevitably miss the mark, fall short of showing what desire feels like *inside* our bodies.[3] Indeed, the sighted often block out the visual during times of sexual intimacy: turning off lights, closing our eyes, both to connect with our partner(s) and to retreat from the regime of the visible. It seems, in fact, that a representative schema that imagined the visible as only one source among many (and not necessarily the most informative), that relied much more heavily upon other senses, might get closer to communicating the textures of sexuality.[4]

For this reason, S/M pornography comes the closest to capturing what sex feels like, since it so often works outside the limits of what is in front of participants' eyes and instead heavily depends upon sensation and the sublimity of sensory extremes. Sadomasochistic writing pays minute and exquisite attention to the maelstrom of experiences playing along the surfaces of the body, so often invisible (the feeling of restraint, the exchange of energy from arm to whip to back).[5]

S/M writing is more successful on its own terms than most lesbian representations of our sexuality, because it takes for granted that the visible can often be an obstacle to the realities of desire.[6] S/M requires that the participants ignore the seemingly inescapable fact that they are, perhaps, secretaries or bus drivers or college professors, and asks them to locate their fantasy lives in the sensual world,[7] disregarding what might otherwise be obvious. That's not to say that those fantasies are more true than the visible evidence of their bodies nor that secretaries or bus drivers or college professors might not constitute someone else's fantasy; it's instead to imagine that sensation can reveal a "truth" otherwise inaccessible to the regime of the visible, a truth that's all about inhabiting a narrative very different from our own (that is, that we're not just cogs in the service economy but governess and child, Marine sergeant and recruit, man and boy).[8]

S/M recognizes that sexuality is an activity, not an ontology—indeed that "sadomasochism, or any kind of 'perverse' sex is about *doing*" (Hart, 1998, 148; emphasis in original). Sadomasochism does not pretend to be real except to the extent that it accurately plays out fantasy. But at the same time, the fantasy is always understood as such, as being brought into material existence by the efforts of two or more people, as a collaborative process that can only exist through discussion, analysis, trust. Reality is beside the point: what matters is the world that the lovers create together, however temporarily.

This may seem like a strange way to begin a discussion of sexuality in the writing of Audre Lorde. Lorde herself was a contributor, as an interview subject, in the classic anti-S/M text, *Against Sadomasochism* (Linden, Russell, and Pagano 1982) and has long been championed as the embodiment of a sexuality far removed from the nastiness of S/M—earthy, physical, and resolutely natural, the Ur/earth mother of lesbian sexuality.[9] Lorde herself had a canny critique of S/M, arguing that sexual fantasy could not be disarticulated from the "larger economic and social issues surrounding our communities," and that there's a political reason that people get a kick out of the intensification of power difference that cannot simply be romanticized or explained away through sexual libertarianism. At the same time, Lorde emphasized that "*I speak not about condemnation* but about recognizing what is happening and questioning what it means" (Star 1982, 67).[10]

In this chapter, Lorde and her interviewer, Susan Leigh Star, often seem to be talking at cross purposes: Star wants Lorde to condemn S/M as unwomanly, unfeminist, and unlesbian, and Lorde wants to talk about the structural inequalities in U.S. culture that shape our imaginations, sexual and otherwise, a deep critique that does not exactly serve the purposes Star (1982) clearly planned for this discussion. As Anna Wilson has argued, white feminists in particular have used Lorde as the figure of a nonthreatening black/lesbian presence, despite Lorde's own best efforts to unseat them from that comfortable position (her "Open Letter to Mary Daly" is a sharp and still fresh example of that project, climaxing in Lorde's arresting question "Mary, do you ever really read the work of Black women?" [1984c, 68]). But Lorde's deep explorations of lesbian sexuality render impossible the liberal feminist fantasy of her as dyke mammy. Indeed, her persistent focus on the embodiedness of lesbian sex and her attempts to represent in language the world-making (and breaking) power of that sex is inextricable from her latter-day persona as griot to the lesbian nation.

So the analogy between the writing of Audre Lorde and writings on S/M is not as far-fetched as it initially might appear. Both recognize sexual desire as constitutive of meaningful lesbian identity—as "a well of replenishing and provocative force to the woman who does not fear its revelation"(Lorde, 1984d, 54)—an assumption that was hardly commonplace as Lorde was writing her most celebrated work. Indeed, Ti-Grace Atkinson's declaration that "I do not know of any feminist worthy of that name who, if forced to choose between freedom and sex, would choose sex," (1982, 91) has been much critiqued both explicitly and implicitly[11] (as though freedom did not automatically include sexual freedom) but is a potent reminder that too often anti-S/M feminists implicitly or explicitly separated feminist or lesbian identity from sexuality.[12] By contrast, both S/M participants and Lorde understand sexuality as a full-body experience and an experience that can embrace bodies of a variety of sizes, shapes, colors, and abilities. Both represent sexuality as a palette of desire enacted through a series of activities that bodies engage in alone and together. And both push the limits of the representation of sexuality, trying to get onto and inside the skin, while recognizing the impossibility of total representability.

I'd like to argue here that Lorde reimagines and represents lesbian sexuality in ways that profoundly challenge her readers, as sited on the surfaces and in the crannies of the body, as floating up into nostrils and ears, as myrrh—a fragrant, viscous scent absorbed into the skin. Moreover, for her, sexual connection between women is always in process, always being negotiated, much like sadomasochistic sexual exchange, which, in the words of Lynda Hart, "is an acting out of commitment, a willingness to be transformed through the recognition of the other" (1998, 80). Lorde bypasses the debate over feminist sexuality dominant during the period she wrote *Zami* (the text I'll be focusing on in my discussion), replacing struggles over objectification and sexual freedom with a sexual language that represented lesbian bodies as sacred, communicative, instrumental, textured, difficult. Lorde's theory of sexuality does not reject the visual but instead reformulates it as one possible way of knowing another person, and a comparatively poor way at that. Ultimately, Lorde represents lesbian sexuality as a conduit for entering into some kind of communion with an other, a way to authentically love others and oneself.

"There is Power in Looking"

In large part Lorde achieves this reformulation by reorienting lesbian sexuality away from the realm of the visual. The challenge of representing female sexuality, let alone lesbian sexuality, has long been a matter of concern for feminists, as the appearance of a volume such as *Against Sadomasochism* (Linden, Russell, and Pagano 1982) suggests and the visual figures as a central problematic. In the mid–1970s, as Laura Mulvey was formulating her psychoanalytic theory of "the gaze" —that is, the psychic mechanism that reshapes male fear of castration by objectifying women on the screen—a conceptual tool that would be so influential in film theory and feminist theorizing more generally, feminist activists were analyzing and attacking the objectification of women through the visual representation of women's bodies and women's sexual pleasures. The "pleasure in looking" offered by the intensely visual medium of film, combined with male control of the means of film production, constructed for Mulvey a world in which "the gaze of the spectator and that of the male characters in the film [and by extension, that of the camera itself] are neatly combined" to fix women on the screen as objects of male visual pleasure (Mulvey 1975/1989, 19). Women are to be looked at and men get to look.[13] Or, as Linda Williams succinctly put it a few years later, "to see is to desire" (1988, 13)[14] Moreover, as Georgina Kleege (1999) acerbically shows in her survey of films featuring blind women, to be looked at but not to be able to see may be a recipe for idealized female movie characters, but it also accentuates the male/sighted viewer's pleasure in women's vulnerable helplessness that is ancillary to the power of the gaze.

In the more than twenty-five years since the publication of Mulvey's groundbreaking work, the debates over the visual and the role of real sexual autonomy have not abated, particularly given the (slight) increase in the numbers of women producing images of women in film, on television, in pornography, and so on. The focus of the debate has only occasionally shifted. That is, the idea that control over women's sexuality is wielded through visual representation has remained a centerpiece.[15]

Moreover, visual power as a theoretical construct has pervaded the intellectual landscape in the United States, from Michel Foucault's statement that "[o]ur society is one . . . of surveillance" (1977, 217) to Jonathan Crary's (1998) observation that in the mid-nineteenth century, vision was separated from other senses, particularly that of touch, to bell hooks's asseveration that "[t]here is power in looking" (1992a, 115). The converse argument, that privilege empowers one to look, is made by Trinh T. Minh-ha (1989) in her critique of colonialist anthropology, which she sees as shading imperceptibly into voyeurism, the rawest expression of the sexualized desire for visual mastery. Visibility is somewhat more vexed in theories around sexuality. For example, the goal of "gay/lesbian visibility" that has been intrinsic to the liberal gay rights movement takes for granted that to be seen by the dominant power structure is a cultural and political advantage. At the same time, queer theory has worked with the gaze, often playfully, moving between a belief in the policing, disciplining power of the gaze, and in the liberatory potential of making oneself visible. Informed by psychoanalytic, particularly Lacanian, theories of the gaze, queer theorists have punned on looking with book titles such as *How Do I Look?*, a collection of essays on film, or *Novel Gazing*, an anthology of queer readings of modern fiction, even as projects informed more by liberalism have imagined queerness as *Hidden From History*, according to the title of one collection. Sally R. Munt (1998) has written with moving eloquence of the double-edged sword of lesbian visibility vis-à-vis the gaze, identifying the lesbian flâneur and the butch in relation to looking/being looked at.[16]

In disability studies, too, the gaze—or, as Rosemarie Garland-Thomson (1997, 26) has reformulated it, "the stare"—has been theorized as a vehicle of able-bodied mastery and, when reversed, of liberatory potential. Freaks, crips, gimps are objects in the able-bodied world, forced to endure the silent (or occasionally vocalized) stares of the normate majority; indeed, the stare was not so long ago a reliable source of income for those visibly disabled people recruited into freak shows and carnivals.[17] The "spectacle of the extraordinary body"(55) extended to the visibly disabled, racial and ethnic others, the very tall, short, thin, or fat, even the spectacle of the body out of control (as Ellen Hickey Grayson explores in her analysis of laughing gas demonstrations of the first half of the nineteenth century [1996]), as normates measured themselves against, and (dis)identified with the people on display.

Moreover, sexuality has often been folded into this process of objectification. The display of Saartje (or Sarah) Baartman, the "Hottentot Venus," in the 1810s focused on Baartman's buttocks and genitalia and extended beyond her death, as her labia were preserved for "scientific study.[18] Similarly, if more benignly, in 1863 P. T. Barnum arranged a wedding between midget performer Charles Stratton, who became "General" Tom Thumb, and Lavinia Warren (with equally small best man and maid of honor). The wedding and marriage both downplayed Stratton's sexuality by constructing a "wedding that looked like children imitating adults" and foregrounded it by producing a baby as the supposed issue of the marriage (although Warren was, in fact, infertile) and proof of Stratton's sexual potency (Merish 1996, 193). Barnum's display of "Circassian Beauties" on the one hand and Julia Pastrana, a hirsute Mexican woman whom he dubbed "the Ugliest Woman in the World," on the other, explicitly linked a freak identity with the (putatively male) viewer's sexual desire and standards of female pulchritude.[19]

The equation of freakery and sexual difference works in both directions, too. As Joshua Gamson (1998) has eloquently shown, today's "freaks" are embodied by sexual and/or racial and/or class difference: the poor and working class lesbians, gay men, bisexuals, and transgendered people, both white and of color, who are the objects of the gaze on television talk shows. Although Gamson argues forcefully that these "freaks" "talk back" to their audiences, to authority figures, and to each other, he acknowledges that the power of the medium to "freakify" can often overwhelm the desire of objectified Others to transform themselves into speaking subjects.

It can seem, then, that the gaze is, if not omnipotent, certainly omnipresent. Its power works both affirmatively—to render an other hypervisible—or negatively—to ignore the other and behave as though she is invisible. The desire in U.S. liberation movements to construct new images has been grounded in this double bind of the hyper/invisible Other, and the belief that the only way to escape the imperious gaze of the mainstream is create new audiences and new ways of looking: a visual economy controlled from the grassroots.[20] In the discussion that follows, however, I would like to try to unseat the visual from its perceptual throne. Rather than imagine a utopia in which the oppressed get to create ourselves "in our own image," I want to explore, through my reading of Lorde, a sense of self outside visual imagery, an eyes-free sexual vocabulary, a literally blind desire.

Blind Girl, Lesbian Woman

Audre, the narrator and protagonist of Audre Lorde's "biomythography" *Zami: A New Spelling of My Name* (1982), and a version of Lorde herself, is, as she reminds us several times, "legally blind" for the first five years of her life and functionally so until she gets glasses at the age of three. Through Audre's eyes, the visible world is refracted and nonspecific to the point of incomprehensibility, full of "strange lights and fascinating shapes" (31). Even the brightest, most direct light is transformed into diffuse "starburst patterns" (31). So Audre's earliest and most immediate childhood memories are organized around feel, sound, taste, smell. Certainly, her formative experiences of her mother are about sensation, not sight: the pain of her mother's fingers pinching her upper arm, the "warm milky smell" of her mother's sleeping body (34), her mother's combing of her hair, all occur outside the realm of the visible. Her memory is dominated by the extravisual, which extends into the universal, as hair combing is defined by "the radio, the scratching comb, the smell of petroleum jelly, the grip of her knees, and my stinging scalp" which "all fall into—*the rhythms of a litany*, the rituals of Black women combing their daughters' hair" (33).

In *Zami*, the mythical place of "*home*" itself is understood not by sight, because neither Audre nor her sisters has ever seen her mother's home island of Carriacou but through taste, touch, and smell: "the fruit smell of Noel's Hill" and of "the heavy smell of limes" (13), the taste of guava jelly and "chalky brown nuggets of pressed chocolate," the "sweet-smelling tonka bean" (14). In fact, the visible world fails Audre again and again in her search for her mother's homeland. Although she has heard about it, touched its fruit and artifacts, smelled and tasted it, Audre does not *see* Carriacou on a map until her mid-twenties. Ironically, the cultural marginalization of the Caribbean to the mapmakers of the United States, the social marginalization of Caribbean-Americans in this country, and the perceptual marginalization of the nonvisual senses (can you prove a place exists just because you have smelled and tasted it?) all come together in this moment of invisibility

Audre's childhood nearsightedness shapes her relation to the world even after she gains the ability to see through glasses. Her first encounter with the written word, rather than subordinating other senses, depends upon them for meaning. Audre learns to read "at the same time I learned to talk," establishing an equivalency between written and oral language (21). More tellingly, in her first encounter with a book, Audre "traced the large black letters with my fingers," absorbing written language as much through touch as through sight (in contrast to the confidence of that tracing, Audre can only "peer" at the "beautiful bright colors of the pictures" [23]).

Reality itself is measured through touch, as we see in the brief encounter between a four-year-old Audre and the evanescent little girl Toni. Encased in a wool snowsuit, Audre experiences her own body as sweaty and itchy—all too real. Toni, on the other hand, is a vision, in all senses of the word. Lorde describes in loving detail every stitch of Toni's outfit, from the "wine-red velvet coat" to the "white cotton knickers" (40). But it is Toni's visualness that makes her seem incorporeal, like a vision indeed. Sight must be confirmed by touch, so Audre "reached out my hands and lightly rubbed the soft velvet of her frock-coat up and down" (38). She feels the "soft silky warmth" of Toni's fur muff and begins to "finger the small shiny gold buttons on the front of her coat" (38). This erotically charged foreplay soon gives way to the main event: "I wanted," Audre says, "to take off all of her clothes, and touch her live little brown body and make sure she was real" (40). Touch is the guarantor of the real, because eyes couldn't necessarily tell the difference between a "real and warm" fleshly bottom and the "hard rubber, molded into a little crease" of a doll (40).[21]

All of the moments I have described so far are, following Lorde's defini-tion, erotic. That is, they exist in that space between "the beginnings of our sense of self and the chaos of our strongest feelings" (1984b, 54). They speak to a role the body plays that is larger than function but that does not participate in a fantasy of transcendence from the body. Moreover, they are about a sensory con-nection with others, "[t]he sharing of joy, whether physical, emotional, psychic, or intellectual" that embraces the entire body, that "flows through and colors . . . life with a kind of energy that heightens and sensitizes and strength-ens all . . . experience" (56–57). The erotic infuses and intensifies the experi-ence of the body, links the sensory with the spiritual.

This is a far cry from the usual language about representations of women's sexuality, particularly the eroticism of African American women. As numerous black feminist critics have observed, black women have long been in a precari-ous space in discussing and describing their sexuality.[22] More often than not, women of African descent have been objectified as sexual playthings, Jezebels, or scarlet women, or desexualized as Topsies and mammies. Only very rarely have black women been given cultural space to express themselves as the au-thors of their own desire and even then too often within the narrow bounds of male-defined sexual parameters. Critiques of this rough treatment have rightly looked to theories of the gaze as a way to understand the representation of black women's sexuality.

In her descriptions of lovemaking in *Zami*, Lorde opens up to us the erotic world of the extravisual that connects to Audre's formative sensory experiences. I am not trying to argue here that lesbian sexuality is somehow linked to child-hood and the connection to the mother, although that certainly was an argument about the etiology of lesbian relationships that connected theoreticians writing at the same time that Lorde was producing *Zami*.[23] In her profoundly influen-tial object-relations based 1978 study, *The Reproduction of Mothering*, Nancy Chodorow convincingly argued that women's primary role in rearing children meant that girls learned emotional connection as a female bond. Although Chodorow's thesis almost exclusively dealt with heterosexual women, her single mention of lesbianism affirmed that "[l]esbian relationships do tend to recreate mother-daughter emotions and connections" (1978, 200).

Adrienne Rich took this logic one step further in her essay "Compulsory Heterosexuality and Lesbian Existence." Rich speculated that women's role as "the earliest sources of emotional caring and physical nurture for both female and male children" raises the question of "whether the search for love and tenderness in both sexes does not originally lead toward women [and] *why in fact women would ever redirect that search*" (1980, 35; emphasis in original). For Rich, women's "emotional and erotic energies" must be "wrench[ed]" away from other women in order to serve patriarchy (35).

Rather than siting an idealized mother-daughter bond that is the grounding of the lesbian self, Lorde problematizes Audre's relationship with her mother, Linda. Far from the stereotypical mother of the middle-class nuclear family, Linda is tough, "different from other women," something of which young Audre is proud, but which also, she notes, "gave me pain and I fancied it the reason for so many of my childhood sorrows" (1982, 16). Audre does not learn how to love from her mother: instead, she learns how to fight, a skill that is certainly useful but hardly ensures a harmonious home life (indeed, Lorde characterizes Audre's teen years as "resembl[ing] nothing so much as a West Indian version of the Second World War. . . . Blitzkrieg became my favorite symbol for home" [82–83]). The feelings of nurturance and tenderness that Chodorow and Rich associate with motherhood are not absent from Linda Lorde's mothering, but they exist in a complex admixture with helplessness at racism, rage at her powerlessness in the white American world, harsh protection of her children, and fierce loyalty to and love for her husband.

Audre comes to understand (indeed, to authentically experience) her love for her mother when she embraces lesbian sexuality. The power of touching other women erotically allows her to connect with her mother, to empathize with her. Lorde reverses Rich's and Chodorow's logic, eroticizing Audre's relationship with her mother as though it could be another of her loving relationships as an adult woman. Audre's deep and enraged connection to her mother can be understood through her later lesbian consciousness, which can make sense of the sensory. The memories of smells, sounds, tastes, touches, all fall into place as part of a larger lesbian sensorium, an array of stimuli that the younger, prelesbian Audre could only experience as unrelated and episodic. For Lorde, then, lesbian (erotic) identity makes sense of the world both present and past.

An excellent example of this is narrative of Audre's first period. Pounding garlic, onion, salt, and pepper for a family meal, Audre feels "a new ripe fullness just beneath the pit of my stomach" (1982, 78). Connecting for the first time with the complexity of her sexuality (the smell of garlic combined with her sweat, the "jarring shocks of the velvet lined pestle," the thunk of pestle striking the bowl and her own humming [79]), Audre does not understand the implications of these new feelings—invoked in a very different context in her affair with Kitty—or of her encroaching adulthood, in her pre- or protolesbian identity. It is only as a lesbian adult that Audre/Lorde can form a narrative around her experience that interweaves the spicy fragrances of the contents of the mortar and her own sexed blood into a deeper understanding of how her sense of herself as a woman came into being.

All of the representations of sex between women in *Zami* exclude the visual as a primary way of knowing the other. Audre's first sexual experience with a woman, her first night with Ginger, is almost wholly about smells, tastes, and feelings. As Audre puts her arm around Ginger, "through the scents of powder and soap and hand cream I could smell the rising flush of her own spicy heat." Ginger tastes like "a winter pear" and like "myrrh"; Ginger's body "fill[ed] my mouth, my hands, wherever I touched" (1982, 139). Ginger's skin and hair are described by touch as "silky" and "crispy." Indeed the darkness of the night, rather than closing down connection through invisibility, opens up the exchange of energy between the two women, achieved as it is through the shifting touch of mouths, hands, and cunts.

Even when the visible seems to be at a premium, in the scene in which Eudora, Audre's lover during her sojourn in Mexico, reveals the scar that remains from her excised breast, Lorde interlaces the visual and the tactile. Eudora is visually alienated from her postmastectomy body: about her scars she says "I don't much like to look at them myself" (1982, 164). And Audre responds to Eudora's logic, looking hard at her chest, "with its rosy nipple erect to her scarred chest. The pale keloids of radiation burn lay in the hollow under her shoulder and arm down across her ribs." But Audre's focus is not on how Eudora's body looks. She tells us, "I had wondered so often how it would feel under my hands, my lips, this different part of her." Her desire for Eudora resembles the sunbursts of her life before glasses, "like a shower of light surrounding me and this woman before me" (167).

Audre falls back on the tactile to understand this new experience: "I bent and kissed her softly upon the scar where our hands had rested. I felt her heart strong and fast against my lips" (1982, 167). But she also acknowledges the crucial role visibility plays in Eudora's being able to integrate her own body into her sense of self. By on the one hand transferring the focus of their connection beyond the visual and on the other hand refusing to turn the light off, Audre gives Eudora both the opportunity to understand her body on her own terms and a new set of terms in which to experience herself as a sexual actor.

Later in life (although in a text written before *Zami*), as a survivor of a mastectomy herself, Lorde thinks back to her time with Eudora in similar terms: "I remember the hesitation and tenderness I felt as I touched the deeply scarred hollow under her right shoulder and across her chest" (1980, 35). More significantly, Lorde's anxieties about her own mastectomy deal primarily with questions of touch, as she imagines how her lover will approach her body and how their bodies will feel together, wondering "[w]hat is it like to be making love to a woman and have only one breast brushing against her? . . . What will it be like making love to me? Will she still find my body delicious?" (43).

This explicitly lesbian concern is in marked contrast to the anxieties the dominant culture, as represented by the woman from the American Cancer Society's Reach for Recovery, imagines mastectomy survivors' experience. Wielding a pink "flesh colored" prosthesis, the woman's focus is on breast cancer survivors' appearance—"Her message was, you are just as good as you were before because you can look exactly the same. . . . 'Look at me,' she said. . . . 'Now can you tell which is which?'" (*1980,* 42). Lorde rejects the prosthesis not only because it does not look the same (not least because of its racially inflected pinkness) but, more important, because "not even the most skillful prosthesis in the world could . . . feel the way my breast had felt, and either I would love my body one-breasted now, or remain forever alien to myself" (44).

Moreover, the physical and psychic pain that Lorde experiences seems to have little relationship to how severe her wound appears to be on the outside. She looks down at her chest, "expecting it to look like the ravaged and pitted battlefield of some major catastrophic war. But all I saw was my same soft brown skin, a little tender looking and puffy from the middle of my chest up into my armpit. . . . The skin looked smooth and tender and untroubled" (1980, 44–45). That same night, Lorde reports that "I hurt deep down in my chest and couldn't sleep, because it felt like someone was stepping on my breast that wasn't there with hobnailed boots" (45). In this experience, seemingly opposite to the pleasures of the erotic chronicled in *Zami,* Lorde learns the same lesson: that our bodies feel and are felt outside solely visual perception, that the dimensions of pleasure and pain are experienced through a complex of the senses.

It is in her relationship with Afrekete/Kitty that Audre becomes deeply immersed in an erotic vocabulary that extends beyond the visual and into what she calls the biomythographical. Afrekete, the goddess into whose hands Lorde entrusts herself and all of us, is translated into Kitty, a singer, sometime supermarket clerk, Southern migrant, mother, lesbian, and "tough and crazy" proto-lesbian feminist (1982, 250). The text moves in and out of narrative and dream, New York city reality and pan-Africanist myth, roman and italic fonts, just as the plantains, avocados, bananas, cocoyams, and cassava Kitty buys under the bridge move over, around, in and out of their bodies. The sexual and edible become inseparable, scent and taste and touch intertwine—the "deep undulations and tidal motions of [Kitty's] body slowly mashed ripe banana into a beige cream that mixed with the juices of [her] electric flesh" (249).

Indeed, Kitty herself is in part the source of Audre/Lorde's ability to recognize these intersections of the senses, since "Afrekete taught me roots, new definitions of our women's bodies—definitions for which I had only been in training to learn before" (1982, 250). The sensual and the visual combine in a moment of sacred synaesthesia as "I remember the moon rising against the tilted planes of her upthrust thighs, and my tongue caught the streak of silver reflected in the curly bush of her dappled-dark maiden hair" (252). Light itself, the sine qua non of the visible, has become a solid (liquid? ethereal?) substance to be tasted and swallowed, like the guavas and tonka beans of Carriacou. Audre's and

Kitty's bodies are reduced and amplified into "elements erupting into an electric storm, exchanging energy, sharing charge, brief and drenching" (253), most abstracted where they are most embodied.

The culmination of Lorde's implicit meditation on how we might reimagine lesbian sexuality both represents and has been made representable by Afrekete through the sensorium of the body. It is imprinted upon the skin itself, just as Afrekete's "print remains on my life with the resonance and power of an emotional tattoo" (1982, 253), just as "every woman I have ever loved has left her print on me" (255). Kitty herself disappears—indeed, it is never clear in the text whether she ever actually existed or, rather, how much of Audre and Kitty's encounter was autobio- and how much mythographical—but her touch has a half-life that endures beyond her visible presence.

It is no coincidence that the encounter with Kitty is the last episode in *Zami*, for the text as a whole seems to have been leading up to this life-changing interchange of power. Audre's initiation into lesbian sexuality (and a tentative black consciousness) with Ginger; the lesson she learns partly from Eudora, partly from Muriel, the lover with whom she lives after her return to New York (but whose ground was laid by her intense teenage friendship with her schoolmate Gennie, whose suicide shattered her), that sexual love might palliate but cannot heal a profoundly damaged person; her intense, improvisatory, ultimately disastrous relationship with Muriel, consummated in the meals of "strange succulent vegetables and peculiar fragrant pieces of dried meat" (1982, 201): all of these connections contain seeds of Audre's transformation through her intersection with Kitty.

These lessons serve her well. A crucial part of Lorde's recovery from a mastectomy years later is being able to reconnect with herself through erotic feeling, through feeling herself, in all senses of the phrase. As Jay Prosser observes, "feeling one's body as one's own . . . is a core component of subjectivity, perhaps its very basis" (2000, 78). Once Lorde can feel herself, both transitively and intransitively, through masturbation and the self-recognition that both issues from and accompanies it, she feels a reigniting of herself, "dim and flickering, but it was a welcome relief to the long coldness" (1980, 25). Ultimately, her appearance as a one-breasted woman is less significant than her ability to *feel* that one-breasted woman as herself. "I did not have to look down at the bandages on my chest to know that I did not feel the same as before surgery. But I still *felt like myself*, like Audre, and that encompassed so much more than simply the way my chest appeared" (57; emphasis added).

Feeling Our Way: New Vocabularies

What understandings about representing lesbian sexuality does Lorde offer her readers in *Zami*, then? Certainly not a narrative of the kind of lesbian exceptionalism that was typical of the years in which Lorde wrote *Zami*, the sense of moral superiority that issues from marginalization.[24] Indeed, *Zami* itself is a testament to the fact that the experience of subordination can warp and distort the lives of the marginalized in direct proportion to the critical distance it provides from the mainstream—oppression can shut people off from each other, lead them to destroy each other and themselves, and lead them to internalize dominant cultural assumptions about themselves and other subordinate people.

Zami is also not a testament to Audre/Lorde's overcoming the adversity presented by her visual impairment nor some kind of heroization of blindness as the key to the other senses. As Naomi Schor has eloquently pointed out, Western literature and culture have long been organized around sight as a master metaphor for comprehension and perception of all kinds. At the same time, Western culture has leaned upon the "myth of the moral blindness of the sighted [. . . and] the moral superiority of the physically blind upon the sighted," a myth that turns disability into a convenient metaphor for the sighted and refuses the complex meanings (let alone the day to day ramifications) of blindness for blind people themselves (1999, 92). Lorde was nobody's token, as her blistering critiques of the "academic arrogance" of white feminists who singled her out as "the" black woman to be on their panels and featured in their conferences amply illustrate (1984b, 110). Nor did she allow what Rosemarie Garland-Thomson (1996) has termed the "benevolent maternalism" of more privileged women to deny her the right to her rage or to her own methods of healing of self and others. As Elizabeth Alexander has observed, in *Zami* Lorde lays out her ethical and philosophical stance that "making love, how the body acts, is a counterpart or antidote to what has been done to it" (1994, 709). For Lorde, lovemaking is not just how the body acts but how it perceives, how it sorts through the welter of sensory information to construct a sense of self based on plenitude.

This sense of self is not strictly phenomenological or psychoanalytic but experiential; it is what Didier Anzieu has called the "Skin Ego"—the self that is constructed through touch and interaction. The Skin Ego, formed in early childhood, requires and contributes to "the construction of an envelope of well-being" (1989, 44). According to Anzieu, a child's first sense of safety is the belief that she shares a skin with her mother; she can separate from the mother when she realizes that she inhabits her own skin—a very different narrative from the heterosexualized trauma of the Oedipal crisis.[25]

More important, unlike the binarized gendering of Freudian psychoanalysis, Anzieu's theory of the Skin Ego acknowledges that identity is constructed through multiple differences, because "the human skin presents a considerable range of differences as regards grain, color, texture, and smell. . . . They allow one to identify others as objects of attachment and love and to assert oneself as an individual having one's own skin" (1980, 103). This is remarkably similar to Lorde's approach to difference—that "there are very real differences between us of race, age, and sex. But it is not those differences between us that are separating us. It is rather our refusal to recognize those differences, and to examine the distortions which result from our misnaming them" (1984a, 115). Difference is not destructive, but constitutive; a meaningful feminism, a meaningful humanity can "devise ways to use each others' difference to enrich our visions and our joint struggles," that is, to "identify others as objects of attachment and love" (122–123).

The source of this connection is the skin, the organ of touch and feeling, "an envelope which emits and receives signals in interaction with the environment; it 'vibrates' in resonance with it; it is animated and alive inside, clear and luminous" (Anzieu, *1989*, 230). In *Zami*, Lorde shows us what it means to truly live inside one's skin—a skin marked by race, gender, sexuality, ability, age, to name only a few ways in which the body interfaces with the world. As Lorde observes at the end of *The Cancer Journals*, "I alone own my feelings. I can never lose that feeling because I own it, because it comes out of myself. I can attach it anywhere I want to, because my feelings are a part of me, my sorrow and my joy" (1980, 77).

Anzieu's theory of the Skin Ego also dovetails with Lorde's understanding of touch in *Zami*. The skin touches and is touched simultaneously; even when I touch myself I am both actor and recipient, reminded of the mutuality of human interaction. This sense of the individual as a collection of self-determined feelings that exist to *attach*, to feel another person, is at the core of Lorde's definition of self and a core perception of disability studies as well. Understanding the contribution of disabled people and perspectives means validating the interconnection and interdependence of all people; Lorde's definition of "zami" as "a Carriacou name for women who work together as friends and lovers" (1982, 255) echoes a central principle of disability activism—that human identity is a phenomenon of self-with-others, not atomized individuals existing only for their own advancement. The ability to see without being seen, to exist removed from and acting upon rather than with others, is one of Western culture's (masculinist and imperialist) fascinations. By contrast, Lorde is interested not in the patriarchal separating power of the gaze but in the lesbian, feminist, and disabled conjoining power of touch.

For these reasons, I am wary of Garland-Thomson's conclusion in *Extraordinary Bodies* that disabled figures in black women's writing such as *Zami* (as well as Ann Petry's *The Street* [1946] and the novels of Toni Morrison) "enable their authors to represent a particularized self who both embodies and transcends cultural subjugation, claiming physical difference as exceptional rather than inferior" (1997, 105). My first unease is with the idea of difference as exceptional. I read Lorde, both in *Zami* and in her theoretical work, as arguing that difference is itself the human condition: this, as Anzieu points out, is the lesson our skin teaches us. My second discomfort is that this analysis steps dangerously close to the philosophy of lesbian superiority that Lorde explicitly rejects, and the traditional trope of the moral insight of blind people about which Schor so eloquently warns us. It does not take into account the powerful narrative of mutuality that *Zami* lays out through its exploration of the sensual.

It is certainly true that "*Zami* denaturalizes the normate viewpoint and protests its dominance," giving its reader an alternative history of the 1950s from the margins of hierarchies race, class, gender and sexuality. Moreover, Lorde consciously challenges and reverses the often unspoken value judgments of a racist, misogynistic, and homophobic world: a particularly arresting example is her mention of U.S. citizens who moved to Mexico when they were "whitelisted out of work" by McCarthyism (1982, 159). But where Garland-Thomson understands the work of *Zami* as transposing the power of the gaze and maintains that "Lorde invites the freak show viewer to leave the audience and stand beside the freak on the platform so that they can gaze together at the normates below with amused superiority and faint contempt" (1997, 133), I would argue that the text instead dips beneath, above, beyond, through the radar of the visual altogether. And far from encouraging "amused superiority and faint contempt," *Zami* acts as a guidebook for all its readers, if willing—lesbian or not, black or not, disabled or not, female or not, working class or not—to feel our own way out of the punishing strictures of the regimes of heterosexuality, white supremacy, male dominance, and visual primacy.[26]

Rather than reversing the gaze, or parodically appropriating it, as Garland-Thomson suggests, Lorde brings to it what is a central wisdom of disability studies: that we are all potentially disabled—none of us, if we live long enough, will maintain our hold on the able bodiedness of normate youth. Once we acknowledge that vision itself, able bodiedness itself, is in the final analysis fungible, the world is radically transformed and so are we. Given this insight, how must our assumptions about the world and our mobility within it be shaken up, redistributed, reordered? What would happen if we abandoned our prostheses of vision (glasses, contact lenses, magnifying glasses, etc.), our prostheses of identity, and moved beyond the visual as a way of organizing not just experience but our sense of self?

This insight is inextricable from the meanings Lorde garners from lesbian experience and lesbian identification. The lessons Audre learns from her body and the bodies of other women allow her to reach back into her childhood, back to her mother, through the language of lesbian desire, which must recognize, for example, her mother's difference from her (Linda would "rather have died" than call herself a dyke, but Audre identifies her as such [1982, 15]), even as it reclaims her mother for her own explicitly lesbian purposes. And she meditates on an epic question: "As a deep lode of our erotic lives and knowledge, how does our sexuality enrich us and empower our actions?" (71).

This is not to say that Lorde believes, to quote Pat Califia in a different idiom but a quite similar spirit, "that pleasure is always an anarchic force for good. I do not believe that we can fuck our way to freedom" (1988, 15); indeed, both Califia and Lorde share this skepticism about the liberatory power of sex per se. Lesbian bodies are not *the* source of knowledge and power; they are, instead a conduit to those forces. In other words, Lorde's project in *Zami* and in her other writing is not utopian but reparative; as Eve Kosofsky Sedgwick has phrased it in another context, Lorde reminds us that "[h]ope, often a fracturing, even a traumatic thing to experience, is among the energies by which the reparatively positioned reader"—the reader Lorde hopes to construct—"tries to organize the fragments and part-objects she encounters or creates" (1997, 54). The power of a politically conscious and socially ethical hope is to readjust the balance among the senses, rework the relationship between body and consciousness, and reforge the broken links shattered by fear of difference. Our work here should not be to "cure" difference but to recognize the multiple subjectivities difference brings into being. As Deaf activists have argued, what the mainstream sees as disability, marginalized people often understand as a parallel and valuable culture that can expand the definitions and parameters of human experience and interaction.

At the end of her essay "Blindness as Metaphor" (1999), Naomi Schor tells her readers that "the time has come for a new body language, one which would emanate from a sensorium that is grasped in its de-idealized reality, in its full range of complexity" (103). *Zami* gives us that language. It teaches us how to recognize ourselves in relation to others, how to feel our bodies ethically, as actors in a profound human drama. More important, in *Zami*, Lorde posits lesbian sexuality as a place to start thinking about how to understand such a language, a source of a new ethics of interconnection from which we can all learn, a new spelling of all our names.

Acknowledgments

Thanks to Robert McRuer and Abby Wilkerson for their insightful comments in shaping and polishing this chapter. My deepest thanks, as ever, go to Kris Franklin, whose love, generosity, and humbling intelligence continue to change me, and to Gabriel and Lea, who have truly taught me the power of touch.

Notes

This article originally appeared in *GLQ: A Journal of Lesbian and Gay Studies*, Volume 9, pp. 181–204. Copyright, 2003, Duke University Press. All rights reserved. Used by permission of the publisher.

1. And that is a big if—the debate over what makes someone a lesbian has been ongoing, and occasionally quite vitriolic, for decades. In her introduction to *The Apparitional Lesbian* (1993), Terry Castle lists the myriad questions facing anyone trying to pin down what makes a woman a lesbian: "Was a lesbian simply any woman who had sex with women? What then of the woman who had sex with women but denied she was a lesbian. What about women who had sex with women but also had sex with men? What about women who wanted to have sex with women but didn't?" (14).

    These questions have a lengthy feminist pedigree. For the radical feminists of the 1960s and early 1970s, for example, lesbian identity had very little to do with sexuality. Monique Wittig (1992) declared that lesbianism was constituted by a resistance to heteropatriarchy, a refusal to be a "woman," "the refusal of the economic, ideological, and political power of a man" (13). Similarly, for the political group Radicalesbians, lesbianism was both a rejection of male dominance and the ultimate expression of "woman-identification." But as Castle argues, this identification of lesbian as a solely political stance participates in what she calls the "ghosting" of lesbians that is a characteristic of Anglo-American modernity.

Moreover, contemporary theorists have taken the concept of identity itself to task. Judith Butler's simultaneous claiming and disavowal of the identity "lesbian" is paradigmatic: in asking "[w]hat or who is it that is 'out,' made manifest and fully disclosed when and I reveal myself as a lesbian?", Butler goes on to question the transparency of the meaning of the lesbian identity therein revealed: "For it is always finally unclear what is meant by invoking the lesbian-signifier" (1991, 15).

But other theorists yoke this unsureness to a kind of decision to forge ahead anyway. As Lynda Hart points out, "[I]dentities are necessary to function in 'reality.' . . . [They are] prosthetic devices, which is not to say that they are any less 'real' than anything else" (1998, 2). Similarly, after working through her own doubts as to the meaning of "lesbian," Judith Roof returns to lesbian identity as pull of sexual desire, acknowledging that a large part of her own sense of lesbian identity is her search for that identity in others and in texts, "for what happens rhetorically to eroticized relations between women, because reading, even academic reading, is stimulated, at least for me, by a libidinous urge connected both to a sexual practice and to the shape of my own desire" (1991, 120). And Sally R. Munt links this primacy of sexual desire to a cultural imperative: "Desire is implicated in all aspects of living a lesbian life; it is the fuel of our existence, a movement of promise" (1998, 10).

Ultimately, I find Audre Lorde's own certainty about her identity as lesbian as grounded in the erotic (about which I discuss in more detail below), her own intense sexual connection to women and to herself as a woman, a convincing index of what "lesbian" means: "a woman whose primary emotional and erotic allegiance is to [her] own sex" (Castle, 1993, 5).

2. For a terrific, and still current, analysis of the mediocrity of representations of sex in lesbian novels, see Bonnie Zimmerman's *The Safe Sea of Women: Lesbian Fiction 1969–1989* (Boston: Beacon Press, 1990). In her survey of twenty years of lesbian novels, Zimmerman was surprised to find that although "lesbian novelists describe sex in greater detail than do most heterosexual female novelists," the quality of this description is "repetitive, predictable, unimaginative, and dull" (99).

3. For a discussion of what it is that pornography *does* represent (i.e., its attempts to represent the "truth" of sex through generic conventions), see Linda Williams, *Hard Core: Power, Pleasure, and the "Frenzy of the Visible"* (Berkeley: University of California Press, 1989).

4. In her study of intercultural cinema, *The Skin of the Film* (2000), Laura U. Marks takes a similar approach. She argues that film marginalized people makes shows the incompleteness of visuality to represent experience, either because that experience has been excised from the visual record (e.g., the assassination of Patrice Lumumba) or because the culture being represented foregrounds other senses (the centrality of taste and smell to the people of the Indian subcontinent). These filmmakers manipulate filmic conventions, play with texture, sound, and time, to make a film that she terms "haptic"—film that shrinks the gap between vision and touch.

5. In Pat Califia's story "Jessie," the narrator is blindfolded and chained by her rockstar idol, the Jessie of the title. Unable to see, the narrator depends wholly on her other senses, only able to tell Jessie's proximity by "some imperceptible heating of my skin, an oh-so-slight stirring of the hairs on my forearms and the back of my neck" (1988, 54). Similarly, in an extended story, "The Calyx of Isis," one character reminds an-

other, "You must remember how good it makes you feel to whip her yourself. . . . How good it feels in the muscles of your arm" (126).

6. "On its own terms" is the operative phrase here. I am not arguing that S/M pornography is the only site in which fantasy and sexuality are at work or that it is the only explanatory schema for an extravisual representation of sex. S/M stands out for its clarity, rather than its uniqueness. Moreover, because of the intense battles waged over sadomasochism and "feminist sex" in the 1970s and 1980s, a broad and deep array of written engagements with S/M by practitioners and theoreticians (and some who bridge that gap) exists, making the example of S/M available for more general theoretical work such as this.

7. To talk about the senses without reference to vision is a kind of sleight of hand, but that's what I hope to do here. So the issue of vocabulary can be tricky. I am using the term *sensual* not only to describe "sensation" (i.e., physical touch) but also as part of a larger collection of sensory experiences of taste, smell, and even hearing, outside the visual domain. Though the word is not necessarily stretchy enough to embrace all the nonvisual senses, it seems the best choice in that it invokes a sensory experience in which "feeling" in its most complex meanings might be understood.

8. This imaginative process is actually quite similar to the psychic work that Jay Prosser argues transsexuals go through to integrate postoperative bodies into a sense of self. Prosser maintains that transsexuals have *already* imagined themselves with post-op primary and secondary sexual characteristics, despite all visible evidence to the contrary, and that the post-op physical body is simply confirmation of what they believed about themselves all along, that "reassignment is the restoration of the body" they always felt themselves having (2000, 88).

9. In her short commentary before the text of the interview with Lorde, Susan Leigh Star comments on the "idyllic" beauty of the Vermont countryside in which the two women met, and "suddenly imagined what it would be like to see someone dressed in black leather and chains, trotting through the meadow, as I am accustomed to seeing in my urban neighborhood in San Francisco." Connecting "radiant Audre" with the "radiant sunshine" of the Vermont summer, Star aligns S/M with the "created culture" of urban life, "sustained by a particularly urban technology," in direct contrast with the bucolic innocence of Vermont and, by association, of Lorde herself (1982, 66).

10. Lorde also implicitly questions the motives behind the foregrounding of S/M as a conflict in feminism, when other, for her more pressing, conflicts such as those around race, class, and sexuality fell into the background. As she put it: "When sadomasochism gets presented on center stage as a conflict in the feminist movement, I ask, what conflicts are *not* being presented?" a critique Star picks up on not at all (Star 1982, 68).

11. See, for example, Joan Nestle, *A Restricted Country* (Ithaca, N.Y., 1987); the entire oeuvre of Susie Bright, including *Susie Sexpert's Lesbian Sex World* (San Francisco: Cleis Press, 1991); Cherríe Moraga and Amber Hollibaugh, "What We're Rollin' Around in Bed With: Sexual Silences in Feminism" in *Powers of Desire: The Politics of Sexuality*, edited by Ann Snitow et al. (New York: Monthly Review, 1983).

12. For a discussion of the intense debate over the role of sexuality in women's liberation among radical feminists, see Alice Echols, *Daring to Be Bad: Radical Feminism 1969–1975* (Minneapolis: University of Minnesota Press, 1990). For documents of

the "sex wars" in which Atkinson lobbed one of the first grenades, see Ann Snitow et al., eds., *Powers of Desire: The Politics of Sexuality* (New York: Monthly Press Review, 1983); Carole Vance, ed., *Pleasure and Danger: Exploring Female Sexuality* (New York: Routledge, 1984); Lisa Duggan and Nan D. Hunter, *Sex Wars: Sexual Dissent and Political Culture* (New York: Routledge, 1995).

13. In a later essay, "Afterthoughts on 'Visual Pleasure and Narrative Cinema' Inspired by King Vidor's *Duel in the Sun*," Mulvey addresses "the 'women in the audience' issue," as well as films in which women are clearly active (such as melodrama). While acknowledging her own pleasure in "women's pictures" like *Duel in the Sun* or *Stella Dallas*, Mulvey concludes on a melancholy note, seeing the "female spectator's fantasy of masculinization at cross purposes with itself, restless in its transvestite clothes" (1989, 37).

14. Williams also argues that the gaze cannot easily be appropriated by women in film—when, as in horror films, women *are* the gazers rather than the gazed upon, their fates are usually death (and grisly, gory death at that) "to demonstrate how monstrous female desire can be" (1989, 97).

   In her later work, Williams moved away from theories of the gaze, and focused on the meaning of hard core pornography, often characterized as the genre most obsessed with the gaze and with fetishizing women as objects. In *Hard Core: Power, Pleasure, and the "Frenzy of the Visible,"* however, she argued that film pornography was a complex product of cultural change, a genre that was shaped as much by material conditions as by Oedipal desires, an analysis surprisingly close to Lorde's.

15. Linda Williams' analysis in *Hard Core* (1989) of women-owned porn studios, like Candida Royalle's Femme Productions, explores how (and how effectively) "woman-centered" pornography takes on the question of visual representation and power.

16. See particularly chapter 3, "The Butch Body."

17. For a rich selection of essays on the mainstream cultural uses of nonnormate bodies, see Rosemarie Garland-Thomson, ed., *Freakery: Cultural Spectacles of the Extraordinary Body* (New York: New York University Press, 1996).

18. For a discussion of the meanings of Baartman's display, see Sander L. Gilman, *Difference and Pathology: Stereotypes of Sexuality, Race, and Madness* (Ithaca, N.Y.: Cornell University Press, 1985).

19. For a full discussion of the history and meanings of the "Circassian Beauties" see Linda Frost's "The Circassian Beauty and the Circassian Slave: Gender, Imperialism, and American Popular Entertainment," in Garland-Thomson, *Freakery*, 248–262. For an analysis of Julia Pastrana, see Garland-Thomson, *Extraordinary Bodies: Figuring Physical Disability in American Culture and Literature* (New York: Columbia University Press, 1997), particularly pages 70–78.

20. See, for example, the feminist art of Judy Chicago that boots the phallus out of its place of primacy, replacing it with the vulvas of *The Dinner Party: A Symbol of Our Heritage* (New York: Doubleday, 1979). See, too (although in a considerably more postmodern vein), the art of the Dyke Action Machine (D.A.M.), which creates lesbian-centered appropriations of media images, from Gap print advertising to fake movie posters to self-help websites.

21. By way of comparison, see Lynda Hart's analysis of the Lacanian "Real": "if the 'Real' is a psychic space that cannot be occupied, it is because it is not ocular. That is, it does not take place in the time or space of the ideological illusion called 'reality' because it exceeds a specular economy" (1998, 161). Similarly, the "Real" of

Toni cannot be seen, only felt; the warmth of the real is representable only as sensual, not visual. Toni's perfection is, in fact, visually deceptive—she's so perfect that she looks like a doll. The only way to find out whether Toni is real (i.e., animate, human, capable of interaction and communion) is to touch her.

22. See, for example, Hazel V. Carby, *Reconstructing Womanhood: The Emergence of the Afro-American Woman Novelist* (New York: Oxford University Press, 1987); and "It Jus Be's Dat Way Sometime: The Sexual Politics of Women's Blues," in *Unequal Sisters: A Multicultural Reader* (New York: Routledge, 1990), 238–249; Deborah McDowell, Introduction to *Quicksand and Passing* (New Brunswick, N.J.: Rutgers University Press, 1986); bell hooks (Gloria Watkins), "Selling Hot Pussy: Representations of Black Female Sexuality in the Cultural Marketplace," in *Black Looks: Race and Representation* (Boston: South End Press, 1992b); Jacquelyn Dowd Hall, "'The Mind that Burns in Each Body': Women, Rape, and Racial Violence," in Snitow et al., eds., *Powers of Desire*.

These critics come at the representation of black women's sexuality from quite different perspectives. For example, Carby (in *Reconstructing Womanhood*) and MacDowell both discuss the perceived need by middle-class black women to distance themselves from myths of hypersexualization, while in "It Jus Be's Dat Way," Carby celebrates the sexual openness of female blues singers such as Bessie Smith and Gladys Bentley, who rejected what they saw as bourgeois pretension. Dowd Hall's essay takes on the holocaust of lynching and its ramifications for African American women, who were constructed as opposites to virtuous white Southern women and, hence, available to the sexual violence that white men projected onto black men.

These perspectives show us how complex the question of reading heterosexual black women's sexuality is, let alone representations of black lesbians, who, as Jewelle Gomez has written, have been covered by a "shadow of repression . . . in literature in direct proportion to [their] invisibility in American society" (1983, 110).

23. Bonnie Zimmerman follows a similar line of analysis in her discussion of *Zami* in *The Safe Sea of Women* (1990), arguing that the text's "female-orientation may be so deeply erotic that in loving the mother, the daughter learns to look for love from other women" (193).

24. Lorde traces the roots of this sense of lesbian political and material superiority back to the 1950s in the denial of racism among her group of "gay girls." "Even Muriel seemed to believe that as lesbians, we were all outsiders and all equal in our outsiderhood. 'We're all niggers,' she used to say, and I hated to hear her say it. It was wishful thinking based on little fact; the ways in which it was true languished in the shadow of those many ways in which it would always be false" (1982, 203).

In the early 1970s, the belief that lesbians were inevitably in the vanguard of the feminist revolution was particularly powerful. The lesbian-feminist group Radicalesbians' assertion that "[a] lesbian is the rage of all women condensed to the point of explosion . . . , the woman who, often beginning at an extremely early age, acts in accordance with her inner compulsion to be a more complete and freer human being than her society—perhaps then but certainly later—cares to allow her" encapsulates this sense that lesbians were more able and more likely to cast off the shackles of heteropatriarchy (1972, 172).

Certainly the battles over "feminist" sexuality were motivated in part by the assumption that lesbian sexuality should be "above" (or at least beyond) issues of power and control. More recently, Alison Bechdel's *Dykes to Watch Out For* (1992) comic strip (a fairly reliable barometer of politically conscious, self-identified, middle-class lesbian culture) featured a discussion between two characters on changes in lesbian political mores that culminated with Lois, the resident bad girl, analyzing the shift away from "lesbian-feminist monoculture" of political superiority and resistance to the mainstream. "After all," she declares, "lesbians aren't all androgynous, vegetarian radicals. Some of us *like* dresses and makeup! Some of us even voted for Bush!" (17).

25. Anzieu also sets himself in opposition to Lacan: "I myself would oppose the formula: 'the unconscious is structured like a language' with a formulation that is implicit in Freud: 'the unconscious is structured like the body'" (*1990, 43*).

26. I would argue, too, that Gloria Anzaldúa's *Borderlands/La Frontera* (1987) plays a similar role. In my experience in teaching both texts, I have found that white students can react quite negatively to the critique of white supremacy, particularly in Anzaldúa's work. However, I see in both texts a desire to show readers alternative modes of perceiving and acting in the world. For Anzaldúa, the key is a connection to the unconscious/supernatural "Coatlicue state," the liminal realm in which a person must relinquish control over self and others. For Lorde it is a trust in the language of the body in connection with others. Both writers emphasize the power of interconnection outside (but acutely conscious of) hierarchy as a place to begin healing the self and a damaged and damaging culture.

Works Cited

Alexander, Elizabeth. 1994. "Coming out blackened and whole": Fragmentation and reintegration in Audre Lorde's *Zami* and *The Cancer Journals*. *ALH* 6:709.

Anzaldúa, Gloria. 1987. *Borderlands/la frontera: The new mestiza*. San Francisco: Aunt Lute Books.

Anzieu, Didier. 1989. *The skin ego: A psychoanalytic approach to the self*. Translated by Chris Turner. New Haven, Conn.: Yale University Press.

———. 1990. *A skin for thought: Interviews with Gilbert Tarrab*. London: Karnac.

Atkinson, Ti-Grace. 1982. Why I'm against S/M liberation. In *Against sadomasochism*, edited by Robin Ruth Linden, Diana E. Russell, and Darlene L. Pagano. East Palo Alto, Calif.: Frog in the Well.

Bechdel, Alison. 1992. *Dykes to watch out for: The sequel*. Ithaca, N.Y.: Firebrand Books.

Bright, Susie. 1991. *Susie Sexpert's lesbian sex world*. San Francisco: Cleis Press.

Butler, Judith. 1991. Imitation and gender insubordination. In *Inside/out: Lesbian theories, gay theories*, edited by Diana Fuss. New York: Routledge.

Califia, Pat. 1988. *Macho sluts: Erotic fiction*. Boston: Alyson Books.

Carby, Hazel V. 1987. *Reconstructing womanhood: The emergence of the Afro-American woman novelist*. New York: Oxford University Press.

———. 1990. It jus be's dat way sometime: The sexual politics of women's blues. In *Unequal sisters: A multicultural reader*, edited by Vicki Ruiz and Ellen Carol Dubois. New York: Routledge.

Castle, Terry. 1993. *The apparitional lesbian: Female homosexuality and modern culture*. New York: Columbia University Press.

Chicago, Judy. 1979. *The dinner party: A symbol of our heritage*. New York: Doubleday.

Chodorow, Nancy. 1978. *The reproduction of mothering: Psychoanalysis and the sociology of gender*. Berkeley: University of California Press.

Crary, Jonathan. 1998. *Techniques of the observer: On vision and modernity in the nineteenth century*. Cambridge, Mass.: MIT Press.

Duggan, Lisa, and Nan D. Hunter. 1995. *Sex wars: Sexual dissent and political culture*. New York: Routledge.

Dyke Action Machine (D.A.M.). Available at www.dykeactionmachine.com.

Echols, Alice. 1990. *Daring to be bad: Radical feminism 1969–1975*. Minneapolis: University of Minnesota Press.

Foucault, Michel. 1977. *Discipline and punish*. Translated by Alan Sheridan. New York: Vintage Books.

Frost, Linda. 1996. The Circassian beauty and the Circassian slave: Gender, imperialism, and American popular entertainment. In *Freakery: Cultural spectacles of the extraordinary body*, edited by Rosemary Garland-Thompson. New York: New York University Press.

Gamson, Joshua. 1998. *Freaks talk back: Tabloid talk shows and sexual nonconformity*. Chicago: University of Chicago Press.

Garland-Thomson, Rosemarie, ed. 1996. *Freakery: Cultural spectacles of the extraordinary body*. New York: New York University Press.

———. 1997. *Extraordinary bodies: Figuring physical disability in American culture and literature*. New York: Columbia University Press.

Gilman, Sander L. 1985. *Difference and Pathology: Stereotypes of sexuality, race, and madness*. Ithaca, N.Y.: Cornell University Press.

Gomez, Jewelle. 1983. A cultural legacy denied and discovered: Black lesbians in fiction by women. In *Home girls: A black feminist anthology*, edited by Barbara Smith. New York: Kitchen Table/Women of Color Press.

Grayson, Ellen Hickey. 1996. Social order and psychological disorder: Laughing gas demonstrations 1800–1850. In *Freakery: Cultural spectacles of the extraordinary body*, edited by Rosemary Garland-Thompson. New York: New York University Press.

Grosz, Elizabeth. 1995. Bodies and pleasures in queer theory. In *Who can speak? Authority and critical identity*, edited by Judith Roof and Robyn Wiegman. Urbana: University of Illinois Press.

Hall, Jacquelyn Dowd. 1983. "The mind that burns in each body": Women, rape, and racial violence. In *Powers of desire: the politics of sexuality*, edited by Ann Snitow, Christine Stansell, and Sharon Thompson. New York: Monthly Review Press.

Hart, Lynda. 1998. *Between the body and the flesh: Performing sadomasochism*. New York: Columbia University Press.

hooks, bell. (Gloria Watkins). 1992a. *Black looks: Race and representation*. Boston: South End Press.

———. 1992b. Selling hot pussy: Representations of black female sexuality in the cultural marketplace. In *Black looks: Race and representation*. Boston: South End Press.

Kleege, Georgina. 1999. *Sight unseen*. New Haven, Conn.: Yale University Press.

Linden, Robin Ruth, Diana E. Russell, and Darlene L. Pagano, eds. *Against sadomasochism*. East Palo Alto, Calif.: Frog in the Well

Lorde, Audre. 1980. *The cancer journals*. Argyle, N.Y.: Spinsters Ink.

———. 1982. *Zami: A new spelling of my name. A biomythography*. Freedom, Calif.: The Crossing Press.

———. 1984a. Age, race, class, and sex: Women redefining difference. In *Sister/outsider: Essays and speeches*. Freedom, Calif.: The Crossing Press, 115.

———. 1984b. The master's tools will not dismantle the master's house. In *Sister/outsider: Essays and speeches*. Freedom, Calif.: The Crossing Press, 110.

————. 1984c. An open letter to Mary Daly. In *Sister/outsider: Essays and speeches*. Freedom, Calif.: The Crossing Press.

————. 1984d. Uses of the erotic: The erotic as power. In *Sister/outsider: Essays and speeches*. Freedom, Calif.: The Crossing Press.

Marks, Laura U. 2000. *The skin of the film: Intercultural cinema, embodiment, and the senses*. Durham, N.C.: Duke University Press.

McDowell, Deborah. 1986. Introduction to *Quicksand and Passing*, by Nella Larsen. New Brunswick, N.J.: Rutgers University Press.

Merish, Lori. Cuteness and commodity aesthetics: Tom Thumb and Shirley Temple. In *Freakery: Cultural spectacles of the extraordinary body*, edited by Rosemary Garland-Thompson. New York: New York University Press.

Moraga, Cherríe, and Amber Hollibaugh. 1983. What we're rollin' around in bed with: Sexual silences in feminism. In *Powers of desire: The politics of sexuality*, edited by Ann Snitow, Christine Stansell, and Sharon Thompson. New York: Monthly Review Press.

Mulvey, Laura. 1975/1989. Visual pleasure and narrative cinema. *Screen* 163: 6–18. Reprinted in her *Visual and other pleasures*, Bloomington: Indiana University Press.

————. 1989. Afterthoughts on "Visual pleasure and narrative cinema" inspired by King Vidor's *Duel in the sun*. In her *Visual and other pleasures*. Bloomington: Indiana University Press.

————. 1989. *Visual and other pleasures*. Bloomington: Indiana University Press, 1989.

Munt, Sally R. 1998. *Heroic desire: Lesbian identity and cultural space*. New York: New York University Press.

Nestle, Joan. 1987. *A restricted country*. Ithaca, N.Y.: Firebrand Books.

Petry, Ann. 1946. *The street*. Boston: Houghton Mifflin.

Prosser, Jay. 2000. *Second skins: The body narratives of transsexuality*. New York: Columbia University Press.

Radicalesbians. 1972. The woman-identified woman. In *Out of the closets: Voices of gay liberation*, 2d ed., edited by Karla Jay and Alan Young. New York: New York University Press.

Rich, Adrienne. 1980. Compulsory heterosexuality and lesbian existence. In *Blood, bread, and poetry: Selected prose 1979–1985*. New York: W.W. Norton, 1986.

Roof, Judith. 1991. *A lure of knowledge: Lesbian sexuality and theory*. New York: Columbia University Press.

Scarry, Elaine. 1985. *The body in pain: The making and unmaking of the world*. New York: Oxford University Press.

Schor, Naomi. 1999. Blindness as metaphor. *Differences: A Journal of Feminist Cultural Studies* 11: 92.

Sedgwick, Eve Kosofsky, ed. 1997. *Novel gazing: Queer readings in fiction*. Durham, N.C.: Duke University Press.

Snitow, Ann, Christine Stansell, and Sharon Thompson, eds. 1983. *Powers of desire: The politics of sexuality*. New York: Monthly Review Press.

Star, Susan Leigh, and Audre Lorde. 1982. Interview with Audre Lorde. In *Against sadomasochism*, edited by Robin Ruth Linden, Diana E. Russell, and Darlene L. Pagano. East Palo Alto, Calif.: Frog in the Well.

Trinh T. Minh-ha. 1989. *Woman, Native, Other: Writing postcoloniality and feminism*. Bloomington: University of Indiana Press.

Vance, Carole, ed. 1984. *Pleasure and danger: Exploring female sexuality.* New York: Routledge

Williams, Linda. 1989. *Hard core: Power, pleasure, and the "frenzy of the visible."* Berkeley: University of California Press.

———. Feminist film theory: Mildred Pierce and the Second World War. In *Female spectators: Looking at film and television*, edited by Deidre E. Pribram, 12–30. London: Verso.

Wittig, Monique. 1992. *The straight mind and other essays.* Boston: Beacon Press.

Zimmerman, Bonnie. 1990. *The safe sea of women: Lesbian fiction 1969–1989.* Boston: Beacon Press.

Disability, Gender, and National Identity in the Painting of Frida Kahlo

⚜

ROBIN ADÈLE GREELEY

Frida Kahlo died in 1954, at the age of forty-seven. She died of complications due to a severe bus accident, when she was eighteen, in which a metal handrail entered her lower body, broke her spinal column and pelvis, and exited through her vagina. This accident, combined with an earlier bout with polio and a possible congenital spinal deformation, left her physically disabled on a number of levels for the rest of her life.

At the time of her death, Kahlo herself was famous—for her communist politics, rather less so for her painting, and for her flamboyant personality and the ongoing, highly public saga of her marriage to muralist Diego Rivera. After her death, her work fell into obscurity until the 1970s. At this point, the confluence of a number of movements and events served to bring her work back to the forefront of national and international renown. In the international sphere, Kahlo's paintings are now more immediately recognizable than any other Mexican artist. In the United States, this sudden interest in Kahlo was first due to the rise of the Chicano movement in the mid–1960s and to the feminist movement. Kahlo was subsequently taken up as a media event, resulting in "Fridamania." A pithy example of this comes from a *New York Times* article in 1990 that claimed Kahlo was only famous because she happened to be: "Hispanic, female and an invalid," not because she made good art.[1]

Clearly, a lot is going on in that quotation with regard to gender, disability, and how the confluence of the two in the body of a talented Mexican woman is characterized within mainstream U.S. society. But I want to look at a rather different situation, in which Kahlo's disability figures in relation to national identity. In Mexico, the reemergence of Kahlo as an important artist occurred under significantly different circumstances having to do with Mexico's violent entry into modernity and its development of a national identity in response. Kahlo was born in 1907—just before the onslaught of the Mexican Revolution. Lasting from 1910 to 1917, the revolution propelled the country precipitously into global modernity under the political rhetoric of socialism. Visual representation was seen as a particularly crucial area in the battle for interpretive power in the years following, in which the Mexican Mural Movement emerged triumphant not only in its home country but throughout Latin America, as the symbolic representor of modern nations fundamentally different from their former colonizers. The Muralists, particularly *Los Tres Grandes* —Diego Rivera, José Clemente Orozco, and David Alfaro Siqueiros—maneuvered to become the primary government-sponsored imagers of modern, revolutionary Mexico largely through a visual rubric of socialism and indigenism.

Despite the government's socialist rhetoric, however, the reality of "progress" was quite different; from the 1940s to the 1960s, the Mexican Revolution, as emblematized by the government of the Institutional Revolutionary Party (the PRI), slowed and stalled. The revolution's promises to narrow the gap of income inequality, to nationalize the economy, and to make internal politics more democratic were viewed by the general Mexican public as ideals betrayed by the PRI. By 1968, political unrest was very high, coming to an explosive head around the Tlatelolco Massacre in which police fired upon a peaceful demonstration, killing some five hundred women, men, and children.[2] Nineteen sixty-eight marks a year of trauma and disillusion in Mexican history, during which any remaining pretensions on the part of the government to revolutionary socialism were revealed to be fraudulent. The Muralists, who had been the cultural representatives of the PRI and its political doctrine of revolutionary nationalism since the 1920s, were discredited as being hand-in-glove with a government willing to slaughter its own citizens to maintain its corporate capitalism status quo.[3]

Yet while Mexican Muralism, as the cultural representative of the PRI, came under severe attack, Kahlo's work attained unprecedented heights of popularity. Unlike her celebrity in Europe and the United States, where she was first taken up by a feminist movement little concerned with issues of race or national identity and then by the mass media as a sensationalist cult object, Kahlo's newfound popularity in Mexico had to do, I argue, with the appropriateness of her representations of her own disability as a metaphor for national identity. In fact, her self-portraits came to stand in the popular imagination for the Mexican nation as wounded, fragmented, and split, as internally tortured and ambiguously figured in relation to its own borders. A new generation of artists took up her images, to be repeated, elaborated, and transformed as a means of interrogating the utopian masculinist and triumphalist rhetoric of revolutionary nationalism the PRI and the Muralists presented. Artists such as Nahum Zenil have reworked Kahlo's imagery to reveal the fictiveness of Rivera's or Siqueiros's heroic fighters, whose perfect and able bodies were the outward sign of an implacable,

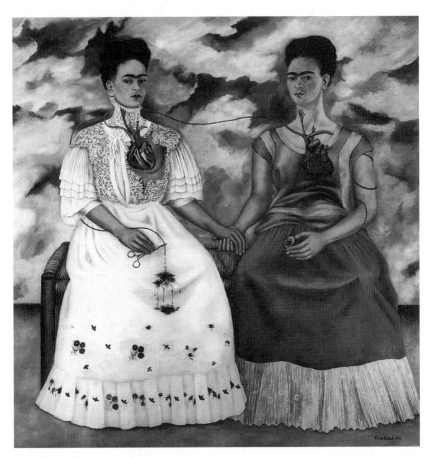

FIGURE 1. Frida Kahlo, *The Two Fridas* (1939) oil on canvas, 173 × 173 cm. Museo de Arte Moderno, Mexico City. © *Banco de México Diego Rivera & Frida Kahlo Museums Trust. Av. Cinco de Mayo No. 2, Col. Centro, Del. Cuauhtémoc 06059, México, D.F.*

single-minded, revolutionary consciousness. Zenil, for example, translates Kahlo's famous double self-portrait, *The Two Fridas*, into a sly commentary on the unassuming humility of everyday Mexican life and the ridiculousness of heroic masculinity (figs. 1 and 2).

Not only does Zenil's substitution of his own self-portrait for one of the Fridas subtly introduce the theme of his own homosexuality—a theme he allows to retain all its troubling, unsettling qualities with regard to the legendary Mexican machismo—but the artist also continues to string the Frida-association along through a further self-portrait to the right that humorously points up how useless the male *herramientos* ("tools") are in their tiny box carefully guarded between the other Zenil-passenger's legs.[4] The split Fridas of Kahlo's

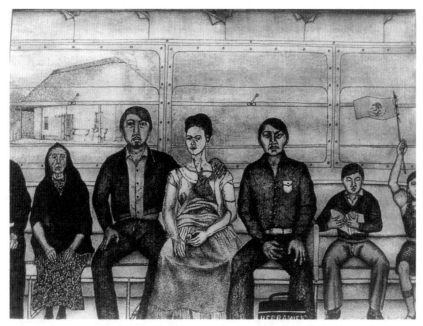

FIGURE 2. Nahum Zenil, *With All Due Respect* (1983) mixed media on paper, 30.5 × 41 cm. *Galería de Arte Mexicano, Mexico City, and Nahum B. Zenil.*

painting, traditionally understood to refer both to her ruptured body and to her dual Mexican-European heritage (her mother was Mexican, her father German Jewish), become under Zenil's hand a black humored critique of the PRI's failure to put its money where its mouth is. As such, Zenil's painting is representative of the best Frida-homages: it conjures up the image of Kahlo's disabled, imperfect body as a metaphor for contemporary Mexican identity but in no way succumbs to the perennial "victim" status all too often accorded Kahlo, Mexico, and its citizens by so-called First World scholarship. Zenil's image is an example of the simultaneous practices of *resistance* embedded both in Kahlo's works and in the popularization of them in post–1968 Mexico. It plays off the complex strategies of visual representation that Kahlo used, which have made her paintings such potent counterproposals to hegemonic ideologies of Mexican national identity.

The importance of Kahlo's work in the post–1968 period gives us an impetus for reevaluating how she dealt with the issue of national identity within the context of other nationalist discourses during her lifetime. The post–1968 response is key, in fact, to avoiding one of the major problems of extant writing on Kahlo: the incessant personalization of her work as some kind of transparent reflection of her identity and artistic intentions. These interpretations view Kahlo's aesthetic intentions as entirely bound up in her "anguish" over the dual "tragedy" of her physical condition and her marriage to Rivera.[5] While these incidents are no doubt central to much of Kahlo's production, to reduce the meaning of her images to this simple reflection of her immediate circumstances does nothing to register Kahlo's intricate social and cultural interactions with any number of larger issues. The complexity and variety of the post–1968 Mexican response to Kahlo's work cannot adequately be explained through simplistic interpretations of her imagery as a direct reflection of her personal difficulties. What this chapter intends, therefore, is to focus on contextualizing Kahlo's work within other visual languages of Mexican national identity of the 1930s and 1940s. It is only by elucidating this context, at least partially, that the effectiveness of Kahlo's perspective on the disabled female body, in relation to the national body, can be understood.

One place to start is with the work of Kahlo's own husband, Diego Rivera, and the mural cycle he painted in the Ministry of Education throughout the late 1920s. The mural *Distributing Arms*, of 1928, is one of the most famous of the cycle, largely because of the portrait of Kahlo included in its middle (fig. 3). It is an upbeat and positive image of social change, taking on the role of women as well as the role of the proletariat and the peasantry in their struggle for social equality. It is a Marxist view, with a particularly Mexican bent, in that it posits an active role for white-clad peasants alongside workers in revolutionizing Mexico.[6] It is very unusual in its central image of a strong female protagonist, dressed in masculine worker's clothing and engaged in armed struggle. No place for a woman, most would have said, despite the overwhelming evidence of women's participation in the Mexican Revolution of 1910–1917.[7] Certainly no place for a woman whose right leg had been so badly affected by polio and by her bus accident that she only walked with difficulty and always with a pronounced limp. Nor for a woman who underwent some thirty operations to fix her spine and pelvis, both broken and deformed by the accident. Yet Rivera bucks convention and paints her, red shirted, short haired and active, at the center of the melee preceding an upcoming class battle.

Nevertheless, Kahlo is only shown helping rather than herself taking up a gun, and significantly she stands directly below the real protagonist—the idealized figure of the male worker who directs the entire scenario. Despite this mural's atypical aspects, in the end Rivera's work upholds a more general gender dichotomy in which it is always men who lead, women who follow and serve. One feels, in fact, that Rivera only found it possible to insert Kahlo's portrait after he had masculinized and proletarianized it, and utopically abled her disabled body. The revolution, in the hegemonic narrative, had no room for the less-than-perfect, the weak, or those whose bodies prevent them from being part of the labor force. Rivera, like so many others, ultimately subscribed to the dominant view that equated social transformation with masculine virility and helplessness with femininity.[8]

The tensions within Rivera's unusual depiction of female activism, and its ultimate capitulation to normative concepts of gender difference, open up several possible avenues of investigation in relation to Kahlo's own works and the

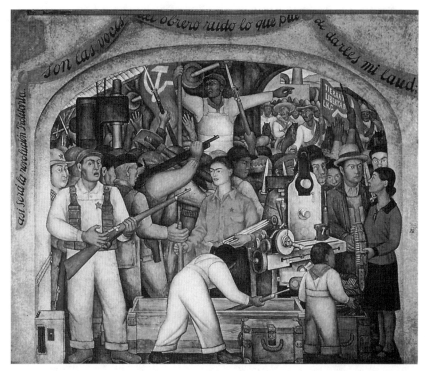

FIGURE 3. Diego Rivera, *Distributing Arms* (1928) Secretaria de Educación Pública, Mexico City. © *Banco de México Diego Rivera & Frida Kahlo Museums Trust. Av. Cinco de Mayo No. 2, Col. Centro, Del. Cuauhtémoc 06059, México, D.F.*

question of disability. One of these is motherhood, in which women's ability to bear children is far too often transformed into a form of servitude. Rivera decidedly does not depict Kahlo as a traditional mother but does translate the image of woman-as-caretaker from family to social class grouping; she becomes the central female caretaker of the proletariat. Despite the masculinization and perfection of her body, Kahlo functions in *Distributing Arms* completely in line with the postrevolutionary rhetoric of the new regime. In fact, much postrevolutionary discourse in Mexico focused on reminding women of their duties as self-effacing caretakers of the family and on transforming what had previously been a Catholic religious discourse of women as individual mothers into a secularized discourse of women as members of "a new holy family in which women accede voluntarily to their own subordination not to a biological father but to a paternal state."[9]

I find this redirection of a very old gender inequality toward upholding the modern nation-state fascinating but nonetheless relatively well researched.[10] While more work needs to be done on how Kahlo undermines the version of motherhood and the patriarchal nation extant in Mexico during the 1930s and

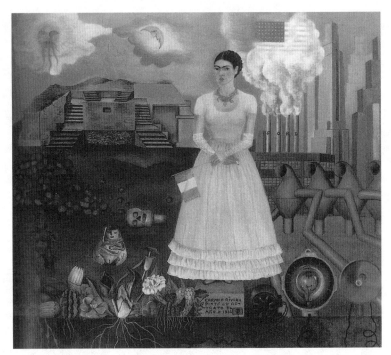

FIGURE 4. Frida Kahlo, *Self-Portrait on the Borderline between Mexico and the United States* (1932) oil on tin, 11³/4 × 13¹/2 in. Collection of Mr. & Mrs. Manuel Reyero, New York. © *Banco de México Diego Rivera & Frida Kahlo Museums Trust. Av. Cinco de Mayo No. 2, Col. Centro, Del. Cuauhtémoc 06059, México, D.F.*

1940s, particularly as she challenges it through depicting her own physical dis-abilities around childbearing, I nevertheless want to take up a slightly different aspect of the issue: Kahlo's critique of the confluence of Mexican nationalism, technology, femininity, and disability. The literature on female disability in re-lation to medical technologies is fairly extensive; but there is much less writing that examines these as functions of capitalism's control of technology generally or of these in relation to national identity. To explore these issues, I want to com-pare Rivera's image of the new Mexican nation with one of Kahlo's most overtly politicized national images: the 1932 *Self-Portrait on the Borderline Between the United States and Mexico* (fig. 4).

Like Rivera's mural, this picture's narrative unfolds around the central im-age of Kahlo. Also like his, this painting depicts contemporary Mexico in rela-tion to the forces of capitalism that are trying to subdue it. Apart from those two general characteristics, however, *Self-Portrait on the Borderline* is about as different from *Distributing Arms* as is possible. Kahlo's image is tiny and por-table, Rivera's is life-size and fixed to the wall of a public government build-ing. Rivera paints a rousing image of impending confrontation and victory; Kahlo paints desolation. Rivera crowds his mural with a multitude of figures; Kahlo paints only one—herself, staring out at the viewer with her typical emotionless gaze.

Let us go further in the comparison. Kahlo refuses the straightforward association that Rivera makes between race and politics. Rivera constantly confuses race with class in his murals, such that the peasantry is always indigenous, the urban worker is always mestizo, and the evil bourgeois, of course, is always white. *Self-Portrait on the Borderline* makes it clear that Kahlo's own attitudes toward "Mexicanness" and social change are much more complex than her husband's. Unlike Rivera, she places no faith in the idealistic nostalgia for an Aztec past that underlies so much of Rivera's work. Nor does she visualize any contemporary remnants of those indigenous cultures as having the power to withstand the onslaught of Fordist capitalism from *el Norte*. The stark contrast she images between Mexico and the United States is not a contrast between a pristine past and a corrupt industrial present, as it so often is in the work of Rivera and others, but a contrast between a technologized but inhuman U.S. cityscape, and a natural, feminized but ruined and "primitive" Mexican landscape.[11]

I could go on for days about Kahlo's critique of the so-called Indian Question in relation to nation identity here, but suffice it to say that she not only critiques essentialist identity politics but does so in deliberately ambiguous ways through her own mestiza, female, and disabled body located right at the collision point between indigenous and nonindigenous cultures, that is to say, on the border between Mexico and the United States.

Kahlo's disabled body. It is not as much physically in evidence in this picture as in others (fig. 5); rather it emerges in more symbolic form as a response to the stresses of border existence, of being caught between the onslaught of capitalist technologies and what Kahlo saw as the inadequacies of a precapitalist culture. Through imaging the effects of capitalist technology on her own body, Kahlo theorizes identity through disability in such a way as to critique both capitalism *and* utopian ideologies of Mexican-ness. Here's how she does it:

Although Kahlo acknowledges the power of industrial capitalism, she does not exhibit the fascination with machine culture that plagued so many of her compatriots, from Rivera to Siqueiros, the *Estridentistas*, the *Partido Comunista*, and others, all of whom imagined that technology was inherently a good thing that the working class could make revolutionary use of. Instead, she sees technology as a function of social, political, and economic power—as something in itself sometimes helpful but frequently indifferent to the plight of the weak and far too often a repressive tool in the hands of the powerful.

A comparison with another Rivera mural will help delineate this issue: Kahlo painted *Self-Portrait on the Borderline* while in Detroit alongside her husband, who had been commissioned by Edsel Ford to paint the Ford industry plant. Unlike Kahlo's unpeopled version of the Ford plant, Rivera's enormous mural, *Portrait of Industry*, is jammed with workers in a tense but nonetheless productive relationship with machinery (fig. 6). Rivera reveals the drama of the factory floor. He paints the curved backs and straining muscles of teams of men

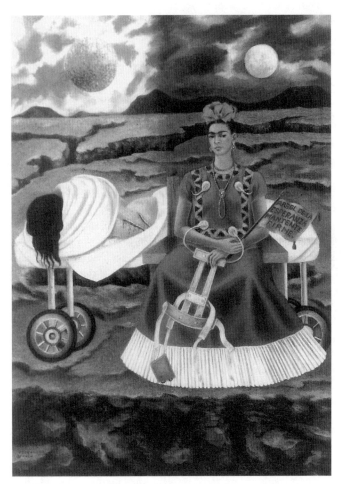

FIGURE 5. Frida Kahlo, *Tree of Hope* (1946) oil on masonite, 22 × 16 in. © *Banco de México Diego Rivera & Frida Kahlo Museums Trust. Av. Cinco de Mayo No. 2, Col. Centro, Del. Cuauhtémoc 06059, México, D.F.*

toiling in unison to control the monstrous machinery which towers over them. The monster belches fire and stamps steel, as the men carry out their task under the panoptic eye of the factory overseer. Everywhere in the mural's many panels, we see working men uniting in struggle, productively with the machines and combatively with their bourgeois bosses. In good 1930s communist fashion and to the dismay of his capitalist patrons, Rivera argued in *Portrait of Industry* that without human (male) work, the machines would not run—a counterproposal to Fordism, which subjected human motion to machine rather than the reverse. Rivera was convinced that, even in the belly of the capitalist beast, the proletariat would triumph and turn modern factories to the benefit of the workers.[12]

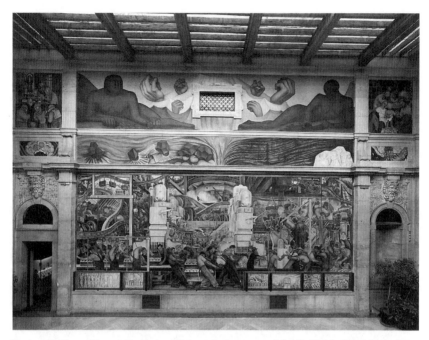

FIGURE 6. Diego Rivera, *Portrait of Detroit Industry*, north wall (1932–1933) Detroit Institute of the Arts, Detroit. Gift of Edsel B. Ford. *Photograph © 2000 The Detroit Institute of Arts.*

Kahlo's relationship to technology was rather less utopian. It bridged from her own misfortunes at the hands of medical technologies—none of which could cure her and many of which made her worse—to a sophisticated critical analysis of the relationship between technology and capitalism. In addition to *Self-Portrait on the Borderline*, Kahlo also produced *Henry Ford Hospital* during her 1932 sojourn in Detroit, after she had suffered a miscarriage that almost killed her (fig. 7). It is in many ways a companion piece to *Self-Portrait on the Borderline*, also evoking Kahlo in relation to the desolate inhumanity of the Ford industrial landscape. Her pathetic, naked body lies helplessly exposed in the very center of the picture to the penetrating gaze of the viewer; indeed, the bleakness of the landscape means we have little to focus upon *except* Kahlo's miserable condition. Barren-ness of landscape is equated visually with Kahlo's own infertility, a maneuver which, to paraphrase Margaret Lindauer, refashions a "private incident" into "public discourse."[13] Thus, this painting is not merely an image of Kahlo's anguish at not being able to bear children, as is often claimed, but functions as something much more—as an analysis of the particular conjunctions between the female body, medical technologies, and assembly-line Fordism.[14] It is not merely working men who are trapped in a battle with capitalist technologies, but women too; Fordist control of technology negatively

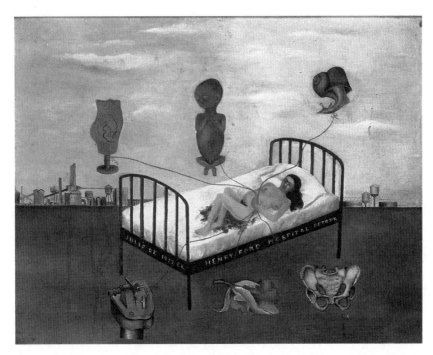

FIGURE 7. Frida Kahlo, *Henry Ford Hospital* (1932) oil on tin, 30 × 38 cm. Museo Dolores Olmedo Patiño, Mexico City. © *Banco de México Diego Rivera & Frida Kahlo Museums Trust. Av. Cinco de Mayo No. 2, Col. Centro, Del. Cuauhtémoc 06059, México, D.F.*

affects not only men on the factory floor but also women's ability to survive the life-threatening process of childbirth. Kahlo underscores this by including a series of floating emblems symbolizing various aspects of sexuality and childbirth; one of these, in the lower left, is a factory machine that looks suspiciously like the medical illustration of pelvic bones to the lower right and like the model of a woman's reproductive organs just above.[15] Fordism has taken control not only of the production of cars but also the production of babies, such that the risks of childbearing and assembly-line factory conditions seem not all that far apart. *Henry Ford Hospital* is a rare picture of the human tragedy of Fordism triumphant as it insidiously affects women in the domestic sphere.

    In fact, Kahlo's image of modern technology not only sharply diverges from Rivera's (and also from Siqueiros's and the other Muralists[16]) in its emphasis on the complete alienation, physical and cultural wreckage that such machine culture produces. Her images also have much in common with the only Muralist to equate machine culture directly with imperialism—José Clemente Orozco.

    Orozco's 1939 mural of Cortés at the Cabañas Institute in Guadalajara shows the great conquistador as a modern Terminator figure, half-man/half-

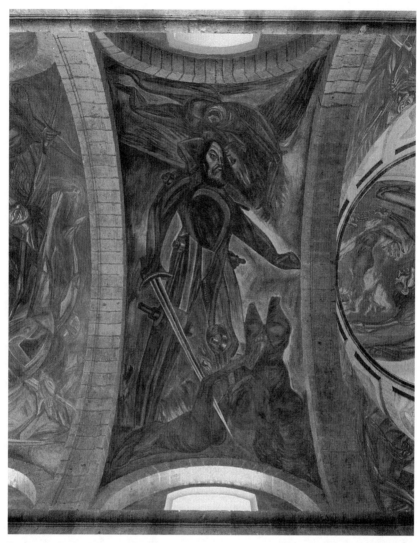

FIGURE 8. José Clemente Orozco, *Cortés* (1939) Hospicio de Cabañas, Guadalajara. © Instituto Nacional de Bellas Artes, Mexico City. Photo: Bob Schalkwijk, Mexico City.

machine (fig. 8). Cortés's metal armor has metamorphosed into the skin itself of his body, his indestructible arms, torso, and legs pinioned together by huge machine bolts. Figured as a giant engine of destruction, he heeds the whispers of the angel of Death as he brings his sword crashing down upon a helpless Aztec man. Cortés is a figure of terrifying power whom the cowering figure under his sword cannot hope to resist. Like Orozco's *Cortés*, Kahlo's *Self-Portrait on the Borderline* embodies the dehumanization and alienation enforced by modern technology. But she refigures the terrifying imperialist masculinity of Orozco's *Cortés*, in which a technologized body *acts upon* another all-too-human body, into a feminized mechanical body *being acted* upon by the technologies of Fordist capitalism. Cortés's body is a machine; so is Kahlo's. But rather than emanate power and invincibility, she stands like a petite wind-up doll, pinioned to her pedestal, plugged into an electric generator that lies at her feet on the U.S. side.

This image of the wind-up doll brings up the issue of Kahlo's physical disabilities. Think how her body would move if you were to flip the switch and see this picture in motion. It wouldn't have the languid human grace of a María Félix or a Dolores del Río—two other famous feminine incarnations of "Mexicanness" of this era.[17] Nor would it have the smooth Terminator machine moves one expects of Orozco's *Cortés*. Instead, one feels it would flop stiffly and awkwardly about, much like Kahlo herself when walking. Kahlo also deftly utilizes the purported "naivete" of her painting style to underscore the stiff fragility of her vulnerable body. The strokes of paint flatten rather than evoke three-dimensionality; the posture is deliberately frontal and rigidly vertical—again, tactics Kahlo purloined from untrained naivist artists who weren't comfortable painting a complex contrapposto. That these are deliberate ploys on Kahlo's part can be seen if we compare her flat figure with the much more convincingly rounded figures of the fertility goddess to the left or the very three-dimensional ventilation ducts to the right. But rather than being simply a personal physical disability due to an unfortunate accident or a mere lack of artistic skill, Kahlo's awkward, half-functional physicality here is figured as a direct product of the clash between Mexico's archaic precapitalism and U.S. Fordism. It is a clash that denies Kahlo any control over either her own bodily movements or her representation of herself.[18] *Self-Portrait on the Borderline* figures Kahlo's disabled body as a mechanical "failure" of Mexico's clash with its northern neighbor. She becomes a living emblem of technological imperialism, showing up the lie in any utopian belief that technology could be ideology- or politics-free. In 1932, before Mexico's 1938 nationalization of its oil industry which so angered the United States, and well before NAFTA was ever even thought of, this was a radical argument. By 1968, however, after the systematic corporatization of the Mexican economy to curry favor on the U.S.-dominated global market, after the promises of modernity and the PRI had revealed their hollowness, Kahlo's view made a lot more sense to the masses of Mexicans impoverished by their government's sellout.

Lina Abu-Habib points out the ways in which disability, especially in relation to women's bodies, can become a metaphor for underdevelopment forced on so-called Third World countries by the First World.[19] In one sense, Kahlo's painting presages the effects of NAFTA on border life between the United States and Mexico; as Ciudad Juárez's mayor, Gustavo Elizondo, recently stated, "The reality of Juárez is the reality of the whole border. . . . Every year we get poorer and poorer, even though we create more and more wealth."[20] Like *Self-Portrait on the Borderline*, Elizondo describes a flow of energies that crisscrosses the border in the form of natural resources, labor, and consumer products but that ultimately produces ruin for Mexico.

In conclusion, however, I would like to argue that Kahlo's image goes even further than this, and perhaps further than any other painting of her time, not only in questioning the "triumph" of the new Mexican nation but also of interrogating even the possibility of positing some essential Mexicanness that might withstand co-optation by the global market. In Kahlo's view, there is no such thing; any "Mexicanness"—or any identity—that can be conjured up is nothing more than a "set of effects" pulled haphazardly, defensively together, always subject to forces beyond our control.[21] To think otherwise is to open oneself to delusion.

Notes

1. I paraphrase a *New York Times* review, which described Kahlo as "the perfect woman for our time" because she was an "Hispanic woman, bisexual, an invalid and an artist—all the qualifications for a cult figure. Even Madonna is a fan." "Why Frida Kahlo Speaks to the 90s," *New York Times*, October 28, 1990, 1, 41. Quoted by Anthony Lee, "The Personal Is Political: Frida Kahlo's Construction of Female Space," unpublished talk, U.C. Berkeley (1991). On "Fridamania," see Margaret Lindauer, "Fetishizing Frida," in *Devouring Frida: The Art History and Popular Celebrity of Frida Kahlo* (Hanover, N.H..: Wesleyan University Press, 1999).

2. See especially Elena Poniatowska, *La noche de Tlatelolco; testimonios de historia oral* (México D.F.: Ediciones Era, 1971).

3. A particularly galling example of this occurred in 1970, when Siqueiros accepted public honors from President Echeverría at the opening of his last mural. It was Echeverría's immediate predecessor, President Gustavo Díaz Ordaz, who had been responsible for the Tlatelolco Massacre, while under Echeverría himself the PRI continued to hunt down and "disappear" thousands of people opposed to the PRI dictatorship. See Leonard Folgarait, *So Far From Heaven: David Alfaro Siqueiros' The March of Humanity and Mexican Revolutionary Politics* (Cambridge: Cambridge University Press, 1987), 54–56.

4. Zenil's painting also references another Kahlo work, *The Bus* (1929).

5. Martha Zamora, *Frida Kahlo: The Brush of Anguish* (San Francisco: Chronicle Books, 1990), 9, flyleaf. This problem, rampant in Kahlo scholarship, badly affects not only Zamora's book but also the otherwise useful biography by Hayden Herrera, *Frida: A Biography of Frida Kahlo* (New York: Harper & Row, 1983) as well as the work of other writers. Oriana Baddeley and Margaret Lindauer have provided a solid critique of this debilitating tendency and have begun to open up Kahlo scholarship to the myriad issues not yet adequately discussed, some of which include the relationship between Kahlo's communist politics and her art, her relationship to indigenism, to nationalism, to the burgeoning feminist movement in Mexico, to modernism, to surrealism, to technology and machine culture, to other members of the Mexican avantgarde, and so on. See Oriana Baddeley, "Her Dress Hangs Here: Defrocking the Kahlo cult," *Oxford Art Journal* 14, 1 (1991); and Margaret Lindauer, *Devouring Frida*.

6. For a variety of views on Rivera's Marxism, see Rivera, *Arte y política, selección, prólogo, notas y datos biográficos por Raquel Tibol* (Mexico City: Grijalbo, 1979); Anthony Lee, *Painting On the Left: Diego Rivera, radical politics, and San*

Francisco's public murals (Berkeley: University of California Press, 1999); and Leonard Folgarait, *Mural Painting and Social Revolution in Mexico, 1920–1940* (Cambridge: Cambridge University Press, 1998). Rivera, like Emiliano Zapata, Che Guevara, and Mao (and unlike Lenin or Trotsky) was very aware that the peasantry provided as much if not more revolutionary impetus as the proletariat.

7. See Anna Macías, *Against All Odds: The Feminist Movement in Mexico to 1940* (Westport, Conn.: Greenwood, 1982); and Shirlene Soto, *The Emergence of the Modern Mexican Woman: Her Participation in the Revolution and the Struggle for Equality, 1910–1940* (Denver: Arden Press, 1990).

8. Jean Franco, *Plotting Women: Gender and Representation in Mexico* (New York: Columbia University Press, 1990), 102. It is actually to Rivera's great credit that he was able to paint an image like *Distributing Arms* at all, given the strength of the general masculinist tendencies both in Mexican art and society. The 1947 painting, *Proletarian Mother*, by the artist María Izquierdo indicates, for example, that it wasn't only men who conceptualized the public sphere as masculine and the domestic sphere as feminine. By showing a desperate and despondent working-class mother, left alone to care for her hungry children, Izquierdo clearly protests the class and gender injustice of women's lot but does not picture the mother as actively resisting her fate. In this, Izquierdo thus upholds the dominant view.

9. Franco, *Plotting Women*, 147–148.

10. In the case of Mexico, interesting work has been done, for example, on the role of women such as Gabriela Mistral as teachers. See, for example, Jean Franco, *Plotting Women*; and Mary Kay Vaughan, *Cultural Politics in Revolution: Teachers, Peasants, and Schools in Mexico, 1930–1940* (Tucson: University of Arizona Press, 1997).

11. It is useful to read Roger Bartra on the issue of the "primitive" in relation to uses of Precolumbian culture in contemporary efforts to define national culture. Bartra writes that "the invention of the Mexican character" is ironic, because it necessitates a continual "search for that barbaric Other which we [Mexicans] carry within us as our ancestor, our father; it fertilizes the natural *mother* country, the land, but at the same time stains it with its primordial savagery." Bartra, *The Cage of Melancholy: Identity and Metamorphosis in the Mexican Character* (New Brunswick, N.J.: Rutgers University Press, 1992), 32, quoted in Margaret Lindauer, *Devouring Frida*, 133. Lindauer goes on to give an intelligent analysis of the role of the "primitive" in Kahlo's painting.

12. For more on this argument, see Terry Smith, *Making the Modern: Industry, Art, and Design in America* (Chicago: University of Chicago Press, 1993); and Anthony Lee, *Painting on the Left*.

13. Margaret Lindauer, *Devouring Frida*, 25.

14. Writing about *Henry Ford Hospital*, Hayden Herrera describes Kahlo as "seized by fits of despair at the thought that she might never have children" (*Frida*, 141). Throughout the book, Herrera writes of Kahlo's "desolation" and "grief" over her inability to have a child and of her "longing" for children. Yet Kahlo herself, in a letter from Detroit to Dr. Eloesser, asks him in detail if he thought it would be better for her health to abort (Kahlo was two months pregnant) or to continue the pregnancy and have a Caesarian operation. Kahlo's language in the letter is calm, reasoned, and frank—not emotional or anguished as Herrera claims—and Kahlo's primary concern is her own health not her ability to bear a child. She states quite explicitly, "I do not know whether it would be good or not to have a child, since

Diego is continually traveling and for no reason would I want to leave him alone and stay behind in Mexico, there would only be difficulties and problems for both of us. . . . " See Herrera, 137–139.

15. Also, *Henry Ford Hospital* is the first painting Kahlo did on sheet metal. Although this technique is usually interpreted as a reference to Mexican traditions of *retablo* painting, there seems an added reference in this case to the use of sheet metal in the fabrication of cars in the Henry Ford Rouge Plant.

16. See especially the use of technology in Siqueiros's mural, *Portrait of the Bourgeoisie* (1939).

17. See Ana M. López, "Tears and Desires: Women and Melodramas in the 'Old' Mexican Cinema," and Carlos Monsiváis, "Mexican Cinema: Of Myths and Demystifications," both in *Mediating Two Worlds: Cinematic Encounters in the Americas,* edited by John King, Ana López, and Manuel Alvarado (London: British Film Institute, 1993).

18. Significantly, too, she signs her name as "Carmen Rivera" rather than Frida Kahlo—a linguistic maneuver that suggests an uncertainty in her ability to control her own naming and identity. Kahlo's full name after marriage was Magdalena Carmen Frida Kahlo y Calderón de Rivera.

19. Lina Abu-Habib, *Gender and Disability: Women's Experiences in the Middle East* (Oxford: Oxfam, 1997):3.

20. Gustavo Elizondo, quoted in the *New York Times* (February, 11, 2001):6.

21. I paraphrase Terry Smith in order to take his very interesting observations in a somewhat different direction. Here is the full quotation: "Kahlo is facing the fearful realization that, despite the history of her country, despite the relatively recent Revolution of 1910, there may well be no deep or essential Mexicanness, only the isolated, random, leftover signs of it. Not just that she, or Rivera, or whoever, has yet to find the imagery of the new Mexico but that there is none to be found, there is nothing there, there is only the searching and the surviving. . . . Kahlo's self-portraits are . . . images of woman constituted as a set of effects. And this is the basis of their resistance: they are an assertion of self and nation—always, importantly, together—against perennial fears of nothingness but specifically against the increasing (and increasingly "modern") forces working actively to deny women and Mexico." Terry Smith, *Making the Modern*, 278.

Bibliography

Abu-Habib, Lina. 1997. *Gender and disability: Women's experiences in the Middle East.* Oxford: Oxfam.

Baddeley, Oriana. 1991. Her dress hangs here: Defrocking the Kahlo cult. *Oxford Art Journal* 14 (1): 10–17.

Bartra, Roger. 1992. *The cage of melancholy: Identity and metamorphosis in the Mexican character.* New Brunswick, N.J.: Rutgers University Press.

Folgarait, Leonard. 1987. *So far from heaven: David Alfaro Siqueiros' The March of Humanity and Mexican revolutionary politics.* Cambridge: Cambridge University Press.

———. 1998. *Mural painting and social revolution in Mexico, 1920–1940.* Cambridge: Cambridge University Press.

Franco, Jean. 1990. *Plotting women: Gender and representation in Mexico.* New York: Columbia University Press.

Herrera, Hayden. 1983. *Frida: A biography of Frida Kahlo*. New York: Harper and Row.

Lee, Anthony. 1991. The Personal Is Political: Frida Kahlo's Construction of Female Space. Unpublished talk, University of California, Berkeley.

———. 1999. *Painting on the Left: Diego Rivera, radical politics, and San Francisco's public murals*. Berkeley: University of California.

Lindauer, Margaret. 1999. *Devouring Frida: The art history and popular celebrity of Frida Kahlo*. Hanover, N.H.: Wesleyan University Press.

———. 1999. Fetishizing Frida. In *Devouring Frida: The art history and popular celebrity of Frida Kahlo*. Hanover, N.H.: Wesleyan University Press.

López, Ana M. 1993. Tears and desires: Women and melodramas in the "old" Mexican cinema. In *Mediating two worlds: Cinematic encounters in the Americas*, edited by John King, Ana López, and Manuel Alvarado. London: British Film Institute.

Macías, Anna. 1982. *Against all odds: The feminist movement in Mexico to 1940*. Westport, Conn.: Greenwood.

Monsiváis, Carlos. 1993. "Mexican cinema: Of myths and demystifications." In *Mediating two worlds: Cinematic encounters in the Americas*, edited by John King, Ana López, and Manuel Alvarado. London: British Film Institute.

Poniatowska, Elena. 1971. *La noche de Tlatelolco; testimonios de historia oral*. México D.F.: Ediciones Era.

Rivera, Diego. 1979. *Arte y política, selección, prólogo, notas y datos biográficos por Raquel Tibol*. Mexico City: Grijalbo.

Smith, Terry. 1993. *Making the modern: Industry, art, and design in America*. Chicago: University of Chicago Press.

Soto, Shirlene. 1990. *The emergence of the modern Mexican woman: Her participation in the Revolution and the struggle for equality, 1910–1940*. Denver: Arden Press.

Vaughan, Mary Kay. 1997. *Cultural politics in revolution: Teachers, peasants, and schools in Mexico, 1930–1940*. Tucson: University of Arizona Press.

Zamora, Martha. 1990. *Frida Kahlo: The brush of anguish*. San Francisco: Chronicle Books.

"But, Mother— I'm—crippled!"

TENNESSEE WILLIAMS, QUEERING DISABILITY, AND DIS/MEMBERED BODIES IN PERFORMANCE

♪♪

ANN M. FOX

Tennessee Williams, as creator of one of *the* oft-invoked disability stereotypes from literature, might initially seem an unlikely subject of study for anyone reinterpreting canonical works of American drama from a disability studies perspective. His Laura Wingfield, the self-proclaimed "cripple" from *The Glass Menagerie* (1945) who is quoted in this chapter's title, is an obvious first-place winner for Myth Disability as she clutches her blue roses and retreats into the dark recesses of the stage by play's end. Judging from the omnipresence of disability here and elsewhere in Williams's plays, one might reasonably read his drama as preoccupied with it for its more negative metaphorical uses. Indeed, Williams's most memorable characters seem to slip repeatedly into the use of disability that disability studies scholars David T. Mitchell and Sharon L. Snyder have defined as "narrative prosthesis," observing that

> while literature often relies on disability's transgressive potential, disabled people have been sequestered, excluded, exploited, and obliterated on the very basis of which their literary representation so often rests. Literature serves up disability as a repressed deviation from cultural imperatives of normativity, while disabled populations suffer the consequences of representational association with deviance and recalcitrant corporeal difference. (2000, 8)

This literary use of disability at best advances narrative and metaphor without addressing the lived experience of disability itself and at worst cycles disability back into a cultural lexicon that perpetuates the rejection and repression of disability identity.

Disability, as it has appeared onstage in American drama in characters such as Laura Wingfield, has amounted to a sort of gentrified freak show, allowing audiences the opportunity to look at disabled bodies metaphorically and voyeuristically. Theater artist and disability studies scholar Victoria Ann Lewis further defines the highly predictable nature of these visual metaphors as they have been used in Western drama as a whole:

> The old moral and medical models of disability continue to dominate theatrical depiction, not only because they fill a deep human need to define ourselves as "normal" against some standard of abnormality, but also, in terms of theatrical practice, because they are dramaturgically useful. For example, under the moral or religious construction of disability, physical difference usually connotes evil, a punishment for sin, or, to the contrary, designates beatitude, a blessing from the gods. . . . The medical model, the historical successor to the moral model, views disability as an illness. The disabled person is either charitably removed from society, i.e., institutionalized, or cures himself, or at least "passes" as cured. The possibility of societal prejudice and discrimination is never considered in the medical model. (Lewis 2000, 94)

When audience members define these social constructions of disability as normal, their collective stare[1] restages what happens outside the theater walls in everyday life. There, so-called abnormal bodies may be appropriated by the looks of strangers and regarded as fitting embodiments of innocence or infamy or simply erased altogether by virtue of social policies promoting institutionalization, selective abortion, or the "right" to die.

That Williams furthermore links disability and homosexuality in many of his plays seems to be simply reinforcing the depiction of these identities as parallel pathologies. Also, the time when Williams's best-known plays were produced, there was a widespread panic over and persecution of queerness in America in the late 1940s and 1950s. Disability images were taken up in the service of homophobia: "The pens of right-wing ideologues transformed homosexuality into an epidemic infecting the nation, actively spread by Communists to sap the strength of the next generation" (D'Emilio 1992, 60). Contemporary poet and essayist Eli Clare has commented on the similarities in experience still existing between the queer and disabled communities in this regard:

> The ways in which queer people and disabled people experience oppression follow, to a certain extent, parallel paths. Queer identity has been pathologized and medicalized. Until 1973, homosexuality was considered a psychiatric disorder. Today transsexuality and trans-

genderism . . . are considered psychiatric conditions. Queerness is all too frequently intertwined with shame, silence, and isolation. . . . Queer people deal with gawking all the time: when we hold hands in public, defy gender boundaries and norms, insist on recognition for our relationships and families. . . . Queer people have been told for centuries by church, state, and science that our bodies are abnormal. (Clare 1999, 96)

Both queer and disabled bodies, seen as violations of natural masculinity and femininity, defy a heterosexist ideal of sexuality and its attendant gender roles, although while the queer body is read as deviant, the disabled body is rendered completely asexual.[2] Queer and disabled bodies not only violate economies of gender but also the capitalist economy upon which our society's identity is largely premised.[3] Homosexual ties between men, for example, are seen as a misappropriation of the homosocial bonds that form the underpinnings of capitalism, while disabled people, either explicitly or implicitly regarded as unfit to work by nondisabled people, are left outside a streamlined model of productivity altogether. The fact that so many disabled individuals continue to be underemployed and live on incomes below those of the general population is less a function of their own ability than the view of impairment as dysfunction, resulting in a refusal to see workplaces as anything other than the province of those who need not be accommodated. Is this place of ostracism the only place these cultures can meet? And why should we pursue a connection at all? Of what use is it in understanding Williams, and in turn, this particular presence of disability in American drama beyond the specter of Laura Wingfield?

Laura Wingfield notwithstanding, I contend that Williams's work gradually merges critiques of those social assumptions about sexual and physical straightness circumscribing queer and disabled bodies across his plays. By midcareer, he eventually uses that juxtaposition to strengthen and broaden a critique of normalcy, that presumption of sexual or bodily norms that labels as deviant all those who exist in opposition to it.[4] From my perspective as a scholar who writes both on modern drama and disability studies, considering Williams in this way is an important model for how literary critics might begin to reevaluate the canon of American drama from a disability studies perspective. Such a reconsideration is important not only so that we might catalog the more problematic representations of disability that have crossed the stage again and again over the course of its history but also that we might more fully understand the complexities of how disability is employed as literary and visual trope within dramatic literature. As Mitchell and Snyder emphasize in their discussion of narrative prosthesis, there is an importance in "attend[ing] to the nuanced relations of literary and social responses to disability" rather than "condemn[ing] the literary as bankrupt with regard to disability" (2000, 9). Disability studies scholar Rosemarie Garland-Thomson's essay, "Seeing the Disabled: Visual Rhetorics of Disability in Popular Photography"[5] (2001) is an example of such

it seeks to uncover the more complicated exchanges surround-
visual production, although this work focuses on disability as
mercial photography.[6] As a live medium, theater has the poten-
he visual and linguistic codes that have worked to construct the
disabled person in society and to collapse the distance between performer and
audience.

In considering how this process unfolds for Williams, I first briefly sketch
how we might begin to see evidence of his increasing interrelation of disability
and queerness across the well-known plays *A Streetcar Named Desire* (1947)
and *Cat on a Hot Tin Roof* (1955). I then closely focus on *Suddenly Last Summer* (1958), placing extended emphasis on this play as a revolutionary merging
of queerness and disability on the American stage. It can be deceptive upon a
first reading. After all, its representation of transgressive bodies seems to cul-
minate in a grandiose freak show, featuring a gay poet who becomes the house
special and a woman whose brain is about to be lobotomized to destroy the truths
she "babbles" about her cousin's sexual proclivities. Disability and homosexuality seem set against one another as destructive forces; when Catharine outs
Sebastian by recounting that the boys whose sexual favors he purchased have
cannibalized him in revenge, her aunt, Violet Venable, can then insist that this
knowledge be in turn outed from her niece, excised by the lobotomy that must
protect the Venables' good name. Like her name saint (who was decapitated when
she refused to stop her version of truth telling, preaching Christianity), Catharine
is imperiled, threatened with permanent disability because she refuses to remain
silent.

Before we consider his plays, it is useful to examine where Williams's own
biography suggests points at which the playwright might have felt the connection between disability and queerness in his own life. When he was only six
years old, Williams contracted diphtheria; it gave rise to a complication, Bright's
disease, which left Williams weakened and unable to walk normally for almost
two years. Because he spent much of this period playing solitary games or reading, this was a time where Williams (by his own account) began imaginatively
to set himself apart from others, making him a "decided hybrid, different from
the family line of frontiersmen-heroes of east Tennessee" (Williams 1975, 12).
What is interesting about how Williams casts this disability experience, however, is not only its connection to his emerging literary gift, but his own linking
of it to a nascent queer identity: "During this period of illness and solitary games,
my mother's overly solicitous attention planted in me the makings of a sissy,
much to my father's discontent" (11–12). Williams's physical inferiority to other
children because of his illness, coupled with the rich imaginative life he culti-
vated during his time of recuperation, was read by Williams (and subsequently,
by some of his biographers) as intrinsically connected to a construction of masculinity that violated key precepts of heterosexual identity.

Williams also witnessed the tyranny of the medical model of disability
through its effect on his sister. Rose Williams, upon whom the character Laura

Wingfield is based, suffered from severe depression and was lobotomized when she was only a young woman. Williams was not informed of the procedure until it was completed and blamed his mother bitterly for its disastrous aftereffects. Edwina Dakin Williams later wrote in her own memoir that she had come to see the lobotomy as a mistaken decision, one she made upon the advice of doctors:

> I now think the lobotomy for Rose was a grave mistake. We all believed at the time that this operation might completely cure Rose, as we relied on the advice of a local psychiatrist. We had no idea of the permanent damage it is now known to do to the personality. During those days, some psychiatrists looked on the operation as a wonderful new discovery that would control madness. But now they do not perform it except on the very old and the very hopeless, realizing it destroys something essential in a person's character. (Williams 1963, 85)

The deadening effect of this unnecessary attempt to cure his sister had haunted Williams all his life. In his eyes, Rose had been butchered. Williams wrote a poem upon hearing the news of his sister's lobotomy that suggested his despair:

> Grand, God be with you.
> A cord breaking.
> 1000 miles away.
> Rose. Her head cut open.
> A knife thrust in her brain.
> Me. Here. Smoking.
> My father, mean as a
> devil, snoring—1000 miles
> away. (Leverich 1995, 482)

The presence of mental illness in his own family caused Williams to be tortured throughout his life by fears of insanity and institutionalization; from his own sister's example, he was keenly aware of the body as a battleground and the punishments society might exact on bodies perceived to be transgressive. This was reinforced during the time when Williams was composing *Suddenly Last Summer*, during which he underwent intense psychoanalysis: "His analyst, Dr. Lawrence Kubie, tried unsuccessfully to wean him from drugs, stop his writing and change his sexual orientation, and Williams ended the analysis later in 1958" (Parker 1998, 308). The psychoanalyst's insistence on curing Williams of a perceived disability through urging him to become heterosexual is a curious corollary to the attempts made to erase queerness through Catharine's proposed lobotomy in *Suddenly Last Summer*.

While Williams was familiar with the disability experience, queer and disability interests clearly diverge in his early plays. Certainly *The Glass Menagerie*'s famous successor, *A Streetcar Named Desire*, does not suggest that ableism will be challenged, even as the destructive power of homophobia is attacked. *A Street-car Named Desire* contains eerie echoes of *The Glass Menagerie* in its presentation of erasure as the ultimate fate of the disabled body; heroine Blanche DuBois, like Laura Wingfield, is separated from society by play's end by disability: Blanche's madness, triggered by her brother-in-law Stanley's sexual assault and her sister Stella's refusal to believe that it has happened. The earliest glimmerings of this madness, of course, are in the guilt that haunts Blanche about her own moment as the enforcer of sexual norms. Earlier in the play, she reveals that her rage at discovering her closeted husband with his lover drove the former to suicide. Her own despair drives her in turn to heterosexuality with a vengeance, as she becomes a creature of excess, infamous for her promiscuity and for preying on young boys. And yet, when confronted with that ultimate symbol of virility himself, Stanley, she quails, and is vanquished.

Blanche's character has been read as part of what critic David Savran (1992, 115) has called a "transvestite poetics," in which Williams hides gay identity in plain sight on stage by transposing the character of a gay man onto the body of a woman. Blanche's madness, read in this light, is the outcome of and metaphor for the mistreatment of gay identity in the face of hypermasculinity, the latter being equated with compulsory heterosexuality. Blanche's retreat into madness compounds, in a sense, the tragic depiction of Laura Wingfield: we may sympathize but are still helpless as Blanche is led away to the mental institution. That bodies are disabled by compulsory heterosexuality in this play (first her husband Alan's, then Blanche's) effects social critique but likewise perpetuates the opposition between disability and desirability, still allowing disability identity to become instead the vehicle for pity and the illustration of destruction. The critique of enforced heterosexuality itself becomes a type of "compulsory able-bodiedness."[7]

Despite its own use of predictable disability metaphors, *Cat on a Hot Tin Roof* (1955) begins to suggest that the prejudice circumscribing disabled and queer bodies may have similar origins. The play opens with the birthday celebration of Big Daddy, the patriarch of a Mississippi Delta plantation, who is dying of bowel cancer. Although his family is successful for a time in convincing him he is not ill, we eventually learn that he is truly dying. Who will inherit the plantation is a question contested by Big Daddy's two sons, Brick and Gooper, although Brick, an alcoholic who has broken his ankle and is pictured on crutches throughout the play,[8] is losing the battle, estranged from his wife and his family and tortured at the thought of his repressed homosexuality.

Queer identity, however, gets a sympathetic treatment within the world of the plantation. The estate is Big Daddy's inheritance not from traditional Southern gentry but from a gay couple, Peter Ochello and Jack Straw. The play thus establishes a line of inheritance and continuity for gay men, because the possession of "twenty-eight thousand acres of the richest land this side of the Valley Nile," has passed from Straw and Ochello to Big Daddy, whose own queer identity I shall discuss in a moment.

Queer interpretations of the play such as Savran's have remarked upon how the play destabilizes masculinity, as "Williams flaunts and magnifies the contradictions on which masculinity, and patriarchal relations generally, are founded" (1992, 101). And indeed, the pivotal scene between Big Daddy and Brick, in which the father confronts his son, is based on an ironic premise. Big Daddy anticipates visiting his sexual appetite—now that he is seemingly cured—on the bodies of women younger and more beautiful than his wife. Likewise, he assures his son, "You're my son and I'm going to straighten you out; now that *I'm* straightened out, I'm going to straighten out you!" (Williams 1955, 75)[9] Yet ironically, Big Daddy "straightens" his son out by pushing him to avoid pretense, revealing that he himself has "knocked around" in gay liaisons as well, "bummed" around the country literally and figuratively. He accepts the prospect that Brick is gay, remarking that "One thing you can grow on a big place more important than cotton!—is *tolerance*! I grown it" (89).

Through disability, however, this statement is given the lie. Big Daddy's bowel cancer merges the site of his illness and his "knocking around": "Big Daddy is dying of cancer, and it's spread all through him and it's attacked all his vital organs including the kidneys and right now he is sinking into uremia, and you all know what uremia is, it's poisoning of the whole system due to the failure of the body to eliminate its poisons" (Williams 1955, 113). Brick has broken his ankle in a drunken attempt to jump hurdles on a track; this injury, like his alcoholism, becomes a symbolic suggestion of the destructive nature of his internalized homophobia. Despite the fact that those forces circumscribing queerness are criticized and disturbed, disability still appears to be reinforced as metaphor for moral judgment about it. In fact, in the original script, once the lie that Big Daddy is *not* ill is exposed, he literally disappears from the world of the play, erased and silenced.

That Big Daddy disappears, however, is not the quiet exit of Laura and Blanche. Big Daddy, to be sure, exults in health, and has used the supposed near miss of his illness to excuse his renewed sexual license (as a heterosexual man): "I let many chances slip by because of scruples about it, scruples, convention—crap. . . . All that stuff is bull, bull, bull! It took the shadow of death to make me see it. Now that shadow's lifted, I'm going to cut loose and have, what is it they call it, have me a—ball!" (Williams 1955, 70) Big Daddy does seem to understand the fear of fragmentation, however, that underlies the fear of illness: "the human animal is a beast that dies and if he's got money he buys and buys and buys and I think the reason he buys everything he can buy is that in the back of his mind he has the crazy hope that one of his purchases will be life everlasting!—Which it can never be" (67). When Big Daddy finds out he is indeed ill, he rages not at his disease but at "all liars, all liars, all lying dying liars," who try to conceal this truth from him. Brick's sympathetic comment, "Mendacity is a system that we live in. Liquor is one way out an' death's the other," links his fate with Big Daddy's—as mutual victims of a society operating on pretense and an insistence of normalcy (94).

But is Big Daddy's a tragic ending? Brick never moves from his position of self-denial and repression; indeed, the tragedy of the play seems to be that his triumphal reunion with Maggie the Cat so they can have a child to inherit the plantation will replicate the loveless marriage of his parents. Heterosexuality itself is outed as restrictive force and hollow shell. The power of Big Daddy's absence throughout act three, however, opens a space in which audience members may effect a similar critique of physical normalcy. Big Daddy's absence is neither explained nor fetishized; we are denied the spectacle of a descent into the romanticized death. Big Daddy damns pretense and disappears, denying us the opportunity to end his story through conventional means. This leaves our focus not on his withering body but on the claims his heirs make on it as they struggle to grasp their inheritance, using his illness as their own justification for the avarice with which they deny their own mortality. Judging from these early plays for which he was well known, then, we might then consider the playwright's position toward disability as one of contempt at worst, indecision at best.

This mirrors the critical debates over Williams's attitudes toward queerness in these same plays; early readings assert that he had simply internalized homophobia. In his essay "'Something Cloudy, Something Clear': Homophobic Discourse in Tennessee Williams," literary critic John M. Clum posits that Williams's is a "split vision," an "internal conflict that compelled him to write of his homosexuality and, in doing so, to rely on the language of indirection and homophobic discourse" (1992, 153). Clum posits that while Williams does embody queerness in his plays and fiction, it exists framed in a homophobic discourse that seemed to anticipate the audience's response. Indeed, the title of Clum's essay comes from the title of Williams's last work on Broadway, *Something Cloudy, Something Clear*—a title which itself came, as Clum recounts, from a disability metaphor Williams himself used to describe his split gay identity: "My left eye was cloudy then because it was developing a cataract. But my right eye was clear. It was like the two sides of my nature. The side that was obsessively homosexual, compulsively interested in sexuality. And the side that in those days was gentle and understanding and contemplative" (152).

Other critiques of Williams's attitude toward queerness in his plays have given him credit for creating a more complicated discourse around the expectations that society imposes on bodies. These same critics point out that when Williams raises the specter of queerness, it is to show an audience the face of the creator, themselves, rather than the monster. For example, literary critic Steven Bruhm asserts that Williams shows society to be the author of the binaries that separate its so-called normal members from its abnormal ones and that "the ordered society *needs* its 'disordered' Other to give it definition. And so, by pointing this finger, Williams . . . destroys the distinction between the homosexual's self-construction and the social construction which condemns him" (1991, 535). Savran remarks that "Insistently . . . [Williams] underscored the broadly social foundation for the personal tragedies with which so many of his plays are concerned, pointing out that the individual subject is not an isolated monad but a component of a 'society' that insistently 'rapes the individual'" (1992, 79). It can in this way be argued that Williams, who denied that his plays were in any way political, still manages to advocate for the queer bodies that were suppressed from public performance at the time his career hit its zenith in the 1940s and 1950s.

More recently, literary critic Anne Fleche wonders what we are to do with this division among critics on the question of Williams's queer poetics: "Williams's gay critics seem caught in this circular homophobia-phobia, in which the closet is obsessively opened and closed, its limits marked and remarked, its positive and negative charged and recharged" (1995, 258). Fleche chooses to situate herself differently relative to this argument, pointing out that in Williams's case, "we might consider that homosexual identity is conferred spatially by its proximity to the closet rather than its within or withoutness; it is relative to this image, rather than dependent on its placement inside or outside" (265). For Fleche, queerness becomes "the undecidability of where one's identity lies, relative to the structuring principle of identity" (265). Whether Williams is self-hating or shrewdly revolutionary becomes beside the point for Fleche, who instead sees Williams's power in his ability to render unstable the divides that would insist on queer identity existing on either side of a closet door.[10]

I believe that we can look to disability as having an integral role in that dismantling of social constructions of identity that both Savran and Fleche, to different degrees, see present in Williams's work. With *Suddenly Last Summer*, Williams transcends his earlier treatment of individual categories of bodily difference with a more comprehensive critique of the processes of categorizing and normalizing themselves. By shifting the emphasis thusly, and placing side by side the identities "normalcy" tries to erase, Williams makes queerness and disability work in concert to assume a new status in *Suddenly Last Summer*. He addresses the fragility we constantly deny in our own bodies, reminding us that those "divisions whole/incomplete, able/disabled neatly cover up the frightening writing on the wall that reminds the hallucinated whole being that its wholeness is in fact a hallucination, a developmental fiction" (Davis 1995, 130). Williams makes use of poet Sebastian Venable's gay body, literally ripped apart and devoured by the young boys whose sexual favors he purchased, to show he understands figurative dis/memberment all too well. This process of dis/memberment is society's slow dissection of identities into categories that are then re/membered—both recalled and rejoined to the body politic—in a specific and hierarchical way. I want to suggest that Williams not only exposes these constructions as just that but in doing so, makes disability and queerness not partners in exile, but an intersection of identities from which movement beyond binaries and hierarchies can be imagined.

As an aside, I want to point out that the movie version of the play which followed close on the heels of its Broadway production inscribed disability and homosexuality as illnesses, an ironic replication of the very attitudes that

Williams's play is trying to confront. Disability is pictured throughout the film as a fate worse than death, as we get to see firsthand not only through early images from within Lion's View but most memorably at a later moment in film during which Catharine mistakenly enters a psychiatric ward. She escapes only after being mauled by bestial-looking disabled inmates. Disability is allied with ugliness, perversion, and emasculation, as the men who are not ineffectually pawing Catharine are engaged in activities such as embroidery. As in the play, at movie's end, Dr. Cukrowicz doesn't perform the surgery; but in a departure from the play's final moments, he instead goes off into the sunset with Catharine in a revisionist happy ending that doesn't resolve as much as smoothes over the questions of sexual identity in the play.[11] In the movie, the anger Sebastian's mother shows in the play is quite literally transformed into madness; her knowledge of her son's homosexuality literally transforms itself into a disability. That "perversity that kills" is still in the system but just has been transferred from Catharine to her aunt. Violet Venable's madness thus reinscribes disability as a metaphor—and punishment—for moral corruption, both her son's and her own.

There's a constant tension between these social constructions and their own imminent decay in the play itself. Literary critic Lennard Davis defines normalcy, borrowing a term from Foucault, as a "location of bio-power. . . . The 'normal' person (clinging to that title) has a network of traditional ableist assumptions and social supports that empowers the gaze and interaction" (1995, 128). Of course, that bio-power includes not merely assumptions about the whole body as ideal, it also extends to assumptions about race, gender, and sexuality. This network depends on the constant preservation of a power matrix, one, ironically, that is as subject to decay as the bodies it polices. As the play opens, the Doctor and Mrs. Venable walk through Sebastian's garden, a postlapsarian garden of Eden. The natural world eschews labels, literally, from the beginning: "The Latin names of the plants were printed on tags attached to them but the print's fading out" (Williams 1958, 10). The primordial reasserts itself over the man-authored process of knowing, of labeling the "well-groomed jungle," where "nothing was accidental, everything was planned and designed in Sebastian's life and his—" (11). This is a world in which the desperate attempt to hold on to categories, to ways of knowing, slowly eludes the characters, a process mirrored in the fragility of the bodies that have already been destroyed (Sebastian's), the ones in decay (Mrs. Venable's), and the ones in danger (Catharine's). Sebastian's attempts to reorder nature have failed; but if nature is red in tooth and claw, it is a reflection of the predatory model with which humans have constructed the world. Sebastian recognizes this even to the last detail of his garden, the Venus flytrap, whose carnivorous existence can only be maintained through careful tending. It's worth mentioning that the food for this plant, flies used for "experiments in genetics," serves to confirm this read of humankind as determined to be determinist. (It also provides an eerie connection to our own age of genome mapping.)

Everywhere we look in this world, there's hard work going on to maintain what the play regards as "natural"; it is no wonder Violet suggests she is exhausted at the beginning of the play. She cannot accept her own aging and at-tendant paralysis, her own divergence from societal standards of beauty and youth. The Hollys, Catharine's mother and brother, are eager to reinsert them-selves into a framework of social and economic privilege, even at the cost of sister's sanity. Catharine, after all, already has refused her proper place in soci-ety as a compliant debutante and silent witness to Sebastian's atrocities.

Indeed, Catharine is the only character that has turned away from the hard work of fiction writing. As she tells her mother about her story of Sebastian's death: "But, Mother, I DIDN'T invent it. I know it's a hideous story but it's a true story of our time and the world we live in and what truly did happen to Cousin Sebastian in Cabeza de Lobo" (Williams 1958, 47). It is no wonder her fate is one "lonelier than death," for her madness is created in the unbelief of others. Like Cassandra, her sanity and clearsightedness become rewritten as the ravings of a lunatic, and her supposed illness is really her dysfunctionality vis-à-vis this society.

In this light, the doctor becomes less a healer of individual illness and more the guardian of the status quo. Although he purports to be horrified at Mrs. Venable's bribe, his view of health at first also rests on normalcy as the hard-won perpetuation of this society's divisions, as is suggested by the story he tells of his first lobotomy:

> Let me tell you something—the first operation I performed at Lion's View.—You can imagine how anxious and nervous I was about the out-come. . . . The patient was a young girl regarded as hopeless and put in the Drum—. . . . The name for the violent ward at Lion's View because it looks like the inside of a drum with very bright lights burning all day and all night.—So the attendants can see any change of expression or movement among the inmates in time to grab them if they're about to attack. After the operation I stayed with the girl, as if I'd delivered a child that might stop breathing.—When they finally wheeled her out of surgery, I still stayed with her. I walked along the rolling table hold-ing onto her hand—with my heart in my throat. . . . [*We hear faint mu-sic.*] —It was a nice afternoon, as fair as this one. And the moment we wheeled her outside, she whispered something, she whispered: "Oh, how blue the sky is!" —And then I felt proud, I felt proud and relieved, because up till then her speech, everything that she'd babbled, was a torrent of obscenities! (Williams 1958, 18–19)

For the doctor, stopping the "torrent of obscenities" of his patient is a sort of divine intervention, a reordering of the world so that what it has defined as "ob-scene" is hidden. Chillingly, the young woman he describes is realigned through proper mental health with her proper role as a woman: silent and submissive, her gaze on the ethereal plane.

God, as Nature, has been shaped in the human image. This is the real hor-ror of that vision of God from which Catharine had wanted to rescue her cousin.

The doctor, as Sebastian's double, unwittingly allies himself with this vision as he considers operating on Catharine. A blond, the doctor is clothed, like Sebastian, in white and is "glacially brilliant," learning from Mrs. Venable (who says this without a touch of irony) that her son "would have been charmed by you" (Williams 1958, 22). Like Sebastian, he is a consumer; here, he will use the body of Catharine to procure for him, too: her aunt's money. He allows his ethnicity to be erased by offering to be called the literal translation of his Polish surname, "Dr. Sugar," rather than "Cukrowicz," thereby further acceding to a world of saccharine whiteness. The body again becomes a commodity and a site of power plays, and the doctor knows the rules of the game.

By operating on Catharine, he will be stilling a voice that reacted against those same conventions even before her trip with Sebastian. Against the backdrop of a Mardi Gras ball, Catharine shamed her family and ruined her own reputation by publicly accusing a man who had seduced her:

> I didn't stop at the cloakroom to pick up Aunt Violet's old mink stole, no, I rushed right into the ballroom and spotted him on the floor and ran up to him and beat him hard as I could in the face and chest with my fists till—Cousin Sebastian took me away.—After that, the next morning, I started writing my diary in the third person, singular, such as "She's still living this morning," meaning that *I* was. . . .—"WHAT'S NEXT FOR HER? GOD KNOWS!"—I couldn't go out any more.— However one morning my Cousin Sebastian came in my bedroom and said: "Get up!"—Well . . . if you're still alive after dying, well then, you're obedient, Doctor.—I got up. He took me downtown to a place for passport photos. Said: "Mother can't go abroad with me this summer. You're going to go with me this summer instead of Mother." (Williams 1958, 65–66)

She is "making a scene," not only acting up but also acting out in a way that is neither socially sanctioned nor allowed for a woman. She comes to understand her objectification and interchangeability with other women, as she describes herself in the anonymous third person, as if looking on the artificial automaton she has become. Ironically, Sebastian seizes upon her at once for her very difference and allure, yet makes her take on his mother's role as procurer.

It is perhaps surprising that queerness and disability do not ally on the body of the play's one gay character, Sebastian. But Sebastian only understands survival; his tragedy is not that he is homosexual but that in exercising privilege to the extent that he can, he perpetuates the structures that eventually encroach on his own body. His taking Catharine under his wing might be read as a turn toward sympathy with one who has so publicly denied the role she is supposed to assume as dutiful debutante. Her coming out is indeed a coming out into the harsh reality that her body will and can be made available to any man who will reach for it. Still, it is Catharine who has presented Sebastian with another possibility through her truth telling at Mardi Gras. But Sebastian will not replicate her coming out in the quarter. He does not scruple to make use of her body in exactly the same way as the man Catharine confronted, using it for sex figuratively, if not literally; Catharine is thus passed from man to man in the most homosocial of scenarios. Sebastian reifies heterosexual norms to obtain the men he seduces, as he moves around the world with a beautiful female "partner" on his arm as bait. He complies with the strictures of a world that reveres youth, whiteness, wealth, and health; he does not scruple to use that privilege to lay claim to the bodies of young, poor, Hispanic boys. There's more than a little irony at work when Violet proudly shows the doctor two photographs of her son taken twenty years apart and challenges him to identify the older one. Her pride in her son's Dorian Gray-like refusal to age is somewhat poignant, given that her son has refused to allow her to accompany him when her health— and appearance—began to decline.

Sebastian's house is one built on sand, however, for all the categories he thinks he can depend upon shift; their hold is tenuous at best, and Sebastian comes up against their inevitable decomposition. In their instability, they perform their own quality as something extrinsic to the bodies upon which they are imposed. Indeed, Savran has noted that Williams's "plays redefine and reconfigure resistance so that it is less the prerogative of rebellious individuals than a potential always already at play within both social organization and dramatic structure" (1992, 81). Mrs. Holly and Violet both live for their sons in a sort of quasi-incestuous manner. Violet approaches something akin to being her son's husband, alternately impregnating and preparing to deliver her son of his yearly poems after nine months. Mrs. Holly inches toward agreeing to the lobotomy so that George, the "crown prince," can inherit his patrimony: money, comfort, and the connections and prestige of a Tulane education. But the crown prince becomes a clown prince: George is a buffoonish satire of the societal ideal, the white heterosexual fraternity brother, athletic and popular. He is the *reductio ad absurdum* of the societal forces that make him and leave him in borrowed robes, grasping at an elusive inheritance.

Williams initially seems to intimate that the coming together of races is particularly disastrous, for indeed, the "dark ones" devour Sebastian. Yet the dichotomy of light and dark as having any intrinsic hierarchy is done away with, by both the menacing blazing *white* heat of Cabeza de Lobo and the pristine whiteness of the suit in which Sebastian is constantly presenting himself. That the Hispanic boys consume him speaks not to their innate savagery, but their ironic replication of Sebastian's hunger. He speaks of them as a "social disease," yet the satiation of his sexual hunger rests on the continuation of their literal starvation. Sebastian is fragmented with a vengeance, cut into pieces by the detritus of society with scraps of metal. Like Catharine before them, the boys perform on the body of their abuser the wrong that has been done to them.

Williams also tears apart the body of the play, playing with dramatic structure to suggest the interplay of possibility. On the one hand, the play follows the unities of time, place, and action. Yet this play eludes the straightforward narrative of realism; characters take turn giving witness to the doctor, as though he, and we as audience, were being asked to judge. The play's episodic nature and lack of a set resolution reinforce the importance of possibility rather than closure, even when the latter seems a laudable goal.

Williams removes sensationalized bodies; Sebastian is absent, and we never see his murder. This is not the simple erasure of unpleasantness we might suspect at first glance. Instead, we are denied the ability to mark those bodies as other, to identify the manner in which we categorize them as somehow separate from us. Williams never tries to mark Catharine with any of the conventions of theatrical portrayals of disability.[12] Obscenity is not equated with an illness that is intrinsic to Catharine but with Mrs. Venable's attempt to violently suppress the "horrible truths" she cannot confront about her son. It is telling that she insists: "I won't collapse! She'll collapse! I mean her lies will collapse—not my truth—not the truth" (Williams, 1958, 12). Her comment suggests that our own bodies house the destruction and destructive influences we try to flee in a way that is quite different than what society would have us believe. As audience members, we are not allowed to displace our anxieties on, define ourselves against, or voyeuristically look at the bodies that are traditionally sensationalized to be sanitized. Instead, we are denied the binary opposite against which we might elect to define our own bodies as normal and stable. We have come full circle from Laura Wingfield; now Catharine leaves *us*, retreating at play's end into the garden, the jungle of disarray and unknowability.

If the doctor has been Sebastian's double for most of the play, the power of the ending comes in his own disintegration, in his embracing the very fragmentation that he has been trained to avoid and purports to be able to cure. From early on, even as he describes the rewards of his surgery, he also understands there is a cost, although he is not able to name it: "it may be that the person [who has the lobotomy] will always be limited afterwards, relieved of acute disturbances but—*limited*, Mrs. Venable" (Williams 1958, 30). As he listens to Catharine tell her story, the doctor is silent; upon hearing it, he resists his own form of consumption, deciding not to seize on Catharine's body by operating. In the end, the only reply he will make to Mrs. Holly's plea "Doctor, can't you say something?" is the statement "we ought at least to consider the possibility that the girl's story could be true" (93). What may seem like an indecisive statement to us is rather a refusal to replicate the mistakes of the past by naming one version of reality as "fact," as the "truth of the matter," by imposing a label, a diagnosis, a place in the binary of truth/untruth on a body. Truth is contingent, as we are reminded, and the doctor's first tentative motion toward that is noteworthy as such. As Dr. Sugar's statement suggests, possibility—not saccharine sweetness—is the real truth, the entertaining of views beyond those declared to be so and just and normal. At this point, all Mrs. Venable can do is rage impotently; the doctor's is a purposeful moving into the maelstrom that Mrs. Venable so offhandedly dismissed as so much "debris." If Sebastian and his mother carved out each day like "a piece of sculpture," the doctor moves away from the fixity of what they have shaped. Mrs. Venable remains trapped in her definition of difference as disability, led away as she exhorts the doctor to "cut this hideous story out of her [Catherine's] brain," to reproduce the violence that has now been negated.

As I hope the foregoing argument suggests, I think it is absolutely necessary to reevaluate the canon of American dramatic history from a disability studies perspective and to tease out the shades of difference, even within an individual author's work, of approaches to disability. Critics have already identified Williams as a playwright operating to subvert attitudes about queerness: "American gay playwrights [pre-Stonewall] deconstructed the image of American masculinity to show its hollowness and cruelty and reconstructed it to include homosexuality. The history of the homosexual in American drama in the fifties and sixties is in large part the story of the reconstruction of the ideal man, the American dream, as an object of homosexual desire *and* as homosexual. . . . " (Clum 1994, 141). What happens, however, when we consider disability connected to this queer identity? It allows us to see Williams's work as a precursor to contemporary plays that explore the intersection of disability and queerness as both social constructions *and* lived identities, such as Tony Kushner's *Angels in America* (1992). We can therefore subvert the traditionally pathologized definitions of both categories and reimagine depictions of disabled characters that seem, at first glance, extremely problematic. This process also allows us to ask how queer and disability aesthetics of theatre, and their necessary play with heterosexist and ableist conventions, can work mutually and productively to effect social change in a world preoccupied with bodily normalcy based in categories such as sexuality and ability.

Acknowlegments

I want to thank the following for their feedback on earlier versions of this article: Suzanne Churchill, Randy Ingram, Richard Kaye, and the members of the queer theory reading and writing group at the 2000 NEH Summer Institute on Disability Studies: Sumi Colligan, Jim Ferris, Kim Hall, Diane Price Herndl, Cathy Kudlick, Cindy LaCom, Robert McRuer, Donna Ryan, Carrie Sandahl, and Linda Ware.

Notes

1. I use the word *stare* purposefully here, in reference to Rosemarie Garland-Thomson's work on how the stare has been used to objectify the disabled individual (the "object of the stare"), cement the unequal power relationship between the looker and the "to-be-looked-at," and cause the impairment alone to stand for the disabled person. For further exploration of this idea, see Rosemarie Garland-Thomson, "Seeing the Disabled: Visual Rhetorics of Disability in Popular Photography," in *The New Disability History: American Perspectives*, edited by Paul K. Longmore and Lauri Urmansky (New York: New York University Press, 2001), 347.

2. Lennard Davis sees this less as an equal footing, however; he makes the point that in cultural studies, while queer bodies are romanticized as transgressive, "Disabled

bodies are not permitted to participate in the erotics of power, in the power of the erotic, in economics of transgression" (1995, 158).

3. For a more detailed discussion of this "violation" of economic ties as it pertains to Williams's drama, see Steven Bruhm, "Blackmailed by Sex: Tennessee Williams and the Economics of Desire," *Modern Drama* (34) 1991: 528–537.

4. For more on "normalcy studies," an area of disability studies delineated by Lennard Davis that deconstructs the history and definitions of normalcy against which the disabled body has been defined, see Davis's *Enforcing Normalcy: Disability, Deafness, and the Body* (New York: Verso, 1995).

5. This essay is contained in the collection *The New Disability History: American Perspectives*, edited by Paul K. Longmore and Lori Urmansky (New York: New York University Press, 2001).

6. Rosemarie Garland-Thomson distinguishes among different visual rhetorics of disability that have been invoked in photography to create "the disabled figure [as], the to-be-looked-at rather than the to-be-embraced" (2001, 340). These rhetorics, taking advantage of photography's quality of providing a disability presence that is at once viewable yet "safely" distant from the viewer, instruct that viewer to engage disability in one of the following relationships: "the wondrous mode directs the viewer to look up in awe of difference; the sentimental mode instructs the spectator to look down with benevolence; the exotic mode coaches the observer to look across a wide expanse toward an alien object; and the realistic mode suggests that the onlooker align with the object of scrutiny. . . . In representing disability, the visualization of impairment, never the functional experience of it, defines the category of disability" (346).

7. I first heard this term used by Robert McRuer at the 2000 NEH Summer Institute on Disability Studies; see also his essay "Compulsory Able-Bodiedness and Queer/Disabled Existence" in *Disability Studies: Enabling the Humanities*, edited by Sharon L. Snyder, Brenda Jo Brueggemann, and Rosemarie Garland-Thomson (New York: Modern Language Association of America, 2002).

8. It is interesting to note that Sebastian Venable's dismembered body figures him as a reference to St. Sebastian, whose image has been evoked repeatedly throughout the twentieth century as a gay icon. Brick's injury, however loosely, makes him a precursor to this later, more direct, reference.

9. By this time, the word *straight* was being used as slang for heterosexuality.

10. It is fitting that these readings of Williams should move toward a place of more ambiguity, as the theatrical and social milieu of the time itself was punctuated by ambiguity relative to masculinity. The playwrights who were creating some of the most memorable male characters themselves defied traditional masculinity, as Clum points out: "Three of the four most critically acclaimed and commercially successful playwrights of the postwar period were closeted homosexuals whose plays were supported by the critical establishment so long as they maintained the conventions of closet drama. Of the pantheon of Tennessee Williams, William Inge, Edward Albee, and Arthur Miller, only Miller was heterosexual" (1994, 149). Masculinity in the postwar era was in an uneasy compromise with what Susan Bordo calls "pro-domesticity," the masculinities represented by such figures as Ozzie Nelson and Marlon Brando occupying opposite, even warring, ends of the scale.

11. The actor before whom all this played out was himself enmeshed in the social forces Williams is trying to expose. In what was a highly ironic casting choice, the doctor was played by Montgomery Clift, who was gay *and* disabled. An alcoholic, he was

also in the midst of a downward spiral due to his distress over his facial disfigure-ment in a 1956 car accident. Trapped by his own sense of loss as "disfigured" man, he could not come out in a full and public fashion either as gay or disabled. The making of the film version of *Suddenly Last Summer* depended on both identities being minimized. His face heavily made up, shielded although very ill by friends Katharine Hepburn and Elizabeth Taylor (who threatened to quit if he was fired), Clift made the picture.

12. It can be quite legitimately argued that Violet, in contrast, appears to be a reinscription of the very moral model of disability that I argue Williams subverts. Her malevo-lence, it seems, at once springs from and is represented in her disability. While this argument is valid, I would point out that an audience who might agree with this view would simultaneously find itself allied with the fight against masking difference and thus enmeshed in the very instability of boundaries and identity categories I argue exists in the play.

Works Cited

Bordo, Susan. 1999. *The male body: A new look at men in public and private.* New York: Farrar, Straus and Giroux.

Bruhm, Steven. 1991. Blackmailed by sex: Tennessee Williams and the economics of desire. *Modern drama* 34: 528–537.

Clare, Eli. 1999. *Exile and pride: Disability, queerness, and liberation.* Cambridge, Mass.: South End Press.

Clum, John M. 1992. "Something cloudy, something clear": Homophobic discourse in Tennessee Williams. In *Homosexual Themes in Literary Studies*, edited by Wayne R. Dynes and Stephen Donaldson. New York: Garland.

———. 1994. *Acting gay: Male homosexuality in modern drama.* New York: Columbia University Press.

D'Emilio, John. 1992. *Making trouble: Essays on gay history, politics, and the univer-sity.* New York: Routledge.

Davis, Lennard. 1995. *Enforcing normalcy: Disability, deafness, and the body.* New York: Verso.

Fleche, Anne. 1995. When a door is a jar, or out in the theatre: Tennessee Williams and queer space. *Theatre Journal* 47: 253–267.

Garland-Thomson, Rosemarie. 2001. Seeing the disabled: Visual rhetorics of disability in popular photography. In *The new disability history: American perspectives*, edited by Paul K. Longmore and Lauri Urmansky. New York: New York University Press.

Leverich, Lyle. 1995. *Tom: The unknown Tennessee Williams.* New York: Crown Publishers.

Lewis, Victoria Ann. 2000. The dramaturgy of disability. In *Points of contact: Disability, art, and culture*, edited by Susan Crutchfield and Marcy Epstein. Ann Arbor: Uni-versity of Michigan Press.

McRuer, Robert. 2002. "Compulsory Able-Bodiedness and Queer/Disabled Existence." In *Disability Studies: Enabling the Humanities*, edited by Sharon L. Snyder, Brenda Jo Brueggemann, and Rosemarie Garland-Thomson. New York: Modern Language Association of America.

Mitchell, David T., and Sharon L. Snyder. 2000. *Narrative prosthesis: Disability and the dependencies of discourse.* Ann Arbor: University of Michigan Press.

Parker, Brian. 1998. A tentative stemma for drafts and revisions of Tennessee Williams's *Suddenly last summer* (1958). *Modern drama* 41: 303–326.

Savran, David. 1992. *Communists, cowboys and queers: The politics of masculinity in the work of Arthur Miller and Tennessee Williams*. Minneapolis: University of Minnesota Press.

Williams, Edwina Dakin, with Lucy Freeman. 1963. *Remember me to Tom*. New York: Putnam.

Williams, Tennessee. 1975. *Memoirs*. Garden City, New York: Doubleday and Company, Inc.

———. 1955. *Cat on a Hot Tin Roof*. New York: Signet.

———. 1947. *A Streetcar Named Desire*. New York: Signet.

———. 1958. *Suddenly Last Summer*. In *Tennessee Williams: Four plays*. New York: Signet Classic.

PART IV

♫

Citizens and
Consumers

Is There Still a "Double Handicap"?

ECONOMIC, SOCIAL, AND POLITICAL DISPARITIES EXPERIENCED BY WOMEN WITH DISABILITIES

&

LISA SCHUR

To what extent do women with disabilities continue to experience a "double handicap" more than a decade after the passage of the Americans with Disabilities Act (ADA)? How much do their low employment levels contribute to economic and social inequalities, and what role does employment play in their political involvement and perceptions of unfair treatment? This chapter addresses these questions by examining the extent to which women with disabilities continue to face gaps in employment, income, education, access to public services and programs, and measures of psychological well-being compared both with men with disabilities and women without disabilities. It focuses on how the low employment levels of women with disabilities contribute to these gaps and how employment may play an important role in explaining their political participation and responses to discrimination.

Literature Review

Feminist disability scholars called attention in the 1980s to the fact that women with disabilities fared significantly worse economically, socially, and psychologically than either disabled men or nondisabled women (Deegan and Brooks 1985; Fine and Asch 1988). The grim realities facing disabled women included lower employment, education, and income levels, fewer opportunities for vocational training, and lower receipt of disability-income benefits.

Although both gender and disability have contributed to these disparities, the gaps should not be assessed simply by using an additive approach. As Bell,

Denton, and Nkomo (1993) note with respect to black women managers, race and class can affect one's experience of gender, and different aspects of one's identity can become more salient in different social contexts. Similarly, disability may work differently for women than for men. Deegan (1985, 50) indicates that there may be a negative interaction as disability reinforces the stereotypical norm of passivity associated with women or a positive interaction as disability creates less of a stigma regarding physical limitations for women than for men; also, disability may have a stronger positive effect on women's "sense of strength, understanding, compassion, and power" if they overcome the extra barriers they face. Hanna and Rogovsky (1993) found that women with disabilities appeared to face "two handicaps plus" and that their employment rates and educational levels were lower than would be expected by combining the effects of gender and disability disparities. Scholars such as Baldwin and Johnson (1995) found wage disparities due to both gender and disability, and the most severe wage discrimination against women with the most stigmatized disabilities. Other authors have noted that women with disabilities who are employed have remained concentrated in nonunion, low-wage jobs and that their unemployment levels have stayed high, especially among disabled women of color (Stoddard et al. 1998). Women have also remained less likely to receive the main form of public disability income, Social Security Disability Income (SSDI), which is based on predisability work earnings, and those who do receive SSDI tend to get lower payments than do men (Baldwin 1997; Mudrick 1988).

The difficulties women with disabilities face have been addressed by a number of federal antidiscrimination laws, including the 1972 Rehabilitation Act, Title IX of the 1972 Education Amendments, the 1975 Education for All Handicapped Children Act, and the 1990 ADA. How much these laws have improved conditions for women with disabilities remains unclear, however, in part because studies have not used consistent definitions of disability. Gaps in educational attainment between people with and without hearing loss appear to have declined from 1972 to 1991 for both men and women, although women continued to have lower employment and pay levels in 1991 regardless of hearing status (Barnett 1997). Examining trends in employment and household income levels from 1980 to 1999, Burkhauser, Daly, and Heutenville (2001) found that while the gender gaps between men and women with disabilities appeared to shrink, the employment and income gaps between women with and without work disabilities grew over this period.

In addition to economic disadvantages, women with disabilities have also experienced social inequalities. Scholars have found that they are more likely to live alone, are viewed more negatively, and have more negative self-concepts than men with disabilities (Fine and Asch 1988, 23; Hanna and Rogovsky 1993). Fine and Asch (1985) argue that women with disabilities are viewed as unable to fulfill traditional adult social roles, such as that of wage earner or homemaker, and that when they try to identify with traditional female sex roles, their actions only reinforce the stereotype of the passive, dependent disabled person.

In contrast, men with disabilities have more opportunities to distance themselves from the disability role by identifying with the male role associated with independence and self-assertion.[1] Fine and Asch claim that the combination of economic, social, and psychological barriers contribute to the "rolelessness" experienced by many women with disabilities (12).

How can women with disabilities best contend with the economic and social disparities they face? Some authors have focused on forging political alliances between the disability rights movement and the women's movement (Hillyer 1993; Morris 1993; Neath 1997). Others argue that many women with disabilities withdraw from politics because neither the feminist nor the disability rights movement fully addresses their needs. They maintain that while gender issues need to be incorporated into the disability rights movement, disability issues (such as the right to be free from involuntary sterilization) need to be integrated into the feminist agenda (Blackwell-Stratton et al. 1988, 307).

Still other authors focus on the value of helping women with disabilities through assertiveness training programs, some of which are based on the model of feminist consciousness-raising groups. Kasnitz and Doe (1998) claim that women with disabilities often develop along a leadership continuum from self-advocacy to fighting for system change and that counseling and training can play an important role in this process. Kolb (1985) and Saxton (1985) discuss programs to empower women with disabilities and help them become advocates for themselves and others with disabilities. The peer counseling program Saxton describes, for example, combines assertiveness training with political and social analysis of the conditions facing women with disabilities. This type of program can enable participants to experience personal events as relevant to the sphere of politics, a process political scientists have termed "political translation" (Hofstetter and Schultze 1989).

Although she does not focus specifically on women, Anspach's (1979) model of "stratagems for stigma management" provides insights into who translates disability problems into political issues and becomes an activist. She describes disability activists as individuals who maintain a positive self-concept while rejecting society's devaluation of people with disabilities. In contrast, "normalizers" maintain a positive self-concept while accepting the value society places on physical wholeness and attractiveness and emphasize that they are "superficially different but basically the same as everyone else" (769). While normalizers ignore or minimize their disabilities, activists embrace this aspect of their identities. "Disassociators" and "retreatists," however, are people with disabilities who have negative self-concepts and withdraw from society out of anger or fear. These responses Anspach outlined were evident in a study of people with traumatic spinal cord injuries (Schur 1998).

Almost no research has been done on political activism among women with disabilities. Prior research on political participation in general tends to predict that they would have lower involvement. They have fewer resources; experience greater isolation, which decreases recruitment opportunities; and may feel relatively powerless—all of which have been found to discourage political participation in the general population (Verba, Schlozman, and Brady 1995). Women in general remain less likely to engage in campaign activity (though they are now as likely to vote and participate in local politics as men), in part due to lower self-evaluations of internal political efficacy, civic skills, and political interest (Conway 2000). Childhood socialization and traditional adult female roles may help explain these lower self-evaluations (Clark and Clark 1986; Conway 2000). In the case of women with disabilities, the effects are likely to be compounded because many girls with disabilities are socialized with negative messages about their capabilities and may experience rolelessness as adults.

The low levels of employment among women with disabilities may also depress their political participation. Employed women in general are more likely than nonemployed women to develop civic skills that facilitate political involvement (Schlozman, Burns, and Verba 1999). In addition, employed women may be more likely to experience discrimination (e.g., in raises, promotions, or other treatment at work), which can be a catalyst to political action. Although disability discrimination in the workplace may motivate some women to engage in activism, employed women with disabilities may possibly be less likely to focus on disability issues, because their jobs enable them to normalize and identify with mainstream society. In contrast, nonemployed women with disabilities who become politically involved may be more likely to focus on disability rights because of their relatively marginal position and the many economic and social barriers they face.

The limited evidence on political participation and disability indicates that voter turnout is lower among people with disabilities in general, particularly among those who are older, not employed, and have difficulty going outside alone (groups that are disproportionately female; Shields, Schriner, and Schriner 1998; Schur and Kruse 2000; Schur et al. 2002). In addition, better health predicts less anomie, greater political interest and information, and greater political involvement among older women (Peterson and Somit 1992). This chapter adds to the literature by providing a recent picture of the economic and social conditions that women with disabilities face, as well as their political participation and responses to perceived discrimination (referring to some of the evidence from Schur 2003).

Data Sources

This chapter makes use of two datasets. The first is the 1999 disability supplement of the Survey of Income and Program Participation (SIPP), which is used only in table 1 for employment, earnings, income, and poverty comparisons among women and men with and without disabilities. The principal data sources are two national household surveys conducted following the November elections in 1998 and 2000. The surveys, conducted by the Rutgers Center for

Public Interest Polling, had samples of 1,242 U.S. citizens of voting age in 1998 and 1,002 in 2000. To ensure a sufficient sample for analysis of disability issues, the samples were stratified to oversample people with disabilities, resulting in an overall final sample of 1,132 citizens with disabilities and 1,112 citizens without disabilities.[2] Consistent with other figures on the disability population, 57.4 percent of the respondents with disabilities were female.[3]

In the sample of women with disabilities, 68 percent reported some sort of mobility limitation while 35 percent reported a mental impairment and 27 percent reported a visual or hearing impairment—figures that were very similar among men with disabilities (Schur 2003). Women were more likely than men with disabilities to report needing help with any daily activities (36% compared to 24%) and difficulty in going outside alone (30% compared to 21%), which may contribute to greater social isolation.

Economic and Social Disparities

To what extent does the double handicap continue to exist? Tables 1–3 provide comparisons on economic, social, and psychological measures. Each table shows the average levels for women and men with and without disabilities in columns 1–4 and the resulting gaps between women with disabilities and the other groups in columns 5–7.

As shown in table 1, women with disabilities continue to have lower employment and income levels than either men with disabilities or nondisabled women (and much lower than nondisabled men), supporting the idea that both gender and disability contribute to their lower economic status. About two out of five working-age women with disabilities are employed in a given week, compared to half of men with disabilities and three-fourths of women without disabilities. Those who are employed are more likely than their male counterparts and nondisabled women to work part-time, and they also have lower average hourly earnings.

Given their low employment rates, it is not surprising that women with disabilities have the highest poverty rate among the four groups. As shown in table 1, 20 percent are living in poverty compared to 14 percent of men with disabilities, 9 percent of nondisabled women, and 7 percent of nondisabled men. The importance of employment is shown by the finding that less than 8 percent of employed women with disabilities are in poverty, which is just slightly higher than the rates for the other groups (reflecting the fact that their hourly and annual earnings remain lower). Almost one-third of nonemployed women with disabilities are poor, which is substantially higher than the rate among members of the other groups. Contributing to the high poverty rate of nonemployed women with disabilities is the fact that they are less likely than men with disabilities to receive SSDI benefits, which are based on one's previous work history, and that those who do receive SSDI have lower monthly benefits on average. Although

TABLE 1 *Examining the "Double Handicap"—Employment and Income*

| | Women | | Men | | Diff. between Women w/disabs. and: | | |
	With Disability (1)	Without Disability (2)	With Disability (3)	Without Disability (4)	Women w/out Disabilities (5)	Men with Disabilities (6)	Men w/out Disabilities (7)
EMPLOYMENT							
Data from 1999 SIPP survey							
Employed last month (age 18–64)	44.2%	75.5%	49.5%	89.1%	−31.3%**	−5.3%**	−44.9%**
If employed:							
Part-time schedule	30.9%	21.8%	16.5%	7.9%	9.1%**	14.4%**	23.0%**
Annual earnings	$20,224	$25,637	$30,887	$39,548	−21.1%**	−34.5%**	−48.9%**
Hourly earnings	$13.08	$14.16	$16.24	$18.26	−7.6%**	−19.5%**	−28.4%**
Data from 1998/2000 political participation surveys							
Employed last week (age 18–64)	40.9%	73.9%	50.5%	90.2%	−33.0%**	−9.6%**	−49.3%**
If employed, work part-time	38.0%	24.5%	21.4%	7.9%	13.5%**	16.6%**	30.1%**
INCOME							
Data from 1999 SIPP survey							
Personal income (mean)	$13,010	$20,302	$21,971	$36,294	−35.9%**	−40.8%**	−64.2%**
Household income (mean)	$35,011	$59,168	$41,227	$63,204	−40.8%**	−15.1%**	−44.6%**
In poverty	20.0%	9.3%	14.3%	6.6%	10.7%**	5.7%**	13.4%**
If employed	7.7%	5.3%	7.1%	4.7%	2.4%**	0.6%	3.0%**
If not employed	32.5%	22.3%	26.7%	24.8%	10.2%**	5.8%**	7.7%**
Receive SSDI	7.8%	0.0%	12.8%	0.0%		−5.0%**	
Mean amount per mo. if received	$530		$688			−$158**	
Receive SSI	13.6%	0.0%	12.8%	0.0%		0.8%	
Mean amount per mo. if received	$345		$384			−$39**	
Sample sizes							
1999 SIPP survey	7468	21296	5134	19738			
1998/2000 political participation surveys	648	635	481	476			

*Significant difference at p < .10   ** p < .05

Source: Survey of Income and Program Participation (1999 disability supplement) and 1998/2000 political participation surveys.

Note: The disability definitions differ between the SIPP and political participation surveys.

the poverty rate is higher among women than among men with disabilities, the two groups are similarly likely to receive means-tested Supplemental Security Income (SSI), and men generally receive slightly higher monthly benefits.

The findings are more encouraging when education is examined. As shown in table 2, significant gender differences do not exist among people with disabilities in terms of average years of completed schooling (though women with disabilities appear slightly less likely to have a college degree). Nevertheless, people with disabilities continue to lag in educational attainment behind their nondisabled counterparts. More than one-fifth of men and women with disabilities did not graduate from high school, compared to less than one-tenth of men and women without disabilities. People with disabilities are also only half as likely to have graduated from college.

Perceptions of civic skills were measured by asking whether respondents considered themselves better than average on five activities. As shown in table 2, women with disabilities are significantly lower than other groups in self-evaluations of their ability to speak in public and lead a group (which may reflect their lower likelihood of gaining these skills through employment). They are lower than nondisabled respondents, but similar to men with disabilities, in their perceived ability to work with others, compose an effective letter to an elected official, and communicate ideas to others.

Many women with disabilities continue to be isolated, both physically and socially. Table 3 shows that more than one-fourth of women with disabilities live alone, compared with one-fifth of men with disabilities. They are less likely to be married than members of the other groups, and less likely to be able to drive a car, which can contribute to isolation in many regions in the country. In terms of group membership and participation, however, women with disabilities are slightly more likely than men with disabilities to meet regularly with any groups, and they are more likely to attend disability groups and religious services. This lends support to the arguments of Kolb (1985) and Saxton (1985) that peer groups may be particularly important for women with disabilities. Nevertheless, people with disabilities in general are significantly less likely than nondisabled people to meet regularly with groups or attend religious services.

Despite the additional barriers women with disabilities face, there are no significant gender differences among people with disabilities on measures of life satisfaction, depression (feeling "downhearted and blue"), and social role fulfillment (feeling "useful and needed"). Table 2 shows, however, that there are strong disability gaps: women with disabilities report lower levels of satisfaction and role fulfillment and higher levels of depression compared to women and men without disabilities.

How does employment affect psychological well-being and perceptions of competence? Table 3 shows that among women with disabilities, those who are employed are more likely to feel useful and needed, though there is little difference in measures of life satisfaction and depression. Interestingly, life satisfaction among nondisabled respondents is slightly lower among those who are

Table 2 Examining the "Double Handicap"—Education and Civic Skills

	Women		Men		Diff. between Women w/disabs. and:		
	With Disability (1)	Without Disability (2)	With Disability (3)	Without Disability (4)	Women w/out Disabilities (5)	Men with Disabilities (6)	Men w/out Disabilities (7)
EDUCATION							
No high school degree	22.9%	8.7%	26.3%	6.5%	14.2%***	-3.4%**	16.4%***
High school degree	30.5%	23.1%	24.1%	20.6%	7.4%***	6.4%***	9.8%***
Some college/AA degree	31.3%	35.1%	31.3%	35.6%	-3.8%	0.0%	-4.3%
BA degree	8.6%	20.0%	12.5%	23.7%	-11.4%***	-3.9%*	-15.1%***
Graduate degree	6.7%	13.1%	5.8%	13.6%	-6.4%***	0.9%	-6.9%***
Total years (mean)	12.6	14.0	12.5	14.2	-1.4**	0.1	-1.6**
CIVIC SKILLS							
Consider oneself better than average in:							
Ability to work with others	50.3%	65.6%	50.6%	71.5%	-15.4%***	-0.3%	-21.2%***
Ability to speak in public	22.3%	29.0%	30.3%	41.7%	-6.7%***	-8.0%**	-19.4%***
Ability to lead a group	27.9%	40.1%	44.2%	61.4%	-12.2%***	-16.2%***	-33.5%***
Ability to compose effective letter to elected official	33.8%	40.5%	29.7%	48.8%	-6.7%***	4.1%	-15.0%***
Communicating ideas to others	45.0%	52.0%	46.7%	65.3%	-7.0%***	-1.7%	-20.3%***
Sum of above	1.79	2.27	2.02	2.89	-0.48**	-0.23**	-1.10**
If employed	2.39	2.37	2.57	3.00	0.02	-0.18	-0.61**
If not employed	1.59	2.08	1.70	2.45	-0.49**	-0.11	-0.86**
Sample size	648	635	481	476			

Source: All data are from the 1998/2000 political participation surveys.
*Significant difference at p < .10   ** p < .05

TABLE 3 *Examining the "Double Handicap"—Social Isolation, Psychological Well-being, and Political Efficacy*

	Women		Men		Diff. between Women w/disabs. and:		
	With Disability (1)	Without Disability (2)	With Disability (3)	Without Disability (4)	Women w/out Disabilities (5)	Men with Disabilities (6)	Men w/out Disabilities (7)
SOCIAL ISOLATION							
Live alone	28.2%	7.9%	20.0%	7.2%	20.3%***	8.2%***	21.0%***
Married, spouse present	46.5%	65.0%	57.5%	67.6%	-18.5%***	-11.1%***	-21.1%***
Regularly meet with any groups	38.1%	57.3%	37.7%	53.5%	-19.2%***	0.4%	-15.4%***
Regularly meet with disability groups	7.5%		4.1%			3.4%**	
Attend religious services most weeks	38.5%	47.2%	32.2%	37.9%	-8.7%***	6.3%***	0.6%
Can drive a car	63.9%	93.4%	80.2%	97.4%	-29.4%***	-16.3%***	-33.4%**
PSYCHOLOGICAL WELL-BEING							
"Very satisfied" with life in general	46.6%	59.4%	40.3%	60.4%	-12.8%***	6.3%	-13.8%***
If employed	47.9%	55.2%	49.1%	57.1%	-7.3%	-1.2%	-9.2%
Feel useful and needed most of time	56.1%	76.2%	52.1%	72.6%	-20.2%***	4.0%	-16.5%***
If employed	68.8%	74.0%	70.7%	76.6%	-5.2%	-1.9%	-7.8%
Downhearted and blue good part of time	15.8%	1.9%	10.4%	0.2%	13.8%***	5.4%**	15.6%***
If employed	17.8%	1.9%	5.8%	0.0%	15.9%***	12.0%***	17.8%***
POLITICAL EFFICACY							
Personal competence							
Feel well-qualified to part. in pols.	53.9%	63.1%	63.2%	75.3%	-9.2%***	-9.3%***	-21.4%***
If employed	56.6%	63.4%	62.0%	75.4%	-6.8%	-5.4%	-18.8%***
Perceived responsiveness of political system							
Feel that public officials don't care	51.4%	44.1%	57.0%	50.7%	7.3%***	-5.6%*	0.7%
If employed	52.4%	45.9%	57.8%	53.3%	6.5%	-5.4%	-0.9%
Feel that people like me don't have say	46.1%	36.7%	49.3%	39.9%	9.4%***	-3.2%	6.2%*
If employed	39.6%	35.6%	45.9%	40.7%	4.0%	-6.3%	-1.1%
Perceive that people with disabilities:							
Receive equal treatment from public officials	57.7%	68.3%	60.0%	72.1%	-10.6%***	-2.3%	-14.4%**
If employed	54.4%	67.1%	66.8%	71.4%	-12.7%***	-12.4%***	-17.0%***
Have equal influence in politics	70.4%	75.6%	70.7%	78.1%	-5.2%*	-0.3%	-7.7%**
If employed	73.5%	75.7%	74.4%	77.7%	-2.2%	-0.9%	-4.2%
Sample size	648	635	481	476			

Source: All data are from the 1998/2000 political participation surveys. * Significant difference at p<.10 ** p<.05

employed (perhaps reflecting the increased stress and time demands associated with many jobs). The result is that no significant gaps are found in life satisfaction or feeling useful and needed between employed women with disabilities and other employed respondents. Employed women with disabilities, however, still have higher depression levels than nondisabled employed people.

Psychological well-being may be linked to feelings of efficacy and competence. In addition, the belief that one is qualified to participate in politics and that the political system is responsive are generally associated with higher levels of political participation. As shown in table 3, women with disabilities are less likely than both nondisabled women and men with disabilities to say they feel well-qualified to participate in politics. They are also less likely than nondisabled women to report that politicians care about them and are responsive to their interests but slightly more likely than men with disabilities to report this. Strong disability gaps are present in perceptions of the respect and influence politicians accord people with disabilities.

Employment appears to increase perceptions among women with disabilities that the political system is responsive and to decrease the gaps between women with disabilities and the other groups on most efficacy measures. At the same time, employed women with disabilities are less likely than employed people in the other groups to report that people with disabilities receive equal treatment from public officials. This may indicate that employment increases women's sense that they have the ability to influence politicians, while also exposing them to more opportunities for unfair treatment and discrimination.

In sum, in the areas of education, psychological well-being, and perceived responsiveness of the political system, there are large disability gaps but no substantial gender gaps. This contrasts with several findings from studies in the 1970s and 1980s, suggesting that some progress appears to have been made for women with disabilities in these areas. Nevertheless, the persistent gender and disability gaps in employment, income, social isolation, and self-evaluations of ability to speak in public, lead a group, and participate in politics indicate that a double handicap continues to exist.

Political Involvement

Are the continuing disparities faced by women with disabilities reflected in lower levels of political participation? Consistent with prior research showing that resource limitations and social isolation discourage participation, table 4 shows that women with disabilities engage in fewer political activities on average over a 12-month period than the other groups. Nevertheless, no significant gender differences exist among people with disabilities on a majority of the specific measures of political participation. Women and men with disabilities report voting at about the same rates in the 1998 and 2000 elections. Women with disabilities are about as likely as members of all other groups to have written a letter to a newspaper and about as likely as men with disabilities to have written or spoken to a public official, worked with others on a community problem, and otherwise worked to change government laws or policies. Women with disabilities are somewhat less likely to have attended a political meeting and less likely to have contributed money to a political organization or candidate (which accords with their lower average incomes). Interestingly, women with disabilities are more than three times more likely than their male counterparts to have participated in a protest or march in the last year, a finding that goes against the stereotype that women with disabilities are especially docile and passive.

While there is only a small gender gap in overall political participation among people with disabilities, there is nonetheless a large disability gap. As shown in table 4, women with disabilities are significantly less likely than nondisabled women and men to participate in a variety of political activities, such as voting, writing or speaking to public officials, and working with others on a community problem. On average they did 1.73 of the eight activities in the past year, which is significantly lower than the 2.13 and 2.43 averages for women and men without disabilities, respectively.

Employment appears to play an important role in increasing political participation among people with disabilities. No significant differences were found in political participation between the employed women and men with disabilities and employed nondisabled respondents. These results appear encouraging, but it is important to remember that only 41 percent of the working-age female respondents with disabilities are employed, compared to 51 percent of the male respondents with disabilities, 74 percent of nondisabled women, and 90 percent of nondisabled men.

Further analysis of these data show that being a woman and having a disability do not in themselves predict lower levels of political involvement (Schur 2003). Rather, several elements of the double handicap among women with disabilities contribute to their lower levels of overall political participation. In particular, economic and social disparities (in employment, income, and group attendance) primarily account for the participation gap between women with disabilities and nondisabled men and women. Differences in perceptions of the ability to participate in politics, however, primarily account for the smaller participation gap relative to men with disabilities.

What about disability activism? In contrast to some of the results on standard measures of political activity, women with disabilities are as likely as their male peers to have engaged in disability activism. Close to one-tenth did at least one of the political activities described above on a disability issue, and a similar proportion took action against a private organization on a disability issue. Employed women with disabilities are slightly more likely than nonemployed women with disabilities to have engaged in each of these activities on a disability issue—going against the idea that employment greatly increases "normalization" among women with disabilities. Individuals who attend disability groups are the most likely to engage in disability activism. The single most important predictor for disability activism, for both men and women, is regularly

TABLE 4 Political Participation

	Women		Men		Diff. between Women w/disabs. and:		
	With Disability (1)	Without Disability (2)	With Disability (3)	Without Disability (4)	Women w/out Disabilities (5)	Men with Disabilities (6)	Men w/out Disabilities (7)
Number of political activities in past year (0–8 scale^)	1.73	2.13	1.93	2.43	−0.41**	−0.20*	−0.70**
If employed	2.16	2.15	2.15	2.37	0.01	0.01	−0.21
If not employed	1.57	2.11	1.82	2.68	−0.54**	−0.25*	−1.11**
Political activities							
Voted	61.5%	71.9%	62.5%	69.8%	−10.4%**	−1.0%	−8.3%***
Written or spoken to elected representative or public official	28.9%	37.1%	33.9%	46.0%	−8.1%***	−5.0%	−17.0%***
Worked with others on community problem	21.8%	27.8%	22.4%	30.3%	−6.0%***	−0.5%	−8.5%***
Contributed money to org. trying to influence gov't. policy or legislation	14.2%	22.8%	20.3%	25.9%	−8.6%***	−6.1%**	−11.7%***
Attended political meeting	11.3%	15.8%	15.3%	17.4%	−4.5%**	−4.0%*	−6.1%***
Contributed money to political party or candidate	11.3%	14.0%	15.6%	20.9%	−2.7%	−4.3%*	−9.6%***
Written letter to newspaper	8.9%	6.7%	7.3%	11.1%	2.2%	1.7%	−2.2%
Otherwise worked with groups or on one's own to change gov't laws or policies	14.9%	17.3%	15.9%	21.6%	−2.4%	−1.0%	−6.8%***
Participated in protest or march^	5.9%	4.6%	1.7%	6.4%	1.3%	4.2%**	−0.5%
Political activity on a disability issue	10.4%		9.7%			0.6%	
If employed	12.1%		7.2%			4.9%	
If not employed	9.9%		11.2%			−1.3%	
If attend disability group	53.0%		37.2%			15.8%	
Took action against private org. on disability issue	8.4%		8.8%			−0.4%	
If employed	11.8%		8.8%			3.0%	
If not employed	7.2%		8.8%			−1.6%	
If attend disability group	28.7%		25.3%			3.4%	
Sample size	650	636	482	476			

Source: All data are from the 1998/2000 political participation surveys.

* Significant difference from column (1) at p < .10   ** p < .05

^ The protest question was asked only in 2000 and is not included in the overall count of political activities.

meeting with such groups (Schur 2003). This is consistent with the ideas of Kolb (1985) and Saxton (1985) that such groups can provide information on disability issues, mobilization networks, and forums for the development of identity politics. An intriguing finding is that while older women are more likely to engage in political participation in general, they are less likely to be involved in disability issues. One interpretation is that older women were socialized to have more negative views of disability (in the era when President Franklin Roosevelt hid his disability) and more traditional views of femininity that limit confrontational actions (Schur, Shields, and Schriner 2001).

Disability Discrimination

Fighting against discrimination that one has directly experienced is different from other forms of political participation, such as voting, which are less confrontational. One might expect that women would be less likely than men to perceive and take action against disability discrimination, either because they are socialized to be more passive and have internalized negative messages about gender and disability (as several writers have suggested) or because they are less likely to be employed and experience discrimination at work. On the other hand, women with disabilities possibly would be more aware of discrimination because of frequent reminders of their lower economic and social status. This effect may be particularly strong among nonemployed women, who have fewer resources and may be less likely to engage in normalizing behavior.

Close to 16 percent of women with disabilities report that they experienced disability discrimination in the last five years, which is slightly but not significantly lower than the 21 percent of men who did so (table 5). While women with disabilities overall are less likely to report employment discrimination, the employed women are about as likely as employed men to do so. Men and women are also about equally likely to report nonemployment discrimination. Most of the reports of employment discrimination among both men and women concerned the loss or denial of jobs, while women reporting nonemployment discrimination are more likely to report discriminatory attitudes of others (e.g., "verbal abuse," "people making fun of my seizures").

Employed women are more likely than nonemployed women to report any discrimination (consistent with the findings of Schlozman et al. 1999), and they are as likely as employed men to report discrimination. Nonemployed women, in contrast, are less likely than nonemployed men to report discrimination. Further analysis shows that reports of disability discrimination are highest among those who need help with daily activities, attend groups regularly, are more educated, and perceive that people with disabilities receive less respect from public officials (Schur 2003). The fewer reports of discrimination among those who do not attend groups may reflect their greater isolation; they may actually experience less discriminatory treatment because of fewer social contacts or have a more narrow view of what constitutes discrimination (Schur 1998). Those who are age sixty-five or over are much less likely to report disability discrimination,

TABLE 5   Perceptions of and Responses to Disability Discrimination

	Women w/ Disabilities (1)	Men w/ Disabilities (2)	Diff. (3)
Perceived disability discrim. in past 5 yrs.	15.7%	21.0%	−5.3%
If currently employed	20.7%	19.3%	1.4%
If not currently employed	14.2%	21.3%	−7.1%
Perceived job discrim. in past 5 yrs.	6.6%	12.4%	−5.8%**
If currently employed	14.3%	15.9%	−1.6%
If not currently employed	4.1%	9.9%	−5.8%*
Perceived nonjob discrim. in past 5 yrs.	9.2%	8.5%	0.7%
If currently employed	6.4%	3.5%	2.9%
If not currently employed	10.0%	11.5%	−1.5%
If perceived discrim., type perceived			
Job discrimination	41.7%	59.2%	−17.5%
Denied job	14.1%	38.4%	−24.3%**
Lost job	17.2%	12.7%	4.5%
Co-worker attitudes	2.5%	2.2%	0.3%
Other job discrim.	7.9%	6.0%	1.9%
Attitudes of others	18.7%	3.9%	14.8%*
Disability benefits/services	6.4%	4.3%	2.1%
Public accommodations	7.4%	2.9%	4.5%
Cost of medical services	5.9%	2.2%	3.7%
Access to medical services	2.7%	4.3%	−1.6%
Insurance	2.7%	3.9%	−1.2%
Other	14.4%	19.4%	−5.0%
If perceived disability discrim., took some action	49.8%	25.5%	24.3%**
If currently employed	51.8%	11.5%	40.3%**
If not currently employed	48.9%	33.5%	15.4%
Worked with others	73.7%	74.9%	−1.2%
Satisfaction with efforts: mean of 1–10 scale	4.90	4.11	0.79
Score of 7 or above	39.5%	21.6%	17.9%
Likelihood of future action if encounter discrim.			
More likely	53.2%	58.8%	−5.5%
Just as likely	34.6%	33.4%	1.2%
Less likely	5.4%	0.0%	5.4%
If perceived job discrim., took some action	62.2%	18.5%	43.7%**
If currently employed	65.9%	7.7%	58.2%**
If not currently employed	58.2%	29.7%	28.5%
Sample size	236	194	

Source: All data are from the 1998/2000 political participation surveys.
* Significant difference at p < .10   ** p < .05

which fits with the earlier result that they are less likely to be involved in disability issues.

Who takes action against perceived discrimination? Here there is a very noteworthy gender difference: while women were less likely than men to report experiencing disability discrimination, those who did were significantly more likely to take action against it. As shown in table 5, almost half of the women, compared to one-fourth of the men, who perceived disability discrimination did something to combat it. This figure is very similar between employed and nonemployed women, while employed men are the least likely to take action against perceived discrimination (perhaps feeling they had too much to lose by challenging unfair treatment). This pattern is even stronger among those who experienced job discrimination. Almost two-thirds of employed women who perceived job discrimination took some action against it, compared to less than one-tenth of the employed men. Consistent with the pattern on reporting discrimination, action against discrimination is highest among women who need help with daily activities, attend groups regularly, and are younger and more educated.

Among those who took action against discrimination, three-fourths of both women and men report working with others when they fought against unjust treatment. Women appear more likely than men to be satisfied with the results of their efforts, but the sample size is too small to draw firm conclusions. Majorities of both women and men report that their experience made them more likely to take action against discrimination in the future, suggesting that there can be an empowering effect of combating discrimination whether or not one's efforts are perceived as successful.

Conclusion

In important respects, women with disabilities still face a double handicap. Most troubling are their continued low employment and income levels and high poverty rates, relative both to women without disabilities and men with disabilities. They also tend to be more socially isolated than either of these groups, and are less likely to feel well-qualified to participate in politics. On several other measures there are important disability gaps but not gender gaps. Both women and men with disabilities have lower educational levels and psychological well-being scores than their nondisabled peers, but few gender gaps between women and men with disabilities on these measures are found.

Although some researchers have examined the economic and social disparities faced by women with disabilities, almost no attention has been paid to their political participation, how they respond to discrimination, and the role of employment. The evidence presented here challenges the stereotype that women with disabilities are especially passive and acquiescent. Despite having fewer economic resources, and being less likely to feel competent to participate in politics, women with disabilities are just as likely as men with disabilities to engage in a variety of political activities and are more likely to take part in protests. They do, however, engage in slightly fewer political activities overall than men with disabilities. The finding that their lower sense of political efficacy accounts for a substantial share of this gap suggests that many women with disabilities have internalized negative messages about their capabilities and that efforts to empower them through training and peer counseling, as several authors suggest, can help increase their political engagement.

The situation is different with regard to disability activism. Women with disabilities are just as likely as men to take action on disability issues and more likely to combat perceived discrimination. Such action is more likely among younger women and those who meet regularly with disability groups. Disability groups can provide support and help people overcome isolation, develop assertiveness, and become politically mobilized. The more frequent reports of discrimination and disability activism among younger women suggest that they are less likely than their mothers and grandmothers to have been socialized with traditional gender roles and negative views of disability and are less likely to "normalize," which is encouraging for future efforts to improve conditions for women with disabilities.

Employment does a great deal to alleviate the double handicap. In addition to raising income levels and decreasing poverty rates, it also appears to increase women's perceived civic skills, their feelings of being useful and needed, and their perceptions that the political system is responsive. It also appears to have a positive effect on political participation among women with disabilities, both in terms of their overall participation and disability activism (going against the idea that employment encourages their "normalization"). Unlike the situation for men with disabilities, employed women are just as likely as nonemployed women to take action against perceived disability discrimination. Because employment plays such an important role for women with disabilities, it remains especially troubling that their employment levels have remained so low and that their educational gains have not led to more job opportunities and higher incomes.

While employment levels clearly need to be raised among all people with disabilities, specific policies are also needed that focus on helping women with disabilities enter and remain in the workforce. For example, vocational rehabilitation programs, which have traditionally been oriented toward men, should ensure that women have equal access to services and that programs are tailored to their needs and abilities. Similarly, high schools and colleges need to increase efforts to assist young women with disabilities in making school-to-work transitions. At the same time, advocacy and self-help groups for women with disabilities should include employment counseling to help them obtain jobs and gain economic independence. Women with disabilities must be actively involved in developing policies and programs to increase their job opportunities and economic prospects—only if their voices are heard can their needs and interests be fully represented. Increasing their employment and income levels, in turn, will help women with disabilities become full and equal participants in political and civic life.

Acknowlegments

This chapter is a companion piece to the article, "Contending with the Double Handicap: Political Activism Among Women with Disabilities." The surveys upon which this study is based were funded by grants from the New Jersey Developmental Disabilities Council, National Institute for Disability and Rehabilitation Research, Presidential Task Force on Employment of Adults with Disabilities, and Rutgers School of Management and Labor Relations, but none bear responsibility for the analysis and conclusions. Dorothy Sue Cobble and Kay Schriner provided valuable comments. Todd Shields, Douglas Kruse, and Kay Schriner were collaborators on the survey. The author is responsible for any remaining errors or omissions.

Notes

1. Other writers, however, such as Morris (1993), point out that men with disabilities may also experience "rolelessness" if their disabilities render them unable to perform traditional male roles: "To be a disabled man is to fail to measure up to the general culture's definition of masculinity as strength, physical ability and autonomy" (87).
2. In the 2000 survey, five hundred of the 1998 respondents were reinterviewed. Because participation, disability status, and other variables in this study often change over time, these five hundred reinterviews are treated here as separate observations. The disability screening questions were based on the six disability questions used in the 2000 Census, plus two questions from the Harris disability survey. Where more than one person in a household was identified as having a disability, the interviewer asked to speak to the person with the most recent birthday.
3. Women were 55.5 percent of the disability sample age fifteen or over in the 1997 Survey of Income and Program Participation (McNeil, 2001: tab. 1). The procedure used in the current survey ensures a random sample of people with disabilities, while the sample of those without disabilities reflects those who first answered the telephone, which accounts for the high number of women in the nondisability sample (636, or 57.2%, were women). To reflect more closely the overall disability and nondisability populations, results are weighted by gender, region, and household size separately for the disability and nondisability populations (using data from the Survey of Income and Program Participation).

Works Cited

Anspach, Renee. 1979. From stigma to identity politics: political activism among the physically disabled and former mental patients. *Social Science and Medicine* 13A: 765–773.

Baldwin, Marjorie L., and William G. Johnson. 1995. Labor market discrimination against women with disabilities. *Industrial Relations* 34: 555–77.

Baldwin, Marjorie. 1997. Gender differences in Social Security disability decisions. *Journal of Disability Policy Studies* 8 (1/2): 25–50.

Barnett, Sharon. 1997. Gender differences in changes over time: Education and occupations of adults with hearing losses 1972–1991. *Journal of Disability Policy Studies* 8 (1/2): 7–24.

Bell, Ella, Toni Denton, and Stella Nkomo. 1993. Women of color in management: Toward an inclusive analysis. In *Women in management*, edited by Ellen Ferguson, 105–130. Newbury Park, Calif.: Sage Publications.

Blackwell-Stratton, Marian, Mary Lou Breslin, Arlene Brynne Mayerson, and Susan Bailey. 1988. Smashing icons: Disabled women and the disability and women's movements. In *Women with disabilities: Essays in psychology, culture and politics*, edited by Michelle Fine and Adrienne Asch. Philadelphia: Temple University Press.

Burkhauser, Richard, Mary Daly, and Andrew Heutenville. 2001. How working-age people with disabilities fared over the 1990s business cycle. In *Ensuring health and income security for an aging workforce*, edited by P. Burdetti, R. V. Burkhauser, J. Gregory, and A. Hunt, 291–346. Kalamazoo, Mich.: W. E. Upjohn Institute for Employment Research.

Clark, Cal, and Janet Clark. 1986. Models of gender and political participation in the United States. *Women and Politics* 6: 5–25.

Conway, M. Margaret. 2000. *Political participation in the United States*. Washington, D.C.: CQ Press.

Deegan, Mary Jo. 1985. Multiple minority groups: A case study of physically disabled women. In *Women and disability: The double handicap*, edited by Mary Jo Deegan and Nancy Brooks. New Brunswick, N.J.: Transaction Books.

Deegan, Mary Jo, and Nancy A. Brooks, eds. 1985. *Women and disability: The double handicap*. New Brunswick, N.J.: Transaction Books.

Fine, Michelle, and Adrienne Asch. 1985. Disabled women: Sexism without the pedestal. In *Women and disability: The double handicap*, edited by Mary Jo Deegan and Nancy Brooks. New Brunswick, N.J.: Transaction Books.

———, eds. 1988. *Women with disabilities: Essays in psychology, culture, and politics*. Philadelphia: Temple University Press.

Hanna, William John, and Betsy Rogovsky. 1993. Women with disabilities: Two handicaps plus. In *Perspectives on disability*, edited by Mark Nagler. Palo Alto, Calif.: Health Markets Research.

Hillyer, Barbara. 1993. *Feminism and disability*. Norman, Okla.: University of Oklahoma Press.

Hofstetter, C. Richard, and William A. Schultze. 1989. Some observations about participation and attitudes among single parent women. *Women and politics* 9: 83–105.

Kasnitz, Devia, and Tanis Dee. 1998. Leadership and peer support in the independent living disability rights movement. In *Insights and outlooks: Current trends in disability studies*, edited by Elaine Makas, Beth Haller, and Tanis Dee. Portland, Maine: Muskie Institute.

Kolb, Cynthia. 1985. Assertiveness training for women with visual impairments. In *Women and disability: The double handicap*, edited by Mary Jo Deegan and Nancy Brooks. New Brunswick, N.J.: Transaction Books.

McNeil, John. 2001. American with disabilities 1997. Current Population Reports, P70–73. Washington, D.C.: U.S. Bureau of the Census.

Morris, Jenny. 1993. Gender and Disability. In *Disabling barriers-enabling environments*, edited by John Swain, Vic Finkelstein, Sally French, and Mikel Oliver. London: Sage Publications.

Mudrick, Nancy. 1988. Disabled women and public policies for income support. In *Women with disabilities: Essays in psychology, culture and politics*, edited by Michelle Fine and Adrienne Asch. Philadelphia: Temple University Press.

Neath, Jeanne. 1997. Social causes of impairment, disability, and abuse: A feminist perspective. *Journal of Disability Policy Studies* 8 (1/2): 195–230

Peterson, Steven, and Albert Somit. 1992. Older women: Health and political behavior. *Women and Politics* 12 (4): 87–108.

Saxton, Marsha. 1985. A peer counseling training program for disabled women: A tool for individual and social change. In *Women and disability: The double handicap*, edited by Mary Jo Deegan and Nancy Brooks. New Brunswick, N.J.: Transaction Books.

Schlozman, Kay L., Nancy Burns, and Sidney Verba. 1999. "What happened at work today?": A multistage model of gender, employment, and political participation. *Journal of Politics* 61: 29–53.

Schur, Lisa. 1998. Disability and the psychology of political participation. *Journal of Disability Policy Studies*. 9 (2): 3–31.

———. 2003. Contending with the "Double handicap": Political activism among women with disabilities. *Women and Politics*.

Schur, Lisa, and Douglas Kruse. 2000. What determines voter turnout? Lessons from citizens with disabilities. *Social Science Quarterly*, 81:571–587.

Schur, Lisa, Todd Shields, and Kay Schriner. 2001. Growing older alone? Social capital, age, participation, and disability. Presented at the American Political Science Association Meetings, San Francisco, Calif.

Schur, Lisa, Todd Shields, Douglas Kruse, and Kay Schriner. 2002. Enabling democracy: Disability and voter turnout. *Political Research Quarterly* 55 (1): 167–190.

Shields, Todd, Kay Schriner, and Ken Schriner. 1998. The disability voice in American politics: Political participation of people with disabilities in the 1994 election. *Journal of Disability Policy Studies* 9: 33–52.

Stoddard, Susan, Lita Jans, Joan M. Ripple, and Lewis Kraus. 1998. Chartbook on work and disability in the United States. Berkeley, Calif.: Info Use.

Verba, Sidney, Kay Lehman Schlozman, and Henry E. Brady. 1995. *Voice and equality: Civic voluntarism in American politics*. Cambridge, Mass.: Harvard University Press.

Integrating Consumer Disabilities into Models of Information Processing

Color-vision Deficiencies and Their Effects on Women's Marketplace Choices

Carol Kaufman-Scarborough

Today's modern woman has a multitude of roles and responsibilities: caregiver, wife, mother, employee, friend, and volunteer, among others. Twenty-six million of these American women are living with disabilities, varying conditions that make these roles even more challenging because of physical or mental limitations. Various diseases and conditions produce some form of disability, and a number of them disproportionately affect women (National Women's Health Information Center).

I believe I am a fairly classic red-green color-deficient person. However, as a woman, I also believe I have a somewhat different set of challenges than similarly affected men. I tend to have the most difficulty with red, green, or any colors containing them: purple, pinks, olive drabs running to tans, and so forth. (Female 47)

Introduction

An assumption in everyday life is that consumers come to the marketplace daily to evaluate products, make purchases, and attempt to meet their needs for a satisfactory life. Consumers who are female and consumers who are disabled, however, are likely to face a "double discrimination" that is both related to their gender and to the nature of their disabilities (Fine and Asch 1985; Asch 2001; Rousso 2001). This is particularly evident when we consider that consumer roles, values, beliefs, and norms are often linked with gender-based expectations.

Quite simply, men and women within any society are typically assigned specific roles such as breadwinners, nurturers, and caretakers that embody certain skills often assumed to be innately related to gender. For instance, in traditional models of households, females are typically expected to care for home-related concerns ranging from furnishings and décor to daily shopping and childcare. In addition, by virtue of their supposed female interests in beauty and self-image, women are expected to incorporate socially established norms of acceptable body image, fashion, and beauty.

Feminists have challenged the realism and worth of such demands, considering the burdens and psychological pressures placed on women, yet society's icons continue to influence women's perceptions of themselves. Furthermore, socially constructed gender is thought to have a major impact in the marketplace, particularly when one's gender roles are also linked with one's disabilities. In some cases, disabilities can make the enactment of such roles difficult, dissatisfying, and perhaps impossible.

The current chapter uses consumer theories in marketing to enrich our understanding of the experience of disabled women's choices in the marketplace. Because business disciplines have lagged in suggesting frameworks for analysis in disabilities studies, this chapter attempts to bridge the gap. A model is proposed linking the interaction of gender, marketplace roles, and disabilities, using the responses of women with color-vision deficiencies to inform the discussion.

Background

The Census Bureau indicates that more than 54 million Americans are limited in one or more major life activities, including physiological and psychological disorders, amassing approximately one-fifth of the U.S. population. Despite progress through legislation such as the Americans with Disabilities Act (ADA), many disabled persons continue to encounter obstacles and barriers to their consumer experiences (Stephens and Bergman 1995). Persons with disabilities are often viewed as "unexpected participants" in society (Asch 2001) and in many cases, they appear to be unexpected in the marketplace. Quite often, the needs of disabled persons are addressed solely through legally mandated architectural accommodations that often do not recognize subtle psychological and interpersonal needs, especially in the retail setting (Kaufman-Scarborough 1999). As consumers, persons with disabilities are often discounted as retail stores and shopping centers, products, and advertising messages are developed with the able-bodied consumer in mind. In addition, the needs of perceptually disabled persons have lagged behind (Macias and Rucker 1979; Inana 1980), while architectural issues have been at the forefront of ADA guidelines. This is particularly the case when basic consumer information processing assumptions are considered.

Consumer Information Processing

Fundamentally, consumer researchers examine a sequence of information processing steps that are thought to be linked with the successful transmission of marketplace information: exposure, perception, comprehension, agreement, retention, retrieval, decision making, and action (McGuire 1976). These steps provide an information base built through a consumer's lifetime, enabling them to construct, retrieve, or adapt choice heuristics in response to their needs (Payne, Bettman, and Johnson 1988; Bettman, Luce, and Payne 1998). Through experience, consumers become socialized in learning how to identify and use marketplace information, such as coupons, product comparisons, and instructions. Nevertheless, the ways that information is presented can affect the ways that consumers process it and they may restructure information to gain improved insights, transforming their information into a more usable format (Bettman 1970; Bettman and Kakkar 1977; Coupey 1994).

Perceptually disabled persons are generally limited in their abilities to perceive and interpret parts of stimuli in their environments (Reedy 1993). Thus, many cues commonly used in the marketplace, such as printed texts, colors, sounds, scents, and lighting, might only be partially perceptible, distorted, or totally imperceptible. Information relying on such cues may become inaccessible, potentially limiting the perceptually disabled consumer's effective participation in the marketplace (see the following for discussions of these stimuli: Milliman 1986; Adkins and Ozanne 1997; Mitchell, Kahn, and Knasko 1995).

As a result, perceptually disabled persons are not likely to be able to participate in each information processing step as marketplace designers might anticipate. For instance, hearing-impaired consumers cannot be exposed to messages that solely rely on auditory cues, while persons with color-deficient vision may not be able to perceive informational cues presented in colors that they cannot distinguish (Kaufman-Scarborough 2001a). Persons with attention deficit disorder are known to confuse background information with central information, leading to poor purchases and product misuse. Basically, consumer roles can require information processing abilities that are outside the capacity of some perceptually disabled consumers. Such problems are particularly evident when gender roles are considered in the marketplace.

Socially Constructed Gender Roles in the Marketplace

When women are specifically considered in their consumer roles, some very specific types of specialization are likely to be examined, such as caregivers, mothers, nurses, teachers, wardrobe maintainers, and decorators, quite often in a supportive or secondary marital role (Oakley 1974). Decades of home economics research has tracked the output of household production with its parallel to the small factory, producing clean clothing, well-fed families, and attractive homes (see Juster and Stafford 1985; Pleck 1985 for reviews). Family sociologists have also traced changes in family role structures and allocation of tasks (see Roberts and Wortzel 1984 for a comprehensive multidisciplinary review of household theories). The set of expected female roles has been well-articulated as women's work. However, some changes have been noted as women have increased their workforce participation.

For instance, Diekman and Eagly aptly state that "differential role occupancy in the family and occupations fosters gender stereotypes by which each sex is expected to have characteristics that equip it to function adequately in its typical roles" (2000, 1172) leading to gender role changes over time. Women's roles have changed considerably as women have entered male-dominated occupations, and research has documented a perceived increase in women's masculine personality characteristics and with a lesser perceived increase in men's feminine personality characteristics (2000). However, given that women also retain female-dominated roles, many traditionally stereotypically female expectations remain: women have been expected to make things attractive, make themselves beautiful, and create a happy home life for their families.

Despite more current shifts in gender roles to egalitarian household management, societal gender myths still are known to affect the pressures that females face in developing their self-image, enacting their household role allocation, and juggling the multiple pressures of everyday life. Thus, things are supposed to match in the home, while certain women's products are supposed to create beauty and self-image as valued by society.

Disabilities and Women

Women who have disabilities are likely to experience discrimination due to the interactive effects of sexism and ableism (Prilleltensky 1996). This "double handicap" has been documented and discussed in the literature, painting a picture of helpless, dependent, asexual persons who may not be capable of carrying out adult roles in society (Deegan and Brooks 1985; Asch and Fine 1988). In developing a theory of disability and gender, Gerschick argues that three sets of social dynamics must be considered: "the stigma assigned to disability, gender as an interactional process, and the importance of the body to enacting gender" (2000, 1264).

Applying Goffman's (1963) analyses, societies enact and establish sets of attributes that define members of that society into categories such as "normal," "ordinary," "beautiful," and "sexual." Persons in a given society attempt to meet or to exceed such standards in becoming full, participatory members in the societal institutions that they choose. In contrast, persons who are different or deficient in some of these aspects may be stigmatized as inferior or unacceptable, depending upon the criteria and how they are applied. Not surprisingly, persons with disabilities are often included in descriptions of stigmatized groups, may experience stereotypical devaluation, and may be challenged to minimize their differentness and maximize their fit into society's norms (see Taub, Blinde, and Greer 1999; Taylor 2000 for reviews). Women with disabilities instead may enact methods of stigma management that can enable them to minimize the impacts of their disabilities in specific societal roles. For instance, feminist therapy literature has encouraged women with disabilities to accept their bodies while in turn minimizing the impacts of societally defined idealized body images.

Society can also define how a person learns expectations, norms, and roles associated with their gender. Theorists find persons with disabilities may experience gender socialization differently, because parents and others in developmental roles may selectively teach and inform them. Their identities as sexually attractive persons may be undermined, causing them to be less likely to marry but more likely to divorce (Gershick 2000).

Some studies have suggested that on the average, women with disabilities are found to be less educated, have lower earnings, and be less likely to have a partner (Prilleltensky 1996). If these conclusions are accurate, women with disabilities would also be expected to participate less fully in the marketplace as active, satisfied consumers. Unfortunately, consumer inequities are likely to be more subtle and less likely to be studied and documented formally, because the consumer roles of disabled persons have not been examined critically nor empirically investigated.

Disabled Women and Consumer Roles

Only a small number of studies in marketing specifically consider the disabled consumer as their primary focus of study (Reedy 1993; Stephens and Bergman 1995; Burnett and Paul 1996; Gould 1997; Kaufman-Scarborough 2000, 2001a; 2001b; Baker and Kaufman-Scarborough 2001; Baker, Stephens, and Hill 2001, 2002). Virtually none of them focus on gender and disability concurrently. The present chapter attempts to address this gap.

Problem Statement

I have specifically chosen to examine women who have perceptual disabilities. In particular, I have chosen color-vision deficiencies since the nature of the disability suggests that women may experience difficulties in the enactment of their expected gender roles as consumers. While physically able to negotiate shopping environments without the restrictions of persons with mobility impairments, color-deficient females are expected to report problems with access to consumer information related to their consumer roles as women. It is hoped that studies of perceptually disabled women can enrich our understanding of the double jeopardy that occurs in the marketplace.

Color-vision deficiency is a disability that is frequently overlooked in research because it is an invisible disability that can both be congenital or acquired. About 19 million persons in the United States are color-blind or color deficient (Rosenthal and Phillips 1997). Approximately 10 percent of white males in the United States have some aspect of color deficiency, with much less prevalence among females. However, the statistics can be deceiving, since color-vision deficiencies can be acquired, can be temporary, and can vary with conditions in the environment. For instance, color-vision deficiencies can be caused by diseases such as diabetes and macular degeneration, head or eye injury, side effects of medications such as contraceptives and antidepressants, plus the natural process of aging. Though the inability to distinguish between reds and greens is the most common form, color deficiencies of other types can cause people to confuse blues and yellows, confuse yellows and greens, see all objects as yellow, see all objects as blue, or see objects tinged with red. Thus, it is not a uniformly described disability inherited solely by men. Its implications for correct information transmission are significant.

Figure 1 diagrammatically organizes and suggests a framework representing the gender role experiences of color-deficient females in the marketplace. Following the concepts introduced in the discussion above, the figure is made up of four key components: the attributes of the marketplace, the attributes of color-deficient women, the psychological negotiation of consumer identity, and the resultant experience of the color-deficient women in the marketplace. This organizing framework is an adaptation of Kaufman-Scarborough's (2001b) model of the factors affecting mobility disabled consumers in shopping environments.

Methodology

The responses are drawn from the author's larger study of color-deficient consumers that has been ongoing since 1997 (for a full study description, please refer to Kaufman-Scarborough 2000). Responses have been gathered through several methods: unstructured interviews, semistructured interviews, written surveys and free response comments, web page postings and email communications from informants, personal communications from eye care professionals, and personal communications from color designers.

At the time of the current analysis, the total number of respondents is seventy color-deficient individuals plus eighteen other informants, including eye doctors, educators, color design professionals, and professors of vision studies. The current sample is composed of sixteen females and forty-five males with diagnosed color-vision deficiencies. The color-deficient men and women who responded to the survey request did so in several ways: some by filling in the survey independently, others by emailing comments that summarized their reactions. Still others preferred to speak by telephone. Questions throughout the survey requested the respondent to report on problems related to color in using the products that are bought, in advertising, and while shopping.

Results

The responses of men and women were read and re-read in the effort to extract a consistent set of themes emerging from the data (Strauss and Corbin 1998). Specific attention was paid to identify similarities and differences among men's and women's responses.

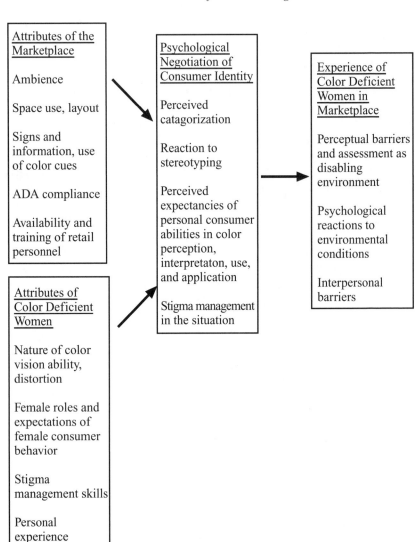

FIGURE 1. Factors Affecting the Experience of Color Deficient Women in the Market-place. *Adapted from Kaufman-Scarborough (2001).*

Gender Differences in Thematic Responses

The sixteen women indicated numerous similarities in problem areas to those reported by men, such as confusion with labels and the impact of poor lighting. However, an important distinction was found in that significant frustrations were faced uniquely by color-deficient women related to the care of their families. The themes found in the women's responses were centered around their homes, their children, their personal self-image, and their hobbies. Examples include the following: children, safety, measurement, makeup, decorating, food labeling, selection of detergents, sewing and needlework, color coordination of towels, sheets, clothing and accessories, matching thread and fabric, and crafting supplies. In contrast, the men's themes centered on problems with the selection of their own personal clothing, most often gaining assistance from their wives. They also mentioned traffic signals and travel information, painting and home repair, and electronics.

Attributes of the Marketplace

Marketplaces ideally provide clear access to product information so that consumers can make the choices that are in their best interests or meet their specific decision criteria. Such environments in turn are ideally supported by well-trained salespersons and informative displays. Color-deficient respondents of both genders, however, reported great difficulty with color-related product choices and unhelpful personnel. Some themes were common across genders, such as wanting a standard color system, with numbered colors or color names that are decipherable. Safety-related perceptual problems included difficulties with reading instructions or warnings printed in red, as well as interpreting product information in which background and textual information are printed in similar colors with low contrast.

The respondents were asked to provide details on types of marketplace characteristics where color vision presented a problem. The female, as well as the male respondents, argued that lighting in stores made a considerable difference in their abilities to perceive, interpret, and process product-information, whether textual or color coded. The women's product-related responses, however, were centered on food labeling and freshness, children's and personal clothing, children's education, makeup, beauty, medicines, detergents, crafts, sewing, and home décor, in contrast to the men's responses that emphasized their own clothing, electronics, paint and home improvement, web pages, and travel and automotive indicator lights. The women's responses reflected the problem of being forced to make a consumer choice in an environment that made it difficult or impossible to access needed information. Some examples include: fresh fruits and vegetables in grocery stores, cosmetics with creative but uninformative names, and instructions and consumer choices indicated solely by color. This perspective is illustrated by the following quotations, with each respondent's age given in parentheses.

> Color-coded instructions are the worst! Being color blind I memorize the product's package. If they change the package in any way or the color I can't find it again . . . clothing and makeup and accessories should have color name tags. . . . I have had sales people laugh at me and walk away. There should be more awareness of this disability. . . . Garanimals was a great children clothing line . . . they had color matching tags . . . saved my child a lot of embarrassment. (Female, 39)

I can't shop for clothes by myself. I often put the wrong product in my carriage because I can't see the difference in the color coding, such as with caffeinated and decaffeinated products; fat-free, low-fat, and regular products; salted and salt-free products, etc. (Female, 53)

Attributes of Color Deficient Women

The female informants had several different types of congenital color-vision deficiencies, including the most common red-green confusions, problems with "cool colors," red-yellow confusion, and rare yellow-green color blindness, plus one 42 year-old female in the sample who acquired color-vision deficiencies due to macular degeneration. In addition, one respondent with achromatopsia was able to perceive only black, gray, and white, describing it in the following way:

My vision difficulty is formally called achromatopsia. To me, this means that any bright light causes me to squint a lot and I wear reddish brown glasses to keep out the glare . . . I have a real problem with fresh produce. Sometimes a bad spot blends in with the rest of the fruit's skin or I sometimes can't tell if bananas are yellow or green. . . . If I weren't wearing my glasses when I'm reading the instructions, then I probably would not be able to pick up the red letters of a warning. . . . (Female, 17)

Such problems appeared to represent frustration and feelings of failure and embarrassment in areas where females are supposed to have special skills, such as selecting fresh foods, decorating homes, teaching their children, and dispensing medications safely. One informant spoke passionately in a telephone interview of her fears of giving her children the incorrect medications due to her color confusions and her children's young ages. Other responses confirm the difficulties and self-discouragement that characterizes daily life:

I can't match my colors, so I can't match clothes, furniture, paint, accessories. It is hard for me on a daily basis to shop and try to get things that look nice. An example is when we were buying a new home, I picked out the prettiest brown carpet (at least that is what I thought). My husband said it was the ugliest green carpet he had ever seen. Without him I would have been stuck with an ugly green carpet. (Female, 38)

I realize that the type of colorblindness I have (yellow-green) is fairly rare, and *very rare* for a female. However, I have a tendency to try to shop where products are labeled. Wal-Mart, for example, does a pretty good job of this, so I will drive an extra twenty miles to shop there instead of a place where I have to ask people all the time. (Female #2, 42; her emphasis)

Psychological Negotiation of Consumer Identity

People learn to be consumers through socialization to the customs and practices of the marketplace. They typically develop strategies that allow them to maximize their benefits and use their resources well. Color-deficient females are no exception. Their negotiation of a consumer identity is, however, much more complex than for other women since it can be related to their self-identities as females. Basically, women are expected to create, to decorate, to match, and to shop, and when they cannot, they are often perceived as disruptive and dishonest:

> Salespersons often don't understand the dilemma and further, they think that I am not being truthful. Being a color blind woman leads to a world of misunderstanding . . . some salespersons direct me to the blue sign or the green shelves or who say to follow the brown arrow. Some colors I don't see at all and so rather than give an impromptu color blind lesson I just go home—very frustrated." (Female, 50)

In another instance, the cosmetics are labeled with colors, but terms are not meaningful to a color blind shopper.

> I frequently have to postpone buying certain items until I can shop with someone I trust—like for cosmetics. Probably the worst, as a woman, is cosmetics. It is impossible for me to buy anything, even when the colors are on the products, because the names of the colors are stupid—"Grey Mist," "Pearl Blue." Huh? I don't want to end up looking like the bride of Frankenstein's monster. (Female, 47)

The Experience of Color-Deficient Women in the Marketplace

The women in the sample had a strong sense of disenfranchisement from many aspects of the marketplace that specifically made use of color as a point of information. They can identify the products, symbols, and environments that distort consumer information in unsafe ways and have developed coping strategies to ensure their safety. They are frustrated, however, and counter to some predominant perceptual theories in consumer research, they report that color is not a reliable cue in providing product information. Color instead was likely to distort information, hide information, or even give cues that were completely incorrect. The women indicated that the marketplace was not designed to communicate to them and they felt uncomfortable and vulnerable, as indicated in the problems that they described:

> Problems when shopping: green beans on cans look blue, spinach looks blue, green on black looks grey, blue-green liquid crystal displays are impossible. I can't read posters with blue or green lettering if background is not bright white. Poison sign is often green face with black lettering; impossible! Should be yellow. (Female #1, 42)

[Problems related to color in products] usually relate to clothing, but I have had problems at work telling the difference between general cleaners (blue?) and glass cleaners (green) if they are not clearly marked . . . trying to find a product someone has described to me (blue "Dawn" dish detergent vs. green). (Female #2, 42)

I must read more . . . to get the information that others get from seeing that a product comes in two colors to distinguish fat free or salt free, etc. . . . I don't rely on color to give me any information . . . if there are warnings which the company relies on color to convey the message, they should not employ this method. Write warnings in larger print than other writing on the label. (Female, 50)

Recommendations

Bridging the Gap between Business Disciplines and Disabilities Studies

The present chapter has proposed a model for examining the experiences of disabled women in their roles as consumers, using color-deficient females as a case example. We have heard the experiences of several women who have given voice to this issue that has long been overlooked by persons in business fields such as marketing.

Implications for Research

Though researchers in management have established solid programs examining human resources issues in disabilities studies, only a scant number of researchers in marketing have done so to date. Many studies in marketing examine the "average" consumer in sampling and theory testing with little to no recognition of the variations in human capabilities. For instance, studies that test reactions to color advertisements versus those in black and white typically recruit participants with no verification of their color-vision capacity. Studies testing reactions to retail layouts and displays typically recruit able-bodied subjects, perpetuating the myth of an ableist society.

The purposeful incorporation of persons with multiple abilities and limitations in our research, however, stands only to enrich our knowledge in the consumer behavior, retailing, and advertising areas. Such an approach can potentially expand and broaden our theories to capture the variations in abilities present in any population, rather than confine our theories to the limited "samples of the average."

Implications for Education

Numerous studies outside of the business disciplines have chronicled the impact of business strategies on persons with disabilities. For centuries, persons with disabilities were assumed not to take part in the marketplace activities of everyday life, and as a result, they were confronted with an ableist environment of shops, products, and consumer messages designed primarily for able-bodied persons.

My premise is that research in consumer and retail marketing must actively integrate disabilities studies into their curriculum in order to affect meaningful change in the created environment. Otherwise, we greatly risk that students will simply be taught to design products for the needs of the average consumer, to create store layouts that assume able-bodiedness and full abilities in all sensory capacities, and to develop promotional messages that can be retrieved by those who have no limitations in their sensory capacities.

Educational curricula must instead inform students when they learn to design such environments. The expectations must be built that persons with disabilities can and will want to participate fully in the marketplace. Thus, we expect them as participants. In contrast, curricula in marketing tend to approach persons with disabilities from a medical model approach, as persons whose inherent limitations may place them outside of the mainstream of consumer life.

In contrast to the medical model that locates disability within the body or mind of the individual, the social model contends that nondisabled persons have created a disabling society as a physical and perceptual environment that effectively isolates and disenfranchises persons with disabilities from the mainstream of life. As a result, responsibility is placed on society to identify barriers and structural inequalities, reconfiguring the environment so that persons with disabilities are expected and welcomed participants. Legislation such as the Americans with Disabilities Act was enacted to address such issues through enforced mandates for accommodations in employment, public services, public accommodations, and telecommunications. While this act has led to great progress, its provisions will still be necessary until both structural and attitudinal barriers are eliminated (Baker and Kaufman-Scarborough 2001).

Note

Author Note: The responses of sixteen color-deficient women are reported in this study. Respondents are distinguished by a gender, age format.

Works Cited

Asch, Adrienne. 2001. Critical race theory, feminism, and disability: Reflections on social justice and personal identity. Plenary session address, Gender and Disability Studies Conference, Institute for Research on Women, Rutgers University, New Brunswick, N.J.

Asch, Adrienne, and M. Fine. 1988. *Women with disabilities: Essays in psychology, culture and politics*. Philadelphia: Temple University Press.

Adkins, Natalie R., and Julie L. Ozanne. 1997. Johnny's mom can't read: The stigma of low literacy in the marketplace. *Proceedings of the 1997 Marketing and Public Policy Conference*, vol. 7, edited by Easwar Iyer and George R. Milne. Chicago: American Marketing Association.

Baker, Stacey Menzel, and Carol Kaufman-Scarborough. 2001. Marketing and public accommodation: A retrospective on Title III of the Americans with Disabilities Act. *Journal of Public Policy and Marketing, Policy Watch Section* 20 (2) (fall): 297–304.

Baker, Stacey Menzel, Debra Lynn Stephens, and Ronald Paul Hill. 2001. Marketplace experiences of individuals with visual impairments: Beyond the Americans with Disabilities Act. *Journal of Public Policy and Marketing* 20 (fall): 215–224.

———. 2002. How can retailers enhance accessibility? Giving consumers with visual impairments a voice in the marketplace. *Journal of Retailing and Consumer Services* 9 (4): 227–239.

Bettman, James R. 1970. Information processing models of consumer behavior. *Journal of Marketing Research* 7: 370–378.

Bettman, James R., and Pradeep Kakkar. 1977. Effects of information presentation format on consumer information acquisition strategies. *Journal of Consumer Research* 3: 233–240.

Bettman, James R., Mary Frances Luce, and John W. Payne. 1998. Constructive consumer choice processes. *Journal of Consumer Research* 25: 187–217.

Burnett, John J., and Pallab Paul. 1996. Assessing the media habits and needs of the mobility-disabled consumer. *Journal of Advertising* 25 (3): 47–59.

Coupey, Eloise. 1994. Restructuring: Constructive processing of information displays in consumer choice. *Journal of Consumer Research* 21: 83–99.

Deegan, M. J., and N. A. Brooks. 1985. *Women and disability: The double handicap.* New Brunswick, N.J.: Transaction Books.

Diekman, Amanda B., and Alice H. Eagly. 2000. Stereotypes as dynamic constructs: Women and men of the past, present, and future. *Personality and Social Psychology Bulletin* 26: 1171–1188.

Fine, Michelle, and Adrienne Asch. 1985. Disabled women: Sexism without the pedestal. In *Women and disability: The double handicap*, edited by Mary Jo Deegan and Nancy Brooks. New Brunswick, N.J.: Transaction Books.

Gerschick, Thomas J. 2000. Toward a theory of disability and gender. *Signs: Journal of Women in Culture and Society* 25: 1263–1268.

Goffman, E. 1963. *Stigma: Notes on the management of spoiled identity.* New York: Simon and Schuster, Inc.

Gould, Steven. 1997. Leveling the playing field for visually impaired consumers: A public policy and research agenda. In *1997 AMA Winter Educators' Conference: Marketing Theory and Applications*, vol. 8, edited by Debbie Thorne LeClair and Michael Hartline. Chicago: American Marketing Association.

Inana, Marjorie. 1980. Grocery shopping: Principles and techniques for the blind consumer. *Journal of Visual Impairment and Blindness* 74: 329–332.

Juster, F. Thomas, and Frank P. Stafford, eds. 1985. *Time, goods and well-being.* Ann Arbor: Institute for Social Research, University of Michigan.

Kaufman-Scarborough, Carol. 1999. Reasonable access for mobility-disabled persons is more than widening the door. *Journal of Retailing* 75: 479–508.

———. 2000. Seeing through the eyes of the color-deficient shopper: Consumer issues for public policy. *Journal of Consumer Policy* 23: 461–492.

———. 2001a. Accessible advertising for visually disabled persons: The case of color deficient consumers. *Journal of Consumer Marketing* 18: 303–316.

———. 2001b. Sharing the experience of disabled consumers: Building understanding through ethnography. *Journal of Contemporary Ethnography* (special issue focusing on marketing, consumer behavior, and ethnography, edited by Eric J. Arnould) 30: 430–464.

Macias, Polly, and Margaret Rucker. 1979. Clothing selection and the visually impaired consumer. *Journal of Visual Impairment and Blindness* 73: 400–404.

McGuire, William J. 1976. Some internal psychological factors influencing consumer choice. *Journal of Consumer Research* 2: 302–319.

Milliman, Ronald E. 1986. The influence of background music on the behavior of restaurant patrons. *Journal of Consumer Research* 13: 286–289.

Mitchell, Deborah J., Barbara E. Kahn, and Susan Knasko. 1995. There's something in the air: Effects of congruent or incongruent ambient odor on consumer decision making. *Journal of Consumer Research* 22: 229–238.

National Women's Health Information Center (NWHIC). [Cited June 22, 2002]. "Women with DisAbilities." Available at http://www.4woman.gov/wwd/.

Oakley, Ann. 1974. *The sociology of housework*. New York: Pantheon Books.

Payne, John W., James R. Bettman, and Eric J. Johnson. 1988. Adaptive strategy selection in decision making. *Journal of Experimental Psychology: Learning, Memory, and Cognition* 14: 534–552.

Pleck, Joseph H. 1985. *Working wives/working husbands*. Beverly Hills, Calif.: Sage Publications.

Prilleltensky, Ora. 1996. Women with disabilities and feminist therapy. *Women and Therapy* 18: 87–97.

Reedy, Joel. 1993. *Marketing to consumers with disabilities: How to identify and meet the growing market needs of 43 million Americans*. Chicago: Probus Publishing Co.

Roberts, Mary Lou, and Lawrence H. Wortzel. 1984. *Marketing to the changing household*. Cambridge, Mass.: Ballinger Publishing Company.

Rosenthal, O., and R. H. Phillips. 1997. *Coping with color-blindness*. Garden City Park, New York: Avery Publishing Group.

Rousso, Harilyn. 2001. Girls and young women with disabilities: What do we know? What do we need to know? Gender and Disability Studies Conference, Institute for Research on Women, Rutgers University, New Brunswick, N.J.

Stephens, Debra Lynn, and Karyn Bergman. 1995. The Americans with Disabilities Act: A mandate for marketers. *Journal of Public Policy and Marketing* 14: 164–168.

Strauss, A., and J. Corbin. 1998. *Basics of qualitative research: Techniques and procedures for developing grounded theory*. Thousand Oaks, Calif.: Sage Inc.

Taub, D. E., E. M. Blinde, and K. R. Greer. 1999. Stigma management through participation in sport and physical activity: Experiences of male college students with physical disabilities. *Human Relations* 52: 1469–1484.

Taylor, S. J. 2000. You're not a retard, you're just wise. *Journal of Contemporary Ethnography* 29: 58–92.

Women and Emerging Disabilities

✑

MELISSA J. MCNEIL AND THILO KROLL

Since the mid–1990s, researchers have noticed and begun to study how social, economic, and the physical environment affect the causes or etiology of disability in the United States. Seelman and Sweeney in 1995 described the impact of these factors as the "new universe of disability." This new universe of disabilities are called "emerging disabilities." In this chapter, we address how sociodemographics, economic impact, and the physical environment are changing the causes of disability.

The "new universe of disability" is based on the observation that "new" causal factors for disability are emerging. Today, we see disabilities that may have different causes or etiologies with the same physical consequences. The "new" causes can be explained using the social, economic, and the physical environment and their interplay with health. These social, economic, and physical conditions that impact disability have been studied but not linked or stated as the *cause* of the disabling conditions. For example, studies that examine uninsurance and underinsurance of women with diabetes have been conducted. However, the role of uninsurance or underinsurance and how it contributed or *caused* an increase in functional limitation is not well documented. The proponents of the emerging disabilities believe that having this kind of information can lend itself to preventable health problems and/or a decrease in disability instead of an increase. Thus, diabetes-related blindness might have a multiple medical implication that needs to be studied for treatment; however, *"lack of eye exams due to underinsurance" blindness* is quite preventable.

Let's review some trends in the emerging disabilities study to further understand how the social, economic, and physical environment contributes to the causes of conditions.

HIV/AIDS survivorship has been made possible through the advent of new potent antiretroviral drugs. Only a decade ago, most individuals in the United States who contracted HIV/AIDS were white homosexual males from middle-class backgrounds or were victims of contaminated blood transfusions. Today's survivors are more likely to be poor and more likely to be from ethnic/racial minority backgrounds—with the major increase in incidence among women and children.

With the availability of improved acute care treatment options for HIV/ AIDS, the focus is shifting from a death sentence to the long-term management of the condition and its often disabling sequelae. In addition, the current focus is not treating HIV/AIDS as a single condition but rather as a complex set of conditions that require a network of clinical management and rehabilitation services beyond the physical health aspects. Frequently, for example, drug addiction needs to be addressed at the same time as the disease itself. For women, other needs occur along with the HIV/AIDS diagnosis, such as unplanned pregnancies, concurrent health conditions such as hypertension and diabetes (Seal et al. 1995), and caregiver responsibilities (Donelan, Falik, and DesRoches 2001). These specific concerns of women must often be addressed in conjunction with managing the sequelae of neurological impairments, cancers, organ failure, pain and fatigue, and diabetes (Seal et al. 1995).

Another example is that health care professionals have recently come to recognize that violently acquired traumatic brain and spinal cord injuries represent a distinct clinical population with unique psychological and social rehabilitative needs. Most of the survivors of these conditions are males under thirty years of age who come from low income and minority backgrounds. While survival of traumatic injuries is mainly the result of improving trauma care, these survivors' continued rehabilitative needs include a complex network of services that extends beyond treatment of their physical impairments.

In other words, violence can be seen as part of the *etiology* of the injury. Spinal cord injury care providers began in the late 1980s and early 1990s to recognize this distinct population as *violently acquired spinal cord injury* or VASCI. Since the inclusion of this in the etiology, rehabilitative units such as The National Rehabilitation Hospital and Rehabilitation Institute in Chicago are addressing the social and environmental factors affecting this population during the restorative treatment process.

As in the examples above, emerging disabilities are known to be associated with race and income inequality. However, not enough attention is being paid to the gender differences associated with these conditions. Various chronic conditions and disabilities affect men and women in different ways. The occurrence of certain chronic conditions such as asthma, diabetes, carpal tunnel syndrome, violently acquired spinal cord injuries and traumatic brain injuries, and HIV/AIDS, appears to be significantly related to gender. These conditions highlight the complex interplay of the social, economic, and physical environment that affects their epidemiology and etiology.

From our study, carpal tunnel and diabetes increasingly affect women at a greater rate than men, while other conditions, such as violently acquired spinal cord and traumatic brain injuries have higher incidence in men. Though the reasons for these incidence patterns are only partially understood, current research provides evidence of some gender-based reasons. Women's position in society puts them at a particular risk for developing disabilities associated with some of these conditions. For example, women are more likely to be un- or underinsured, be the main or single caregiver for children, have low incomes, and have less access to routine and specialty health care services. Women are more likely not to receive services, often because they place the needs of others over their own well being and do not seek services until the problem becomes a crisis. Then, once they develop a serious condition, they are likely to depend on health care services for a much longer time (Office of Women's Health 2001).

By looking more closely into this research, we find that conditions affect men and women differently. For example, though males currently have higher rates of traumatic brain injury (TBI) and spinal cord injury (SCI), reports show that women are more likely to die than men after sustaining the same kind of injury (DeVivo, Krause, and Lammertse 1999; Farce and Alves 2000). Meat packers and individuals operating jack hammers and other vibrating tools have the highest occurrence of carpal tunnel syndrome. Men have traditionally held these jobs. The incidence of carpal tunnel, however, is highest among women (Bureau of Labor Statistics 2000). So, why does this gender differential exist?

Women are a vulnerable population. Though the population of women is highly differentiated in terms of race, income, and educational level, collectively they appear to have needs that must be addressed to decrease the factors that make them more susceptible to disease, injury, and disabling conditions. Issues that disproportionately affect women include higher rates of poverty, unemployment, underemployment, uninsurance or underinsurance, and caretaker responsibilities—which usually decrease their focus on their own health issues.

Other issues may also create barriers to care for women. For example, in the past, women were usually ignored or underrepresented in clinical trials. Thus, some of the medications that are being prescribed for problems that affect women and men may have been proven effective primarily for men. As a result, women may have more persistent and severe health problems in conjunction with chronic conditions. Women are also disproportionately affected by heart disease and are at a greater risk for having a second heart attack compared with men (Office of Women's Health 2001).

Women have the highest rates of disability for the emerging disabilities we examined. Women report higher rates of disability from diabetes, asthma, and carpal tunnel syndrome. Women are also increasingly affected by HIV/AIDS, with the most recent data showing that a rapidly growing number of women are being diagnosed with this disease. To further examine the intersection of gender, race/ethnicity, income, and other sociodemographic variables that contribute to this new universe of disability, we look at two chronic conditions and examine how gender, economic conditions, and the physical environment are associated with these conditions. Last, we look at the incidence of disability associated with these conditions for women.

Diabetes

There are two major types of diabetes—commonly called Type 1 and Type 2. Type 1 diabetes (about 5 to 10 percent of diagnosed cases of diabetes) usually first appears in childhood and is a result of an inability to produce sufficient amounts of insulin. Type 2 diabetes occurs most commonly in adults and is a result of the body's inability to use insulin effectively. Currently, 90 to 95 percent of all cases of diabetes are Type 2. Two other types are less common, including gestational diabetes, which occurs in about 2 to 5 percent of all pregnancies. "Other specific types" of diabetes can result from specific genetic syndromes, surgery, drugs, malnutrition, infections, and other illnesses (Rumrill et al. 1998; Cleveland Clinic 2000; National Institute of Diabetes & Digestive & Kidney Diseases 2001). Diabetes cost the United States $98 billion in 1997. The indirect cost totaled $54 billion as a result of disability payments, time lost from work, and premature death. Direct medical cost totaled $44 billion.

Trends
General Population.   Diabetes is reaching epidemic proportions with more than sixteen million Americans reporting that they have the disease (Centers for Disease Control and Prevention 2000). The World Health Organization (WHO) projects that the number of people with diabetes will double by 2010 (2000). Diabetes is the seventh leading cause of death in the USA (Centers for Disease Control 2001). Diabetes is the leading cause of lower extremity amputations, end-stage renal disease, and adventitious blindness. Diabetes can cause stroke, heart disease, and nervous system disease. Diabetes can make one more susceptible to pneumonia and influenza. Among women, diabetes can cause pregnancy complications and lead to birth defects (Centers for Disease Control and Prevention 2000).

Women.   For women, diabetes is the sixth leading cause of death. Women make up 8.1 million diabetes cases (National Diabetes Data Group 2001). The percentage of women with diabetes increased from 5.6 percent in 1990 to 7.4 percent in 1998, whereas the percentage of men with diabetes increased from 4.1 percent to 5.5 percent (Mokdad et al. 2000)

Disability Associated with Diabetes
Rates of disability are substantially higher among people with diabetes than among those without this disease. A person with diabetes is two to three times

more likely to report disability than their counterparts in the general population. As well, an estimated 20 to 50 percent of individuals with a disability report having diabetes.

Diabetes has been found to accompany other serious forms of disability. In 1983–1985, diabetes made up 2.7 percent of the reported cases of chronic conditions leading to activity limitation, making it the eleventh most commonly cited condition leading to activity limitation in the United States. These numbers appear to continue increasing. The number of persons with diabetes who were limited in activity increased from 3.1 million in 1983 to 4.1 million in 1994, with women having higher limitation rates than men (Centers for Disease Control and Prevention 1997).

Women with diabetes report having higher rates of disability than do men. In 1994, approximately 2.5 million people who have diabetes also reported activity limitations, with women frequently reporting this more than men. In 1996, the number of women with diabetes reporting activity limitations rose nearly to the overall 1994 total, with 2.2 million women reporting activity limitations due to diabetes. Although age and race appear to be more strongly linked to diabetes-related disability, women have higher rates than men in each subgroup, with older and African-American women having the highest rates of disability from diabetes (National Institute of Diabetes & Digestive & Kidney Diseases 2001).

Diabetes-related disabilities in women are associated with increased use of health care services, unemployment, work absenteeism and decreased quality of life (National Institute of Diabetes & Digestive & Kidney Diseases 2000). Current estimates show that approximately 640,000 people with diabetes do not have any form of health care insurance. The percentage of working age people with diabetes without health insurance is 15.6 percent (approximately 93,600). Substantial majorities of uninsured people with diabetes are women (approximately 66,000). Women with diabetes make up 19 percent of the working-age population that have Medicaid and other public programs as compared with 8.2 percent of working-age males with diabetes (National Diabetes Data Group 2001).

Carpal Tunnel Syndrome (CTS)

The carpal tunnel and median nerve is located in the forearm through the wrist. This nerve supplies feeling to the thumb, index, ring fingers, and the nine tendons that flex the fingers and provides function for the muscles at the base of the thumb. CTS occurs when the tissue around the median nerve becomes swollen, causing the nerve to be closed off and the transmission of nerve signals to slow. When this occurs, the individual experiences pain, numbness, tingling in the wrist, hand, and fingers. CTS can become a disabling condition when muscles at the base of the thumb atrophy and sensation is lost. Individuals may experience limitations in performing tasks—including those required for their occupation (Nidus Information Services, Inc. 1998).

Women are at greater risk for getting CTS than men are. Women make up 70 percent of all CTS cases. Current research offers hypotheses to explain the greater prevalence of CTS in women, but the reasons for this gender imbalance are basically unknown. One hypothesis states that women make up a majority of CTS cases due to the intensive hand-wrist motion requirements of housework and other traditionally female occupations. Another hypothesis is that the factors associated with high risk for CTS occur more frequently in women. Such factors are hormonal changes associated with pregnancy, menopause, diabetes, and hyperthyroidism (Nidus Information Services, Inc. 1998).

Trends

CTS and other repetitive motion syndromes make up nearly half of all reported work-related illnesses. CTS accounts for 4 percent of all cases of repetitive motion syndrome. This is expected to increase because of the increased hand-wrist motion used in the service industries and the rapid growth of the information technology sector. As well, women are increasingly moving from welfare to work. Often these programs are geared to move women into the small business industries. Currently, 67 percent of individuals who have moved from welfare to work have moved into small business environments. Although this sector is increasing with more than 53 percent of all jobs in the United States (Association for Enterprise Opportunity 2000), small businesses have shown little awareness of the proper ergonomic needs of their employees (Jeffress 2000). Smaller workplaces report more than 325,000 cases of CTS and other musculoskeletal disorders (MSDs) each year (National Institute for Occupational Safety and Health 1997). Without the proper use of ergonomics—the study of posture, stresses, motions, and other physical forces on the human body at work—to address the causes of CTS (1997), the small business sector will continue to contribute to the increase in the incidence of CTS.

CTS and Disability

CTS-related disability research is not common. One study reported that nearly half of all employees diagnosed with CTS had changed jobs or were absent thirty months after the diagnosis (Nidus Information Services, Inc. 1998). The number of individuals who change occupations due to CTS and the number of individuals having activity-limitation due to CTS is not available. CTS is, however, the work-related injury that accounted for the highest median number of medical days away from work (24 days). The number of days away from work due to CTS increased by 53.3 percent between 1992 and 1996. Women have a higher number of days away from work due to CTS, with a median of thirty days (Bureau of Labor Statistics 2000).

Conclusion

Emerging disabling conditions are widely known to be associated with race and income inequality. Not enough attention is being paid to the gender differences associated with these conditions. These gender differences have implications for advocacy, research, and health policy. Little is known about the intersection of gender, race/ethnicity, income, and disability. Future research is needed to clarify the multiple relationships among these variables to identify particular risk groups in terms of both the incidence and prevalence of disability and access to appropriate prevention, treatment, and rehabilitation services. Specific attention should be directed to low-income women from ethnic/racial backgrounds with caregiver responsibilities. Barriers to timely and appropriate care are yet to be fully understood for this group. By correctly addressing the etiology, a more comprehensive understanding of the specific needs of this population and of the existing barriers to care, prevention and intervention programs can be targeted more effectively. By including the social and physical contributes into the etiology, we can fully address the concerns of women with disabilities. Thus, the uninsurance and underinsurance of women with diabetes or CTS can be added to the etiology of these conditions. By adding these conditions to the etiology, then blindness caused by a lack of insurance to obtain the recommended eye exams or *"lack of exam" blindness* can be addressed through the concerted efforts of activists and advocates for disability and the women's rights community, health care providers, health services researchers, and health plan administrators.

Acknowledgements

Research for this manuscript has been supported by grant H133A990013 from the National Institute on Disability and Rehabilitation Research. The content of this manuscript does not necessarily represent the policy of the Department of Education; endorsement by the Federal government is not to be assumed. The authors would like to thank Suzanne Peake, freelance author of Annapolis, Maryland, for her contributions to the writing and editing of this chapter.

Works Cited

Association for Enterprise Opportunity. 2000 [Cited July 2000]. What is mircroenterprise? Available at http://www.microenterpriseworks.org/microdevelopment/whatis.htm.

Bureau of Labor Statistics. 2000 [Cited June 2000]. Lost-Worktime Injuries: Characteristics and Resulting Time Away from Work, 1998 U.S. Department of Labor. Available at ftp://ftp.bls.gov/pub/news.release/History/osh2.04202000.news.

Centers for Disease Control. 2001 [Cited October 2001]. Deaths, percent of total deaths, and death rates for the 10 leading causes of death in selected age groups, by race, and sex: United States, 1999. *National Vital Statistic Report* 49 (11): 14–49. Available at http://www.cdc.gov/nchs/fastats/pdf/nvsr49_11tb1.pdf

Centers for Disease Control and Prevention. 1997. Disability. *Diabetes Surveillance.* Publication available at CDC's Diabetes Program–Statistics–Diabetes Surveillance. Available at http://wwwcdc.gov/diabetes/statistics/surv197/html/surveill.htm.

Centers for Disease Control and Prevention. 2000 [Cited November 2000]. DATA 2010 . . . the Healthy People 2010 Database-November 2000 Edition. Focus area: 05-Diabetes, data tables generated from CDC Wonder, November 2000. Available at http://wonder.cdc.gov/.

Cleveland Clinic. 2000 [Cited December 11, 2002]. What is diabetes? WebMD Corporation 2001. Available at http://my.webmd.com/content/article/3608.868.

DeVivo, M. J., J. S. Krause, and K. P. Lammertse. 1999. Recent trends in mortality and causes of death among persons with spinal cord injury. *Archives of Physical Medical Rehabilitation* 80: 1411–1419.

Donelan, K., M. Falik, and C. DesRoches. 2001. Caregiving: Challenges and implications for women's health. *Women's Health Issues* 11: 185–200.

Farce, E., and W. M. Alves. 2000. Do women fare worse? A metaanalysis of gender differences in outcome after traumatic brain injury. *Neurosurgical Focus* 8: 1–12.

Jeffress, C. N. 2000 [Cited July 2000]. Statement of Charles N. Jeffress, Assistant Secretary for Occupational Safety and Health, U.S. Department of Labor, before the Subcommittee on Regulatory Reform and Paperwork Reduction of the House Small Business Committee April 13, 2000. OSHA Congressional Testimonies. Available at http://www.osha-lc.gov/OshDoc/Testimony_data/T20000413.html.

Mokdad, A. H., E. S. Ford, B. A. Bowman, D. E. Nelson, M. M. Englegau, F. Vinicor, and J. S. Marks. 2000. Diabetes trends in the U.S.: 1990–1998. *Diabetes Care* 23: 1278–1283.

National Diabetes Data Group of the National Institute of Diabetes and Digestive and Kidney Diseases. 2001. Diabetes in America. 2^d ed. Bethesda, Md.: National Institutes of Health. Available at http://www.niddk.nih.gov/health/diabetes/dia/index.htm.

National Institute for Occupational Safety and Health. 1997 [cited July 2000]. Musculoskeletal disorders (MSDs) and workplace factors. Available at http://www.cdc.gov/niosh/ergtet51.html.

Nidus Information Services, Inc. 1998 [cited November 2001]. Carpal tunnel syndrome. Available at http://www.tifaq.org/articles/carpal_tunnel_syndrome-sep98-well-connected.html.

Office of Women's Health. 2001 [cited November 2001]. Women's health issues: An overview. Available at http://www.4women.gov/owh/pub/womhealth%20issues/inde.htm.

Rumrill, P. D., M. J. Millinton, M. J. Webb, and M. J. Cook. 1998. Employment expectations as a differential indicator of attitudes toward people with insulin-dependent diabetes mellitus. *Journal of Vocational Rehabilitation* 10: 271–280.

Seal, B. F., R. L. Sowell, R. L. Demi, L. Moneyham, L. Cohen, and J. Guillory. 1995. Falling through the cracks: Social service concerns of women infected with HIV. *Qualitative Health Research* 5: 496–515.

Seelman, K., and S. Sweeney. 1995. The changing universe of disability. *American Rehabilitation* (autumn-winter): 2–13.

World Health Organization. 2000 [cited August 2001]. Diabetes. Available at http://www.who.int/ncd/dia/.

The Sexist Inheritance of the Disability Movement

eℐℓℇ

CORBETT JOAN O'TOOLE

This chapter explores some of the inheritance of the disability movement and suggests areas for further analysis within disability studies. I address in particular the lack of analysis within the disability movement, specifically in terms of its diverse membership and how that narrowness has disturbing implications for disability studies.

The U.S. disability movement had many points of origin—from World War II veterans to the 1950s mothers of disabled children to the first Centers for Independent Living in the 1970s. But by 1980, the disability movement presented an image to the world as white people—primarily men, presumably heterosexual—who used mobility devices, most often wheelchairs. This standardized myth is not limited to the United States. Barbara Ryan quotes British writer Carol Thomas, who asserts that "men have dominated the disability movement in Britain, evidenced by a macho-like style in both the political arena and analytical debate. Because the social world is always gendered, a male-led movement centered on structural barriers to accessibility, particularly to work, has left out those related to domestic and family domains. In other words, the social disability movement is sexist" (2000, 4). As the disability movement has aged, the top positions have moved from being primarily white men to primarily white women, but there has not been any systemic interest in analyzing how disability might have a differential impact based on gender.

Furthermore, the U.S. disabled population is racially mixed. Numerous studies have shown us that as poverty increases, so does the number of people with disabilities. Neither poverty nor disability is equally distributed across racial and ethnic lines, and causal relationships exist between poverty (lack of adequate health care, of proper nutrition) and some disabilities. Although only 17.7 percent of the European American population aged 15 to 64 is disabled, 20.8 percent of the African American population and a startling 26.9 percent of the

294

Native American population have disabilities (Bradsher 1996). The staff and leadership of the disability movement in the United States shows a very different pattern—almost completely white, middle class, and until recently, male. In each of the early historical shifts of the disability movement, however, women, people of color, gays and lesbians, and others who did not fit the proffered stereotype were active members. Evident in anecdotal accounts and early writings on the lived disability experience were representatives of all these groups who were important players doing important work for the community without public acknowledgment or equal rewards for their contributions.

The framework of disability during the 1970s produced many great achievements and outcomes—national legislation on disability rights, bringing people with disabilities to the living rooms of America, increasing public access, and increasing integration. These gains are an astounding tribute to years of dedicated hard work. And the hard work of these people, particularly the white men, has been extensively documented (Shapiro 1994). For example, the University of California at Berkeley's Regional Oral History Project undertook a massive effort to document the early history of the disability movement in Berkeley. The principal decision makers were all white and were part of the disability movement of the 1970s and 1980s. In November 2000, a conference was held to announce the completion of the project. Fifty-two people were chosen for this permanent tribute—their oral histories of the disability movement to "live forever as an insider's record of that important time." As Peggy McIntosh (1988) points out, "[white people are] given cultural permission not to hear voices of people of other races or a tepid cultural tolerance for hearing and acting on such voices." Sure enough, of the fifty-two people selected, forty-nine were white, two were African-American, and one was Hispanic. Among these participants, only one spoke about the roles that women played or the presence of lesbians within the early disability movement.

Research shows that those who have benefited the most from these advances have been those whose needs were the most parallel to the mythic disabled man (Fine & Asch 1988; Linton 1998). Citing Elizabeth Minnich, McIntosh writes, "whites are taught to think of their lives as morally neutral, normative, and average, and also ideal, so that when we work to benefit others, this is seen as work that will allow 'them' to be more like 'us.'" Potential funders are still reluctant to include diversity or outreach initiatives in either research or community efforts because of the overriding assumption that what is good for this mythic man is good for all people with disabilities (Garland-Thomson 1999). Research that focuses on, or significantly includes, disabled people of color is often marginalized by both funders and other disability researchers (Glenn 1995; Ford and Corbitt 1999).

The impact of the unwelcome, pervasive, perhaps even insidious, myth of the white, straight man in a wheelchair is evident in personal accounts, essays, and in the professional literature of disability scholars. People who have deviated from this mythic image often found themselves ostracized within the disability movement. One legacy of African American feminist, lesbian, mother, writer, cancer survivor/victim Audre Lorde is to name and claim the multiplicities and contradictions of our lives without shame. As Jim Davis-Rosenthal reminds us in "An Elegy for Audre Lorde" (1995), "The words we are still arguing over including—bisexual, heterosexism, [cancer], erotic; the words so many of us can't manage to include in the names of our organizations, our speech, our writing, appeared in her essays unproblematically [in the 1970s]. Her writing has been so important to so many people because she taught us to transform our silence into power because our fears will not prevent our deaths." Even when collections on disability studies are put into annotated bibliographies, there is no standard format to reference intersecting issues or even a perceived need to inform the reader about the inclusion of diverse perspectives within the original collection. So authors' and editors' hard work is often obscured by subsequent chroniclers of the work—obscuring the depth of the writing that is, in fact, available on intersecting issues.

From my perspective as an activist for nearly thirty years, the disability studies movement has three consistent challenges: bringing the disability rights model into the academy; bringing an academic lens to disability; and providing useful information by, about, and for the disability community. Much of early disability studies focused on the first problem: how to move universities away from a medical model of disability and toward a disability rights paradigm. The writing in this area is extensive. Suffice it for me to say that this is an ongoing battle.

Gaining academic acceptance for the kinds of research encompassed by the term *disability studies* has proved just as problematic. In the early 1990s, Kirk MacGugan was pursuing a second Ph.D., this time in history. Her thesis proposal on the history of the disability rights movement from 1917 to 1947 was rejected because, in the words of her committee, "There is no disability history." Thankfully, subsequent disability studies scholars have proved them wrong. Nevertheless, any review of the attempts to do research on disability—AND having it viewed as a valuable academic contribution—is full of stories of struggle and arm-twisting.

The area that concerns me the most is the third prong: the need for disability studies to provide useful information by, about, and for the disability community. We all undoubtedly have stories from different disciplines about a researcher with an insider's perspective who provided an entirely new lens for challenging what was considered an existing "fact." I believe that any successful reframing of an oppressive idea or practice, without regard to discipline, will have a resounding and ultimately beneficial impact on people with disabilities. In discussing Carol Gilligan, Nancy Rice (2000) writes: "[her] work issued an implicit charge to researchers everywhere: be explicit in what the standard of 'normal' is taken to be and in how this is determined." Gilligan's challenge to "be explicit in what the standard of 'normal' is taken to be and in how this is determined" (2000) has deep resonance with disability studies. Our scholarship is often eager to challenge the medical model's definition of disabled people but is usually less eager to explore the larger tapestry of issues that relate to age, gender, race and sexual orientation.

When I first attended the Society for Disability Studies (SDS) meetings in the early 1990s, both the presenters and the audience were white. At the 2000 SDS meeting in Chicago, most of the presenters and audience were white and about 5 percent were people of color. At some previous SDS meetings, there were some presentations about disabled people of color—but these were almost always done by white, usually nondisabled presenters.

I understood this problem far better when I did a chart of what is being taught under the title "disability studies." It is both very exciting and very troubling to look at the programs and courses offered. Some sound remarkably similar to the courses offered as basic training for service providers in different fields. But there are some remarkable strides being made. Using information from the Winter 2000 issue of the *Disability Studies Quarterly*, and restricting my review to programs based in the United States or Canada, I found this pattern. Of twelve programs offered nationwide, only one has a specific focus to include women and disability issues and only one addresses specific issues related to people of color with disabilities (University of Hawai'i at Manoa). There are fifty-three classes offered at thirty-one universities. Of these, six classes address women and disability, six classes examine disability and race, and two discuss LGBT (lesbian, gay, bisexual, transgendered people) and disability (Kasnitz, Bonney, Aftandelian, and Pfeiffer, 2000). For me as a writer and activist on equity issues in disability, this is not an encouraging head count. It should be noted, however, that programs at Howard University and the Mississippi Institute for Disability Studies at the University of Southern Mississippi, neither of which was included in the *DSQ* article, do have specific goals to increase the participation of people of color in leadership and research roles. It will be instructive to monitor their activities and success in addressing those goals.

There is literature discussing how disability studies is like ethnic or women's studies but surprisingly little discussion of how disability studies is including women and people of color (Preston 2001). As one writer points out, "disability studies borrows from many fields and movements, including cultural studies, area studies, feminism, race-and-ethnic studies, and gay-and-lesbian studies" (Monaghan 1998). However, Rosemarie Garland-Thomson (2000) is often the lone voice reminding us that "disability can be included as a category of analysis that parallels and *intersects* [emphasis mine] gender, race, ethnicity and class." Bodies of literature found in many oppressed communities also document that when people outside the community do research, the results often miss important components of community life that can and often do directly influence the results. Studying disability without looking at the intersections of multiple identities results in a very limited perspective about who disabled people are and what they need. The Howard University Research and Training Center (2001) states:

Very few instruments have been constructed and very little data exists which have utilized African Americans with disabilities as the exclusive data source. Often the research utilizes instruments that contain normative data based upon European Americans . . . This data, at best, is often accepted as generalizable to African Americans and other minorities. However, the validity and reliability of the data is highly questionable and often limited in accurately describing the characteristics of this population.

Feminist disability scholars such as Harilyn Rousso, Rosemarie Garland-Thomson, Simi Linton, and Cheryl Green remind us that it is a mistake to think that the complexity of disability experience can be understood independent of other aspects of our lives.

I had a hard time finding disabled women of color that I admire that you would also know. A few women like Audre Lorde, mostly women who are either perceived as nondisabled or who became disabled later in life, will come to mind. But the voices of these members of my community—African American, Native American, Latina, and Asian American women who have lived with their disabilities for many years and who do not pass, while loud in my ears, are but whispers on the wind for the rest of society.

Do you know LaDonna Fowler, who is leading a struggle for recognition on tribal lands? Do you know Sylvia Walker, who runs a large research and training center that investigates the intersecting issues for disabled people of color? Do you know Atsuko Kuwana, who builds information bridges across the Pacific Ocean so that people in the United States and Japan know about each others' struggles? Do you know Kathy Martinez, who is probably the most successful organizer of disabled women's gatherings worldwide? These women, and thousands others, remain invisible even in disability and women's studies. They are invisible because those of us with access to these academic gatherings have not formally acknowledged their work as vital to the survival and growth of our culture, as vital and as necessary as the efforts that we so passionately and proudly pushed forth in the beginning of the disability movement. We need to look at ways to support them, invite them to speak as equal voices and as keynote speakers, to publish their work widely and to commemorate their contributions to improving our lives and furthering our dreams—not as a one-size-fits-all covering but as a representation of the richly complex community that we are.

One of the great things about the history of disability studies is that it took the basic premises of the early disability movement and built on it. One of the worst things about disability studies is that it took the basic premises of the disability movement and built on it. We have to accept and refer to both aspects of our inheritance if we are to make the necessary changes for the growth of our community and for the future of our disabled children in all their diversity.

I want to end with the wisdom of some quotable women: Peggy McIntosh

(1988) states: "Through Women's Studies work I have met very few men who are truly distressed about systemic, unearned male advantage and conferred dominance. And so one question for me and others like me is whether we will be like them, or whether we will get truly distressed, even outraged, about un-earned race advantage and conferred dominance and if so, what will we do to lessen them." Simi Linton (1998) writes: "We have come out not with those brown woollen lap robes over our withered legs, or dark glasses over our pale eyes but in shorts and sandals, in overalls and business suits, dressed for play and work—straightforward, unmasked, and unapologetic" (3). And the final word from Audre Lorde: "I have come to believe over and over again that what is most important to me must be spoken, made verbal and shared, even at the risk of having it bruised or misunderstood" (Zami 2003).

Works Cited

Bradsher, Julie E. 1996. *Disability among racial and ethnic groups*. Disability Statistics Center, Abstract 10.

Davis-Rosenthal, Jim. 1995 [Cited May 21, 2003]. An elegy for Audre Lorde, 1992. In *Standards* 5 (1). Available at http://www.colorado.edu/journals/standards/V5N1/Lorde/jdrelegy.html.

Fine, M., and Asch, A. (1988). Beyond Pedestals. In M. Fine and A. Asch, eds. *Women with Disabilities: Essays in psychology, culture and politics*. Philadelphia: Temple University Press.

Ford, JoAnn, and Elizabeth Corbitt. 1999 [cited 2001]. Substance abuse: A strong risk, often overlooked. *Window On Wellness* (summer 1999). Available at http://www.windowonwellness.com/back_issues/99summer/subAbuse/subAbuse.shtml. Accessed February 10, 2001.

Garland-Thomson, Rosemarie. 2000 [Cited September 10, 2002]. Incorporating Disability Studies into American Studies. Available at: http://www.georgetown.edu/crossroads/interests/ds-hum/thomson.html.

Garland-Thomson, Rosemarie. 1999 [Cited September 10, 2002]. The new disability studies: Tolerance or inclusion. *ADFL Bulletin*, 31 (1): 49–53. Available at: http://www.adfl.org/ADFL/bulletin/v31n1/311049.htm.

Glenn, Eddie. 1995 [Cited February 10, 2001]. African American women with disabilities: An overview. In *Disability and diversity: New leadership for a new era*. Published by the President's Committee on Employment of People With Disabilities in collaboration with the Howard University Research and Training Center. Available at: http://www50.pcepd.gov/pcepd/pubs/diverse/glenn.htm.

Howard University Research and Training Center for Access to Rehabilitation and Economic Opportunity (HURTC). N.d. [Cited February 10, 2001]. Research Project 7: African Americans with disabilities: An ethnographic study. In *Overview of individual projects* available at http://www.law.howard.edu/HURTC/overview.html.

Kasnitz, D., Bonney, S., Aftandelian, R., Pfeiffer, D. (2000). Programs and Courses in Disability Studies at Universities and Colleges in Canada, Australia, the United States, the United Kingdom, and Norway. *Disability Studies Quarterly* (spring 2000) 20 (2). Center on Disability Studies, University of Hawaii at Manoa, Honolulu, Hawaii, and School of Social Sciences, the University of Texas at Dallas, Richardson, Texas.

Linton, S. 1998. *Claiming disability: Knowledge and identity*. New York: New York University Press.

———. 2000. Trans-Atlantic Commerce. *Disability & Society* 15: 699–703.

Lorde, Audre. 1997. *The Cancer Journals*. San Francisco: Aunt Lute.

McIntosh, Peggy. 1988 [Cited May 21, 2003]. Working paper 189, Wellesley College Center for Research on Women, Wellesley, Mass. Available at http://www.alliancefordiversity.org/resources/article_privilege.html.

Monaghan, Peter. 1998, January 23. Pioneering field of disability studies challenges established approaches and attitudes. *Chronicle of Higher Education*. Available at http://www.uic.edu/orgs/sds/articles.html#chron.

Preston, Paul. 2001. Review of *Illusions of equality: Deaf Americans in school and factory: 1850–1950* by Robert Buchanan. *Disability Studies Quarterly* 21.

Rice, Nancy. 2000. What is disability studies, and what does it have to do with facilitated communication? *Facilitated Communication Digest* 8 (2): 2–8. Available at: http://soeweb.syr.edu/thefci/8–2ric.

Ryan, Barbara. 2000 [Cited September 10. 2002]. Gender and disability from different angles. Review of *Female forms: Experiencing and understanding disability* by Carol Thomas. *Feminist Collections: A Quarterly of Women's Studies Resources* 21 (4): 4. Available at: http://www.library.wisc.edu/libraries/WomensStudies/fcmain.htm.

Shapiro, Joseph. 1994. *No pity: People with disabilities forging a new civil rights movement*. New York: Times Books.

Zami, A Not-for-profit Collective for Lesbians of African Descent. 2003. [Cited May 21, 2003]. Available at http://www.zami.org//lorderquotes.htm.

NOTES ON CONTRIBUTORS

ADRIENNE ASCH is the Henry R. Luce Professor in Biology, Ethics and the Politics of Human Reproduction at Wellesley College. Recent publications include "The Disability Rights Critique of Prenatal Genetic Testing: Reflections and Recommendations" with E. Parens (*The Hastings Center Report*, 29[5] Special Supplement, S1-S22); "Prenatal Diagnosis and Selective Abortion: A Challenge to Practice and Policy" (*American Journal of Public Health*, 89[11], 1649-1657). She is presently at work on a book on the ethical, social, and psychological issues in assisted reproduction.

BRENDA JO BRUEGGEMANN is an associate professor of English, with affiliations also in comparative studies and women's studies, at The Ohio State University. She has helped implement both an American Sign Language program and an interdisciplinary disability studies minor at Ohio State and serves as coordinator for those two programs. She is the author of *Lend Me Your Ear: Rhetorical Constructions of Deafness* (Gallaudet UP, 1999) and co-editor of *Disability Studies: Enabling the Humanities*.

SARAH E. CHINN teaches in the English department at Hunter College, CUNY. She is the author of *Technology and the Logic of American Racism: A Cultural History of the Body as Evidence*, and is currently at work on two projects: a book on immigration and adolescent identity in the United States, and another on the ethics of lesbian reading.

SUMI COLLIGAN teaches cultural anthropology at the Massachusetts College of Liberal Arts. She participated in the first NEH Summer Institute on the New Disability Studies in 2000.

ANN M. FOX is an assistant professor of English at Davidson College, in Davidson, NC. Her teaching and research interests include modern drama, feminist performance, and disability in theater and literature. Her current project is a book examining representations of disability in mainstream American theater across the twentieth century.

ROSEMARIE GARLAND-THOMSON is associate professor in the women's studies department at Emory University in Atlanta, Georgia. Her work focuses on feminist theory and disability studies in the humanities. She is the author of *Extraordinary Bodies: Figuring Physical Disability in American Literature and Culture*, editor of *Freakery: Cultural Spectacles of the Extraordinary Body*, and co-editor of *Disability Studies: Enabling the Humanities*. She is currently writing a book on staring and one on the cultural logic of euthanasia.

ROBIN ADÈLE GREELEY teaches art history at the University of Connecticut. She is author of the forthcoming book, *Organizing Pessimism: Surrealism, Politics and the Spanish Civil War*, and is working on her second book, *Gendering Mexican Cultural Nationalism, 1920-1970*.

ALISON KAFER is a Ph.D. candidate in women's studies and religious studies at Claremont Graduate University. Her dissertation examines academic and popular discourses of science and technology through the lens of disability.

CAROL KAUFMAN-SCARBOROUGH is an associate professor of marketing in the School of Business, at Rutgers University's Camden Campus. Disabilities have been part of her personal life as well as the lives of several family members and close acquaintances. She is particularly interested in bridging the gap between business studies and disabilities studies in the effort to educate business students and researchers in the realities of expected marketplace participation by persons with disabilities.

GEORGINA KLEEGE teaches English at the University of California, Berkeley. She is the author of the novel *Home for the Summer*, and a collection of personal essays about blindness, *Sight Unseen*.

THILO KROLL, Ph.D. is a research psychologist and senior research associate at the NRH Center for Health and Disability Research. He is the project coordinator for the NIDRR funded project on "Rehabilitative Services for People with Emergent Disabilities." Other research areas include the rehabilitative needs of people with violently acquired spinal cord injuries, and research into the access barriers to healthcare for people with physical disabilities.

CATHERINE J. KUDLICK is professor of history at the University of California, Davis. With Dr. Zina Weygand she is author of *Reflections: the Life and Writings of a Young Blind Woman in Post-Revolutionary France* (New York University Press, 2001).

KRISTIN LINDGREN teaches at Haverford College. She is currently completing a study of representations of illness and disability in nineteenth-century women's fiction and autobiography.

MELISSA J. MCNEIL, M.S., LGSW, is a community consultant at the Alabama Coalition Against Domestic Violence engaged in work on projects concerning survivors moving from welfare to work, economic independence, and rural barriers to domestic violence safety. Two recent presentations are "Understanding the rehabilitation experience of individuals with violently acquired spinal cord injuries (VASCI) (with Thilo Kroll) and "Healthcare utilization and expenditure profiles of adults with disabilities" (with Phillip W. Beatty and Gwyn C. Jones).

CORBETT JOAN O'TOOLE is the director of the Disabled Women's Alliance, an organization that provides training and education on the intersections of gender, disability, and queer issues (Corbett@disabledwomen.net). Her articles have appeared in the *Journal of Lesbian Health*, *Disability Studies Quarterly*, *Peabody Journal of Education*, *Sexuality and Disability*, as well as *Disability World* (www.disabilityworld.org). She is a well-known speaker and writer on disabled women's issues.

LISA SCHUR is an assistant professor in the department of labor studies and employment relations at Rutgers University. She received a Ph.D. in political science from the University of California, Berkeley and a J.D. from Northeastern University. Her research focuses on political participation and employment among people with disabilities.

RUSSELL P. SHUTTLEWORTH is currently an Ed Robert's Postdoctoral Fellow in disability studies at University of California, Berkeley. Dr. Shuttleworth has published widely in the areas of disability studies, disability and sexuality studies, and anthropology and disability.

DANIEL J. WILSON is a professor of history at Muhlenberg College in Allentown, Pennsylvania. He has written several essays about the history of polio and is completing a book about the experience of having polio in twentieth-century America.

INDEX

ability/disability system, 76–77
abortion: of disabled fetus, 3, 5;
   selective, 87
Abu-Habib, Lina, 228
ACA (Amputee Coalition of America),
   110, 115n6
accommodation: in employment, 14, 18;
   environmental, 14–16
activism: among women with
   disabilities, 255–256, 263, 265;
   intersex rights movement, 53, 56;
   transgender rights movement, 56. *See
   also* disability rights movement;
   feminist disability theory, activism
   issue in
ADA. *See* Americans with Disabilities
   Act
advocacy, 2–3
"Afterthoughts on 'Visual Pleasure and
   Narrative Ciema' Inspired by King
   Vidor's *Duel in the Sun*" (Mulvey),
   210n13
Against Sadomasochism (Linden,
   Russell, & Pagano), 194, 195
AIDS/HIV, 58n9, 286–287
airline pilot, vision standards for, 19–20
Alexander, Elizabeth, 204
The Alien Within (Ling), 156
Americans with Disabilities Act (ADA),
   9, 13, 58n9, 254, 273, 283; on certain
   immunity of states for violation of,
   32n3–33n3; claimants of, 17;
   definition of qualified individual
   under, 16

Amputee Coalition of America (ACA),
   110, 115n6
amputee-devotee community, 107–108;
   common activities for meeting
   amputee, 115n7–116n7; devotee
   following amputee, 110–111, 112–
   113; gender/disability overview, 108–
   109; on Internet, 107–108, 111, 112–
   113, 116n10; "lady"/"woman"
   difference, 116n8; nontraditional
   gendering in, 113–114; traditional
   feminine gendering in, 111–113;
   traditional masculine gendering in,
   109–111; type of devotee in, 114n1–
   115n1; view of lesbian in, 112,
   116nn8–9
"An Elegy for Audre Lorde" (Davis-
   Rosenthal), 297
Angels in America (Kushner), 247
Anspach, Renee, 255
Anzaldúa, Gloria, 212n26
Anzieu, Didier, 204, 205, 212n25
The Apparitional Lesbian (Castle), 207n1
Appiah, Anthony, 26, 30
Asch, Adrienne, 3, 87, 254–255
ASCOTWorld (Amputee Support
   Coalition of the World), 110, 113,
   115n5, 116n11
asexuality, 50–52, 89, 91
Atkinson, Ti-Grace, 194
autoimmune disease, 154, 286–287

Baartman, Saartje, 78, 197
Baddeley, Oriana, 229n5

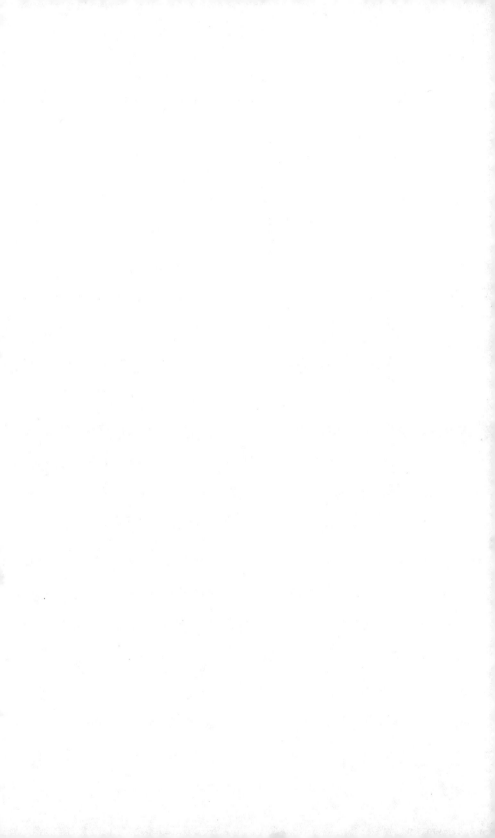